11/28/95
To Cordell + Bernice —
Bon Appétit!
Kathy Walgren

PRESCRIPTIONS *for* GOOD TASTE

A CENTURY OF DELICIOUS RECIPES
FROM OUR KITCHENS, FAMILIES AND FRIENDS

First Edition, First Printing: October 1995

Printed in the United States of America
Crawfordsville Division
RR Donnelley & Sons Company

Copyright 1995 Walgreen Drug Stores Historical Foundation
All Rights Reserved
ISBN 0-9648458-051995

Dedicated to all of the people who worked in the food service division, and to the loving memory of Myrtle R. Walgreen (Mrs. Charles R. Walgreen, Sr.).

Mrs. Walgreen's original, home-cooked meals won the hearts of many a Walgreen customer in 1915. The success of her efforts led to the creation of Walgreens famous soda fountains, and later to a very profitable, nationwide network of cafeterias and restaurants.

Editorial:
Kathleen B. Walgreen
Craig M. Sinclair
Ginger Kay Amirouche
Cathie A. Neumiller-Heller
Timothy Frey
Laura Boerner
Anne Jorndt
Kay Miller

Contributors:
Charles R. Walgreen, Jr.
Ros Nachman
Allyson Mitchell
Gary Grejczyk
Vicki Vacco
Charlie Carter
Marsha Gentile
Phyllis Hudson
Judy Thomas
Julie Jacobs
Adeline Sandberg
Vincent F. Bonsignore

Production:
Wayne E. Shumaker
Erin J. Engelmann
Janice M. Turkowski
Dick Bregenzer
Pamela d. Orlando

Photography:
John Becket
Scott Lanza
Barry Rustin
Bob Schuldt

Set Design:
F. Lynn Nelson
Nancy Backus

Table of Contents

INTRODUCTION	vi
THANKSGIVING at HAZELWOOD	1
APPETIZERS Robin Hood & Briargate	17
SOUPS & SALADS The In-Store Grills	41
FISH & SEAFOOD The Villager Room & The Globe Stores	91
MEATS & MORE Sanborns House of Tiles	121
POULTRY Wag's & Humpty Dumpty	183
WELCOME to WALGREENS HISTORICAL HIGHLIGHTS	213
VEGETABLES The Cafeterias	221
PASTA, GRAINS & POTATOES The Commissaries	251
BREADS Corky's, Plaza Grill & Wigwam Grill	289
DESSERTS & TREATS The Soda Fountains	315
RxCETERA The "Tea Rooms"	
Sauces & Garnishes	381
Beverages	411
WALGREEN FOOD DICTIONARY	419
SPICES, HERBS & SEASONINGS	427
ABBREVIATIONS & EQUIVALENTS	430
COOKING TERMS DEFINED	431
FAT SUBSTITUTES	435
PERSONAL APPEARANCE & CONDUCT	437
ACKNOWLEDGMENTS	440
INDEX	442

We hope you will enjoy this special collection of recipes from the kitchens of Walgreens and members and friends of the Walgreen Alumni Association.

What began as a fun medium for exchanging our own favorite recipes, sparked a very exciting idea...to open up the kitchens of Walgreens former food services, and share the old favorites ~ and a little history "on the side"! *Prescriptions for Good Taste* contains nearly 700 recipes, more than 100 of which are pulled directly from the pages of Walgreens original cookbooks.

You'll find delicious "old standbys" such as Walgreens famous *Double-Rich Chocolate Malted*, invented in 1922 by fountain manager Ivar "Pop" Coulsen (made with Walgreens own extra-rich, homemade ice cream!) And, copied by others, but never duplicated, everybody's favorite, *The Famous Patty Melt* ~ wholesome beef on rye, dripping with melted cheese, garnished with zesty onions and tangy pickle chips!

The history of Walgreens food service division is one of ingenuity and uncompromising quality. This philosophy began in 1901 with the first Walgreens drugstore on Chicago's south side. Walgreens founder, Charles R. Walgreen, Sr., believed in selling only the highest quality products, keeping a spotless store and treating customers with the utmost respect and care. In 1915 he decided to take a chance and cater to the customers who desired the convenience of a bite of lunch at the neighborhood drugstore. This modest effort was taken on by his wife, Myrtle, who actually made the meals in her own kitchen. The Walgreen's son, Charles R. "Chuck" Walgreen, Jr., delivered the freshly-cooked meals to the store!

The "lunch counter" idea spread as Mr. Walgreen, Sr. opened more stores, and grew into the very popular soda fountains, which were supplied by Walgreens first commissary. Ultimately, Walgreens established its own food factories: an ice cream plant, supplied by Walgreens own dairies; a syrup-making facility, a chocolate factory, which made a line of hand-dipped candies; a bakery, which created an award-winning cinnamon-raisin bread recipe; and a coffee plant, for roasting and grinding coffee beans.

Eventually the Walgreens soda fountains of the 1920's became in-store cafeterias in the 1940's, giving way to the freestanding restaurants of the 70's and 80's ~ the most famous of which was Wag's. Although still very profitable for the company, Walgreens sold the food service division in 1988 in order to concentrate on its pharmacy business. Today Walgreens is the nation's largest drugstore chain and the front runner in electronic technology, which includes a nationwide, satellite-linked computer prescription network!

In 1986, the Walgreen Drug Stores Historical Foundation opened a replica of the first Walgreens drugstore at the Chicago Museum of Science and Industry's "Yesterday's Main Street" exhibit. This painstaking re-creation was the realization of a long-held dream for me ~ to give life to an important part of American history. The completion of this cookbook is another ~ to share that history in a very special, and superbly scrumptious way! We hope the recipes and historical accounts contained within this book will help the memory of those wonderful years stay alive and "cookin'" and keep *your* prescription for good eating filled!

All proceeds from the sale of *Prescriptions for Good Taste* will go directly to the Walgreen Benefit Fund. Established by Walgreens in the 1930's Depression Era, the Fund supports Walgreens employees and retirees in catastrophic situations. Over the years, the Fund has benefited those in the most distressed circumstances; including victims of natural disasters, catastrophic illness, violent crime and their orphans.

Kathleen B. Walgreen
(Mrs. Charles R. Walgreen, III)
Chairman,
Walgreen Drug Stores Historical Foundation

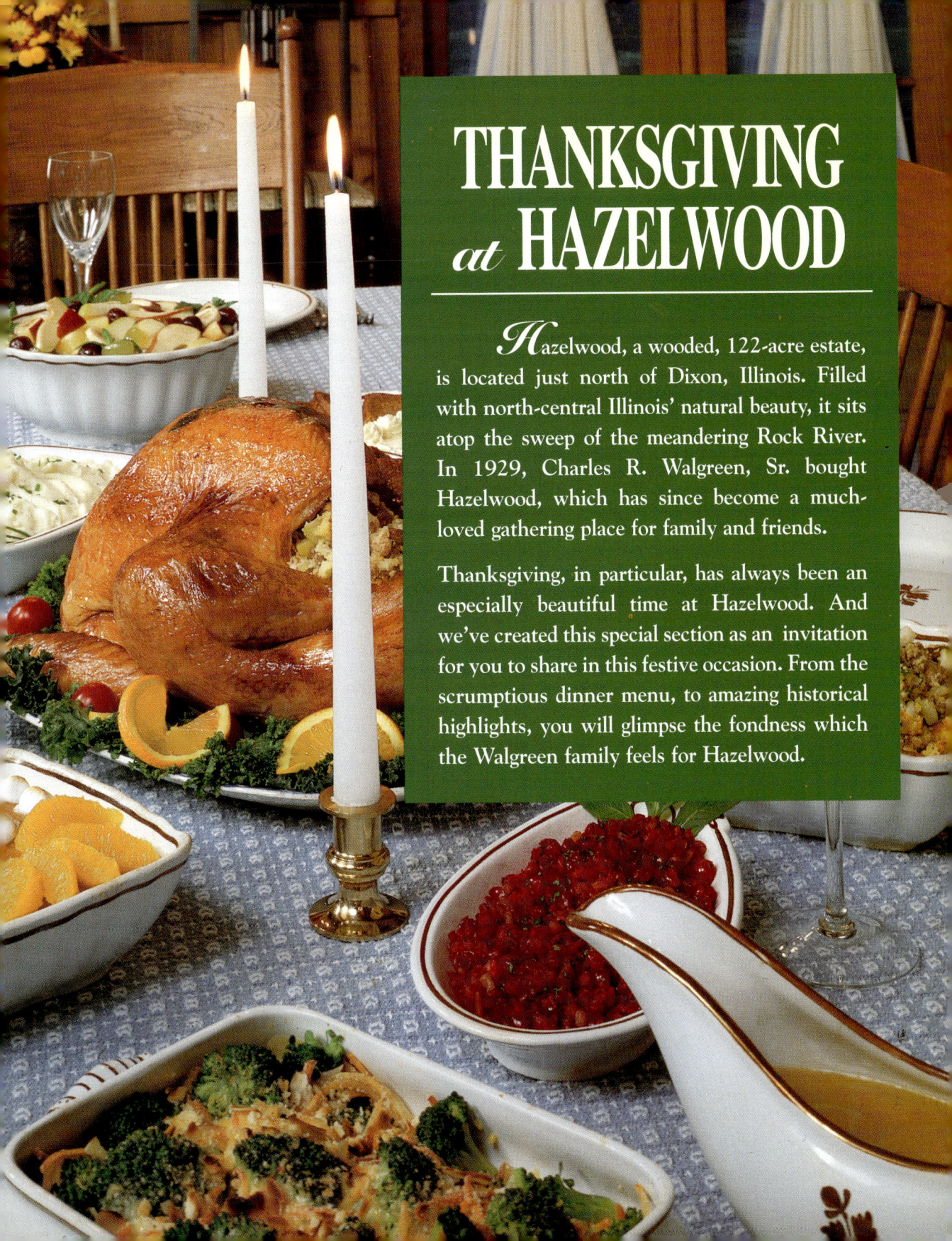

THANKSGIVING at HAZELWOOD

Hazelwood, a wooded, 122-acre estate, is located just north of Dixon, Illinois. Filled with north-central Illinois' natural beauty, it sits atop the sweep of the meandering Rock River. In 1929, Charles R. Walgreen, Sr. bought Hazelwood, which has since become a much-loved gathering place for family and friends.

Thanksgiving, in particular, has always been an especially beautiful time at Hazelwood. And we've created this special section as an invitation for you to share in this festive occasion. From the scrumptious dinner menu, to amazing historical highlights, you will glimpse the fondness which the Walgreen family feels for Hazelwood.

*T*he decades of family gatherings and social events at Hazelwood began with a promise. Early in his marriage (when the Walgreen Company consisted of a couple of stores on Chicago's South Side) Charles R. Walgreen, Sr. promised his wife, Myrtle, that one day they would own a "charming place in the country." At the time, Walgreen, who always planned ahead, already had Hazelwood in mind. In September 1929, a month before the stock market crash, he bought the property, which had captivated him as a young boy growing up in Dixon.

Hazelwood's serene beauty is matched by an equally venerable history. In 1837 Samuel Charter purchased the then 640 acres and built a two-story log cabin (later called the Lincoln Cabin in honor of the president who slept there). A year later his brother, Alexander "Governor" Charter, arrived and named the estate *Hazelwood*, after a park in his native Ireland. Governor Charter, a very popular and successful businessman, built a mansion in which he entertained guests like Abraham Lincoln, Stephen A. Douglas and William Cullen Bryant. During the 1850's he even convinced the Illinois Central Railroad to run its Dixon tracks right through the estate! The mansion later burned in a fire.

By the time Walgreen bought Hazelwood, it was in major disrepair, with grass over two feet high! But the industrious entrepreneur soon turned it into a showplace. Initially the Lincoln Cabin was a weekend home to the Walgreens. However, Walgreen quickly renovated the estate's old barn into new living quarters, which included a billiard room and bar, dubbed the *Cheese and Sausage Club*. Soon his growing family needed even more space, and a year later he added a two-story annex to the house.

The Old Barn

The Cliff House overlooking the Rock River

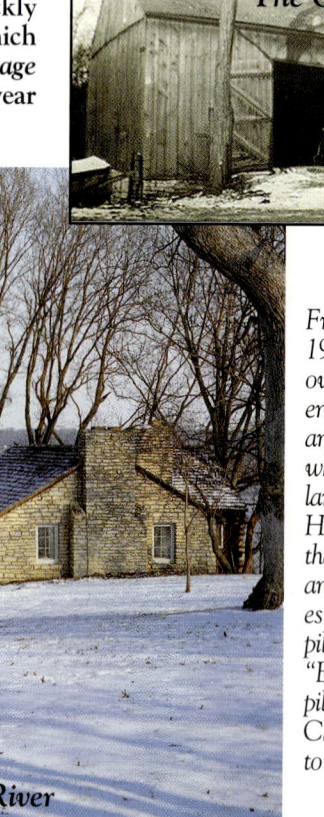

From 1929 to 1933, Walgreen owned a twin-engine Sikorsky amphibious plane which used to land behind Hazelwood on the Rock River, and taxi to the estate. It was piloted by Ira "Bif" Biffle, the pilot who taught Charles Lindberg to fly!

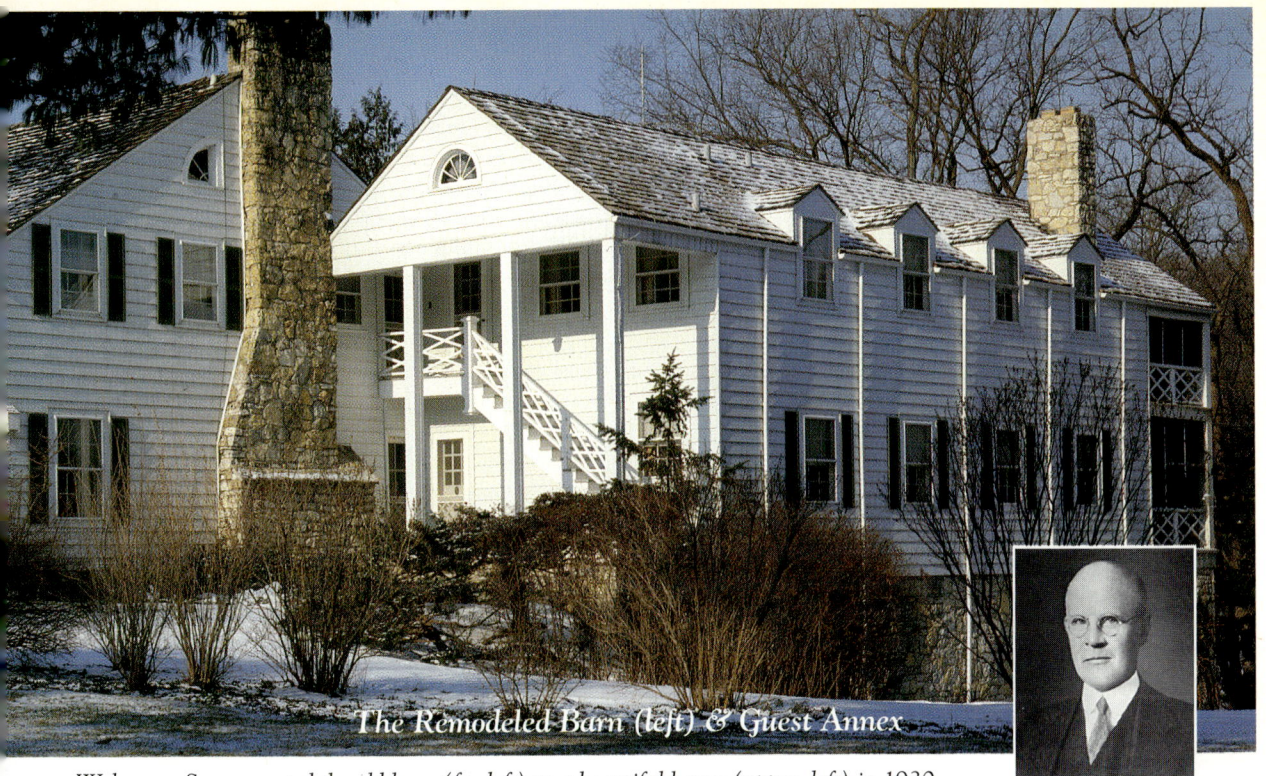

The Remodeled Barn (left) & Guest Annex

Walgreen, Sr. converted the old barn (far left) to a beautiful house (upper left) in 1930. Its hayloft became bedrooms. The Annex (upper right) was added a year later.

Charles R. Walgreen, Sr.

In 1935, a century after Samuel Charter originally purchased the estate, Walgreen built Cliff House. Set into the natural curve of the hill, at the bend of the Rock River, Cliff House was designed by world-renowned architects Zimmerman and O'Brien, and was crafted of native Illinois stones and logs. Walgreen and his son, Charles R. "Chuck" Walgreen, Jr., scoured the area to find the century-old, hand-hewn beams for the home's interior. Walgreen, Sr. delighted in creating theme rooms, like his own "log cabin" room and a "ship's bunk" nursery, complete with bunk beds and portholes! Sadly, however, Charles Walgreen, Sr. only enjoyed Hazelwood for a short time. He died in December 1939, at the age of 66.

An avid gardener and photographer, Myrtle R. Walgreen lived at Hazelwood for many years. She created beautiful gardens, conducted garden walks and captured a photographic record of Hazelwood's beauty on film. She also supported 4-H Clubs nationwide, sponsoring annual awards for home beautification. And, in keeping with tradition, she and Charles Walgreen, Jr. (who succeeded his father as chairman of Walgreens), entertained many important guests. During the 1940's, at a particularly grand event, well-known entertainers Bob Hope, Joe E. Brown and a young Ronald Reagan came to visit. Reagan had grown up in Dixon and had caddied for Walgreen, Sr. on many occasions. During his 50th high school reunion, Reagan returned to Hazelwood, becoming the second President ever to have slept there!

After a long life, blessed with excellent health, Myrtle R. Walgreen died in 1971; she was 92. Charles Walgreen, Jr. and his children (including Charles R. Walgreen, III, the current chairman of Walgreens), grandchildren and great-grandchildren, continue to enjoy Hazelwood.

Walgreen, Jr. donated 45 acres of the property to the Dixon Park District, for nature trails in 1977. In 1979, he gave the remaining 122-acre, seven-building estate, with a trust fund to maintain it, to the University of Illinois Foundation for use as a conference center. Currently, he has exclusive lifetime use. His generous gesture ensures that the Walgreen's avid support of education and the enjoyment of nature, will continue at Hazelwood for many years to come.

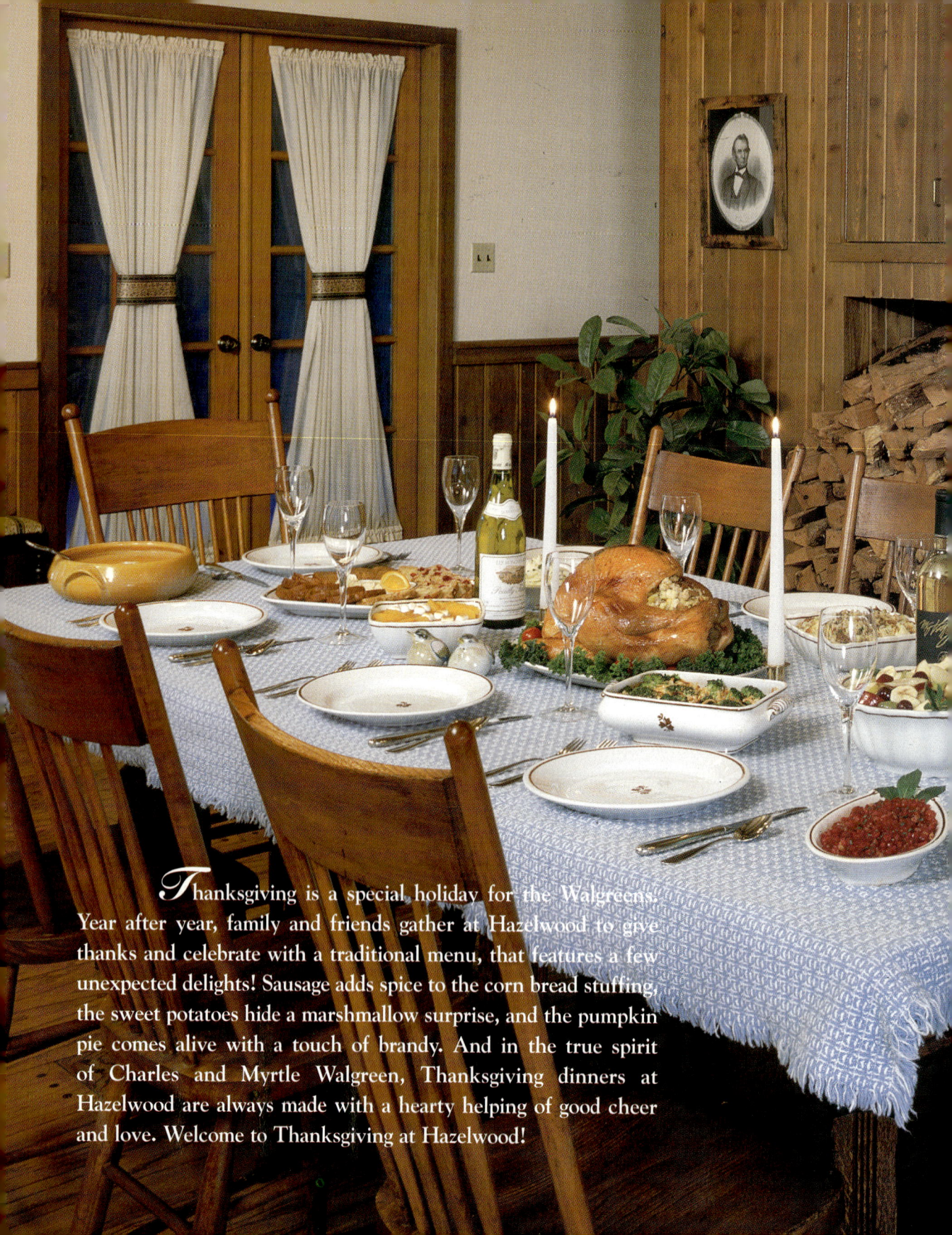

Thanksgiving is a special holiday for the Walgreens. Year after year, family and friends gather at Hazelwood to give thanks and celebrate with a traditional menu, that features a few unexpected delights! Sausage adds spice to the corn bread stuffing, the sweet potatoes hide a marshmallow surprise, and the pumpkin pie comes alive with a touch of brandy. And in the true spirit of Charles and Myrtle Walgreen, Thanksgiving dinners at Hazelwood are always made with a hearty helping of good cheer and love. Welcome to Thanksgiving at Hazelwood!

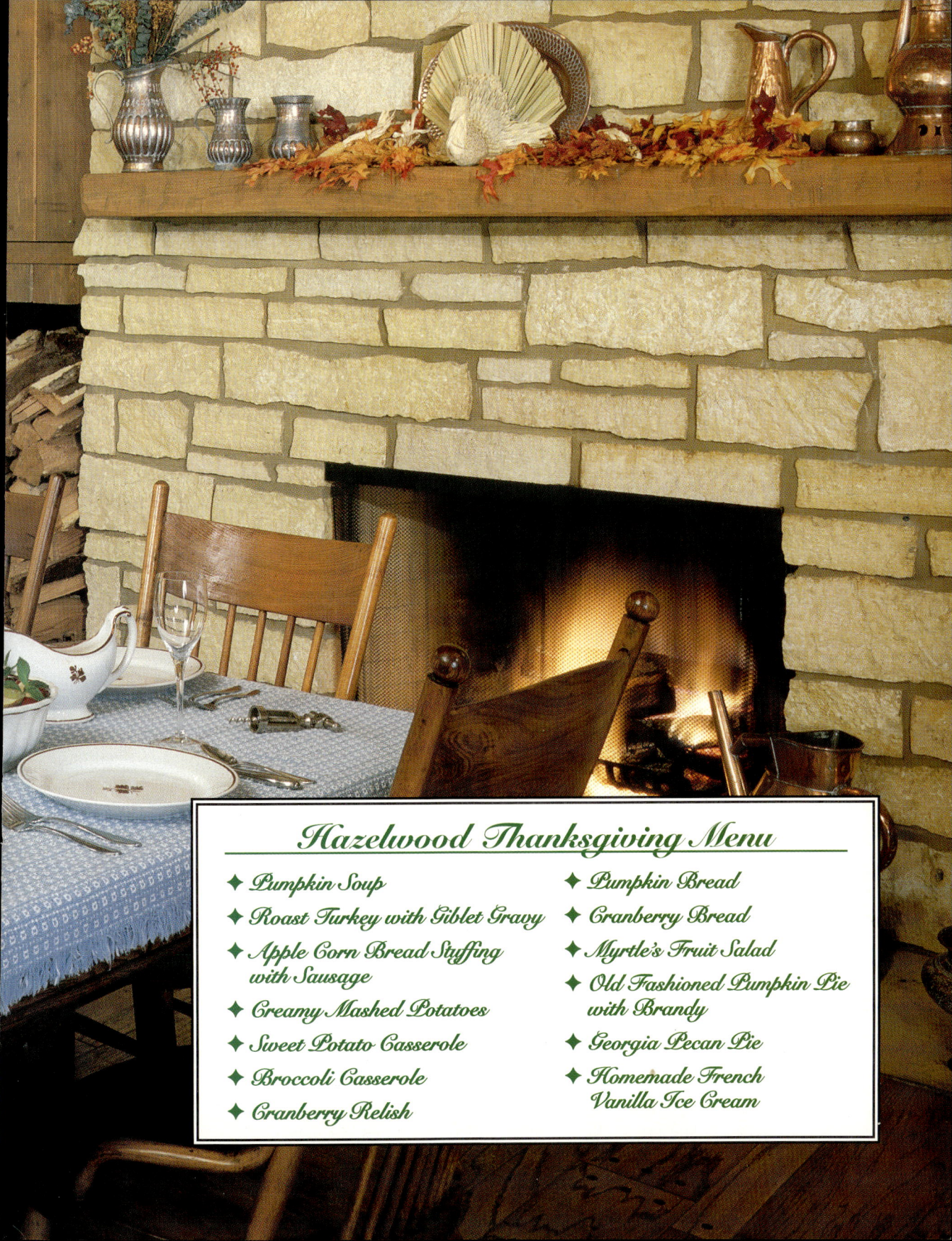

Hazelwood Thanksgiving Menu

- ✦ Pumpkin Soup
- ✦ Roast Turkey with Giblet Gravy
- ✦ Apple Corn Bread Stuffing with Sausage
- ✦ Creamy Mashed Potatoes
- ✦ Sweet Potato Casserole
- ✦ Broccoli Casserole
- ✦ Cranberry Relish
- ✦ Pumpkin Bread
- ✦ Cranberry Bread
- ✦ Myrtle's Fruit Salad
- ✦ Old Fashioned Pumpkin Pie with Brandy
- ✦ Georgia Pecan Pie
- ✦ Homemade French Vanilla Ice Cream

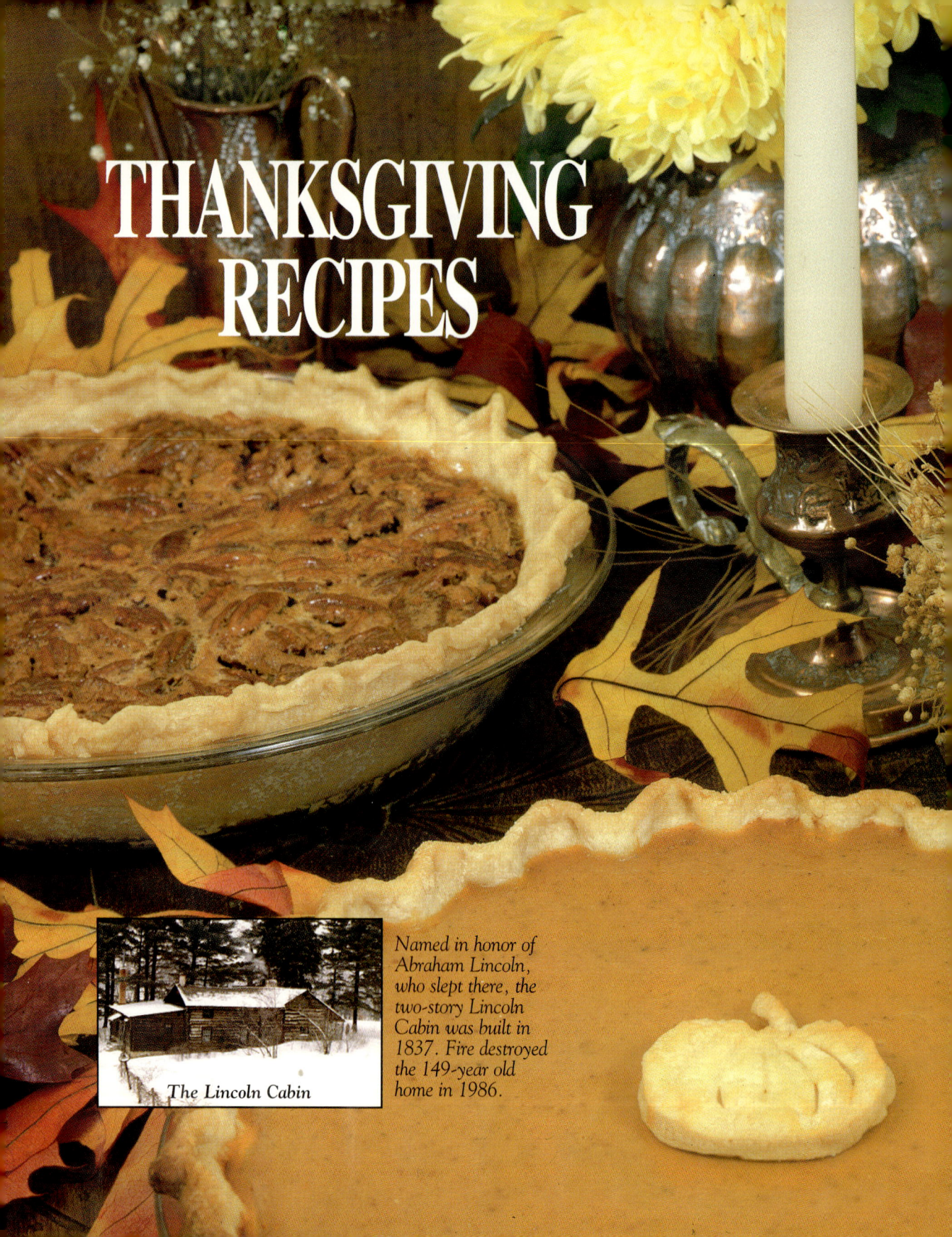

THANKSGIVING RECIPES

Named in honor of Abraham Lincoln, who slept there, the two-story Lincoln Cabin was built in 1837. Fire destroyed the 149-year old home in 1986.

The Lincoln Cabin

Roast Turkey with Giblet Gravy

Serves 12

Turkey:
1   18 to 22-pound fresh turkey
6   fresh sage leaves
4   tablespoons sweet butter, melted
stuffing, if desired

Giblet gravy:
giblets from turkey, cooked and chopped (do not use neck or neck meat)
1   onion studded with cloves
2   sprigs parsley
1   bay leaf
juice and dripping from turkey and roasting pan
2   cups cold water
4   tablespoons flour
salt and pepper, to taste

Preheat oven to 325 degrees. Remove giblet package from inside turkey. Chop giblets into small pieces and place in saucepan; cover with water. Add clove-studded onion, parsley sprigs and bay leaf; cook until tender. Meanwhile, wash inside and outside of turkey. Dry thoroughly. Gently place fingers under breast skin and above breast meat. Wiggle fingers to loosen skin from meat. Place 3 sage leaves in a decorative triangle on left breast; repeat for right breast.

Add stuffing, if desired, to both cavities of turkey. Place turkey breast-side up in roasting pan. Pour melted butter over entire turkey; rub into creases with hands. Tie legs together loosely, to hold shape. Cover legs and wings with aluminum foil; cover roasting pan. Bake 15 minutes per pound of unstuffed turkey, or 20 minutes per pound of stuffed turkey or until meat thermometer registers 175 degrees. Baste every 30 minutes, removing juices that reach more than 2 inches deep in pan; reserve. 1 hour before done, remove pan cover and foil from legs and wings. Continue basting frequently until golden brown. When turkey is thoroughly cooked, remove from roasting pan, reserving juices. Transfer turkey to platter; tent with foil and let stand 30 minutes. Scoop out stuffing, carve and serve with giblet gravy.

To prepare giblet gravy, add water to roasting pan, loosening browned bits and turkey drippings. Strain, if necessary. Add all drippings and juices to saucepan. Cook over medium heat until boiling. Whisk together flour and cold water. Slowly pour flour mixture into boiling drippings, whisking constantly. Reduce heat and cook for 5 more minutes. Add more water, if necessary. Add giblets, salt and pepper, to taste. Cook 1 minute longer. Remove clove-studded onion, parsley sprigs and bay leaf. Serve with turkey.

Apple Corn Bread Stuffing with Sausage

Serves 12

Myrtle R. Walgreen's original recipe!

12 tablespoons butter
2½ cups onions, finely chopped
3 large tart apples, cored and chunked (do not peel)
1 link sage seasoned bulk sausage
3 cups corn bread, coarsely crumbled
3 cups whole wheat bread, coarsely crumbled
2 teaspoons dried thyme
1 teaspoon dried sage
½ cups parsley, chopped
1½ cups pecan halves, shelled
2 cups chicken or turkey broth or stock
salt and pepper to taste

Melt 6 tablespoons butter in skillet. Add chopped onions and cook over medium heat, partially covered, until tender. Transfer to large mixing bowl. Melt remaining butter in same skillet. Add apple chunks and cook over high heat until lightly colored but not mushy. Add to mixing bowl. Crumble sausage into same skillet and cook over medium heat until lightly browned. With a slotted spoon, transfer sausage to mixing bowl, reserving rendered fat. Add remaining ingredients to mixing bowl and combine gently. Add broth; combine to moisten all ingredients. Salt and pepper to taste. Cool completely before stuffing turkey.

Note: Enough stuffing for a 20-pound turkey.

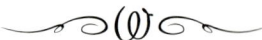

Creamy Mashed Potatoes

Serves 12

8 large white potatoes, peeled and diced
5 tablespoons butter
1 cup milk
1 teaspoon salt
½ teaspoon white pepper

Place potatoes in saucepan, cover with cold water and boil until well done. Drain and return to saucepan. Meanwhile, add butter to milk in measuring cup. Place in microwave for 2 minutes, or until butter is melted and milk is hot. Mix potatoes, salt and pepper in food processor. Slowly pour milk and butter through feeding tube; blend until creamy. Serve hot with giblet gravy.

Sweet Potato Casserole

Serves 12

8 large sweet potatoes
6 tablespoons sweet butter, softened
½ cup half & half
½ teaspoon nutmeg
1 tablespoon cinnamon
1 tablespoon cardamom
1 cup brown sugar
½ cup orange juice
1 large orange, sectioned
1 cup miniature marshmallows

Preheat oven to 350 degrees. Wash and boil potatoes until tender. Peel and mash. With electric mixer beat in butter and half & half. Add spices, brown sugar and orange juice; heat until blended. Place all in casserole dish. Decorate top with orange sections and marshmallows. Bake for 30 minutes.

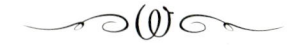

Broccoli Casserole

Serves 12

3 heads (2 pounds) broccoli
12 ounces Velveeta cheese, thinly sliced
1½ sticks plus 2 tablespoons butter, softened
2 cups Ritz cracker crumbs
6 carrots, peeled and cut into 2-inch strips
1 3¾-ounce package sliced almonds

Preheat oven to 350 degrees. Use only 1 head of broccoli and the stems from the other two. Wash and chop the head and stems into very small pieces; steam until crisp, but tender. Drain thoroughly. Cut the two leftover broccoli heads into very small florets. Cook broccoli florets until crisp, but tender. Drain well. Spread chopped broccoli in bottom of lightly greased 10x15x4-inch baking dish, reserving florets. Cover with cheese.

Combine 1½ sticks butter and cracker crumbs. Mixture will be lumpy. Drop large spoonful over cheese and spread evenly. Steam carrots sticks until tender, but crisp; drain. Cover the cracker crumb-butter mixture with a mixture of steamed carrots and broccoli florets, arranging in a decorative pattern. Pat gently into cracker mixture so that vegetables are one-third submerged. Sprinkle with almonds. Dot top with remaining 2 tablespoons butter. Bake for 20 minutes, until crumb topping browns lightly.

Pumpkin Soup

Serves 6

An authentic recipe from The White House Cookbook, *1887!*

6	small pumpkins, hollowed out ~ save tops
1	medium pumpkin ~ peeled, seeded and cut into chunks
2	tablespoons butter
2	tablespoons onions, chopped
¼	teaspoon allspice
½	teaspoon ginger, ground
1	tablespoon flour
2	cups chicken stock or bouillon
½	teaspoon salt
2	cups milk

sour cream

Place pumpkin chunks in kettle and cover with water. Bring to a boil, reduce heat and simmer until soft. Drain thoroughly, mash, and reserve; this should yield 2 cups. Meanwhile, sauté chopped onion in butter; add allspice and ginger. Stir in flour. Add cooked pumpkin and cook mixture slowly for 5 minutes. Gradually add chicken stock, salt and milk. Simmer 5 more minutes. Scoop mixture into pumpkin shells and top with a dollop of sour cream. Place tops on pumpkins, and serve.

Note: For 12 servings, simply double the recipe.

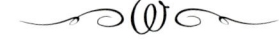

Cranberry Relish

Serves 12
Yield: 3 to 4 cups

1½	12-ounce packages fresh cranberries
1½	cups sugar
2	small oranges, seeded
4	sprigs fresh mint (reserve 1 for garnish)
½	cup walnuts, chopped

Place package of fresh cranberries in freezer for several hours. Blend frozen cranberries, sugar, orange and 3 sprigs fresh mint in food processor until it is the consistency of relish. Remove and add chopped walnuts. Garnish with 1 mint sprig, and refrigerate until ready to serve.

Pumpkin Bread

Yield: One 9x5-inch loaf

- 1½ cups sugar
- 2 eggs
- ¼ cup salad oil
- ½ cup water
- 2 cups flour
- ½ teaspoon baking powder
- ¾ teaspoon salt
- ½ teaspoon cloves
- ½ teaspoon cinnamon
- ½ teaspoon nutmeg
- 1 teaspoon baking soda
- 1 cup pumpkin

Preheat oven to 350 degrees. Cream sugar and eggs together. Add salad oil and water. Sift dry ingredients together and mix thoroughly into creamed mixture. Add pumpkin and mix well. Pour into a greased 9x5x3-inch pan. Bake for 1 hour.

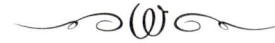

Cranberry Bread

Yield: One 9x5-inch loaf

- 1 egg, beaten
- 2 tablespoons hot water
- 2 tablespoons soft butter
- ½ cup orange juice
- 1 cup sugar
- ½ teaspoon baking powder
- ½ teaspoon baking soda
- 2 cups flour
- 1 cup fresh cranberries, washed and cut in half
- ½ cup chopped nuts

Preheat oven to 350 degrees. Mix eggs, hot water, butter, and orange juice. Sift sugar, baking powder, soda, and flour into first mixture. Add cranberries and nuts and pour into loaf pan. Bake for 30 minutes.

Myrtle's Fruit Salad

Serves 12

Myrtle R. Walgreen's original recipe!

Salad:
- 2 Red Delicious apples, cored and seeded, but not peeled
- 2 Granny Smith apples, cored and seeded, but not peeled
- 2 Bartlett pears, cored, seeded and peeled
- 2 bananas, sliced and dipped in lemon juice
- 2 Honey Bill oranges, peeled, seeded and sectioned
- 1 whole pineapple, peeled, cored and cubed
- 1 large bunch seedless green grapes, halved
- ¼ pound fresh cherries, pitted and halved
- 1 cup walnuts, halved

Dressing:
- 1 pint heavy cream
- 1 pint sour cream
- ½ cup sugar
- 1 teaspoon vanilla

Combine salad ingredients in a large bowl and refrigerate for several hours. Make dressing 1 hour prior to serving. To make dressing, whip cream until it peaks, then fold in sour cream, sugar and vanilla. Mix dressing into fruit salad and refrigerate until ready to serve.

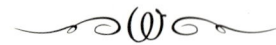

Georgia Pecan Pie

Yield: One 9-inch pie

- 1 9-inch pie pastry
- 3 large eggs
- ½ cup sugar
- ½ teaspoon salt
- 6 tablespoons butter, melted
- 1 cup dark corn syrup
- 1 teaspoon vanilla
- 1 cup pecan halves

Preheat oven to 375 degrees. Roll out pastry. Line a 9-inch pie pan with pastry. Combine eggs, sugar, salt, butter, corn syrup and vanilla. Mix thoroughly and fold in pecans. Spoon filling into pie shell. Place pie on lower oven shelf and bake until bottom crust is golden brown, about 45 to 50 minutes. Cool, or serve warm, with *Homemade French Vanilla Ice Cream*, *(see recipe at right)*.

Old~Fashioned Pumpkin Pie with Brandy

Yield: One 9-inch pie

- 1   9-inch pie pastry
- 1   cup canned pumpkin
- 1   cup evaporated milk
- 3   large eggs
- 1   cup light brown sugar
- 1   teaspoon cinnamon
- ½   teaspoon ground ginger
- ¼   teaspoon ground cloves
- ½   teaspoon ground nutmeg
- ¼   cup brandy

Preheat oven to 400 degrees. Roll out pastry. Line a 9-inch pie pan with pastry. Trim edge even with pie pan. Cover with foil and weigh pastry down with dried beans. Place pie pan on bottom oven rack and bake about 15 minutes.

Remove beans and foil; set partially baked crust aside to cool. Meanwhile, add pumpkin to a large mixing bowl. Add milk and eggs; whip until smooth. Combine sugar with spices and mix well. Beat them into pumpkin mixture, add brandy and mix thoroughly. Spoon filling into partially-baked crust. Place pie on lower oven shelf and bake for 8 minutes. Reduce heat to 350 degrees and continue to bake until a knife inserted in middle comes out clean, about another 35 to 40 minutes. Serve warm or cold with *Homemade French Vanilla Ice Cream* (see recipe below).

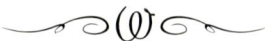

Homemade French Vanilla Ice Cream

Yield: 1 quart

- 3   eggs
- 1   cup sugar
- 2   cups cream
- 2   cups milk
- 2   teaspoons vanilla

Beat eggs and sugar together in a large saucepan. Add sugar. Cook over low heat, stirring constantly until thickened, about 10 minutes. Mixture should coat the spoon smoothly. Cool; then add cream and vanilla. Beat the mixture well, incorporating air, but do not over-beat. Freeze overnight. Serve with *Georgia Pecan Pie* or *Old Fashioned Pumpkin Pie with Brandy* (see recipes, above and at left).

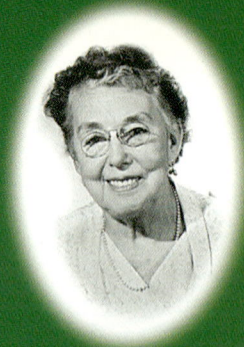

My Daily Prayer

*Heavenly Father, we thank you for
the many blessings bestowed upon us.
We have so much to be grateful for:*

*Our eyes, with which we see all
the beauty surrounding us.*

*Our ears, with which we hear the song
of birds and all other sweet music.*

Our hands, with which we can work.

*Our minds and hearts through
which we gain understanding.*

*And may the great understanding minds of
the world bring us universal peace.*

*Again we thank you for your
countless benefactions. Lead us
and guide us in Thy way.*

This is asked in the name of the Lord, Amen.

Myrtle R. Walgreen

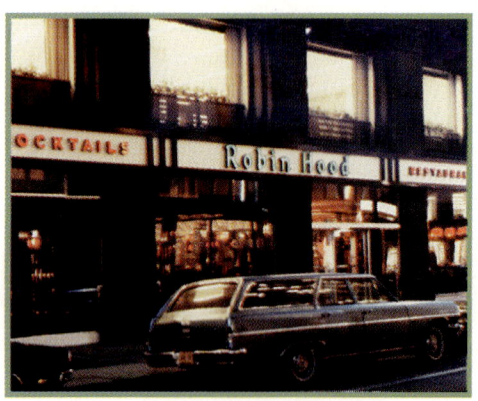

The Robin Hood restaurants in downtown Chicago were very popular after-work meeting spots.

Facing Page: *Bruschetta*
Photo: Scott Lanza, 1995
Stylist: F. Lynn Nelson

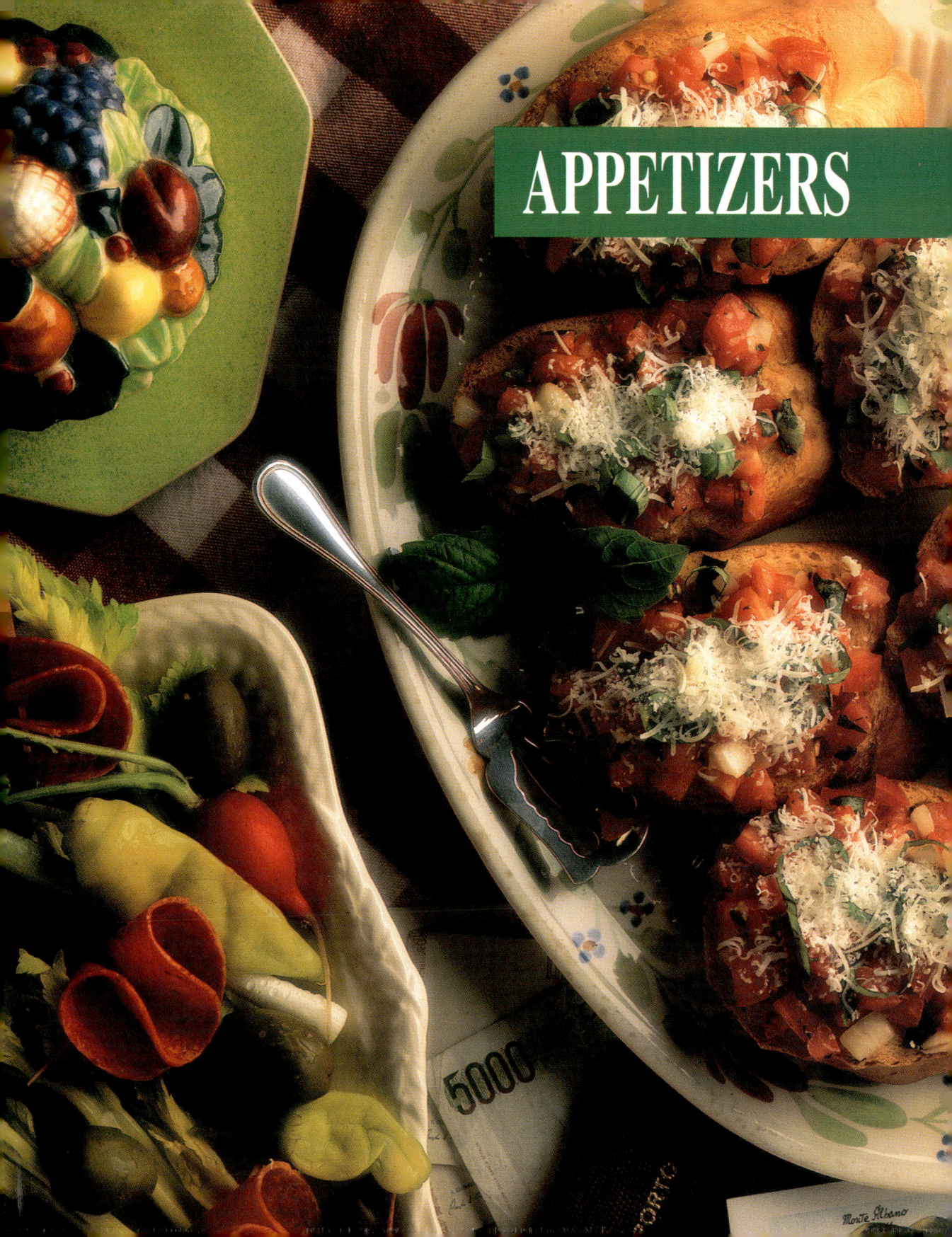
APPETIZERS

Robin Hood & Briargate
Exciting Dining in Sherwood Forest

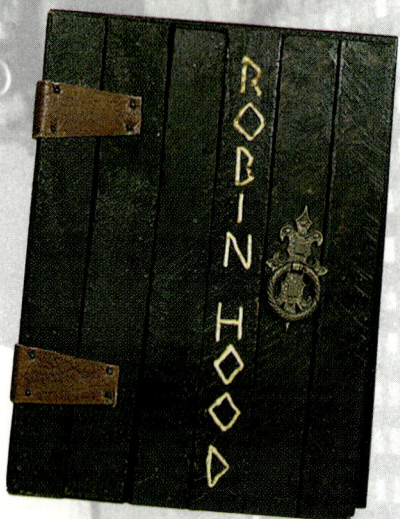

"Robin Hood was a very popular, family-style restaurant with elaborate medieval decor."
Dominic Bandera,
A former head chef & manager of Robin Hood

Go forth ye and eat heartily...! One of the first restaurants anywhere to carry "finger foods," *Robin Hood* (with its counterpart, *Briargate*) was Walgreens first line of freestanding restaurants. Extremely popular from the late 1960's to the late 1980's, much of Robin Hood's claim to fame was owed to its exciting and elaborate medieval ambience! Walking into Robin Hood was like a visit to the Sherwood Forest, from rough-hewn timbers and heraldic shields, right down to authentic carved-wood menu casings ~ complete with brass "door pulls"! Robin Hood was best-loved for its food, however, and its fresh salad bar and delicious house specialties always received rave reviews. But it was the appetizers, Robin Hood's own inventions ~ like sumptuous *Flamed Mushrooms* sautéed in wine ~ that really made the restaurant famous!

Cucumber Sandwiches

Serves 6

Also works well as a light lunch!

1 package Good Seasons Italian dressing mix
½ cup mayonnaise
2 8-ounce packages cream cheese, softened
1 loaf party rye bread, sliced
2 large cucumbers, evenly sliced
dill weed sprigs

Combine dressing mix, mayonnaise and cream cheese, and mix well. Spread ingredients on rye bread, and place 3 slices of cucumber on each slice. Garnish each with a sprig of dill weed.

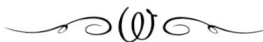

Healthy Fruit Spread

Yields: 2½ cups

1 8-ounce can crushed pineapple, well drained
1 8-ounce container fat-free soft cream cheese
1 carrot, shredded
1 small apple, cored and shredded
2 tablespoons sugar or sugar substitute
½ teaspoon vanilla extract
½ cup pecans, chopped (optional)

6 apples, cored, sliced and dipped in lemon juice (to prevent browning)
Triscuits (optional)

Combine pineapple, cream cheese, carrot, small apple, sugar, vanilla extract and pecans. Spread on apple slices. May also spread on Triscuits.

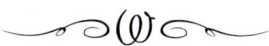

Roasted Garlic Cloves

Serves 4 to 6

1 medium head garlic
2 teaspoons olive oil

1 fresh loaf French bread, sliced

Preheat oven to 400 degrees. Peel away the outer layers of skin from head of garlic. Leave skins on cloves intact. Cut off the pointed top portion (about ¼-inch) with a knife, leaving the bulb intact, but exposing the individual cloves. Place garlic head, cut-side up, in a small baking dish. Drizzle with olive oil. Bake, covered, for 25 to 35 minutes, or until cloves feel soft when pressed. To serve, press garlic paste from individual cloves and spread on French bread.

Cheese on Rye

Serves 12 to 15

12 to 14 ounces cheddar cheese, grated
5 green onions, bulbs and stems thinly sliced
1 4¼-ounce can chopped black olives, drained
mayonnaise, enough to bind mixture together

cocktail rye

Preheat oven to 350 degrees. Mix all ingredients. Spread mixture on rye bread. Place on cookie sheet and bake for 10 to 12 minutes.

Note: Mixture will keep in refrigerator for 12 to 14 days.

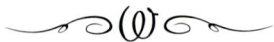

Hungarian Cheese Spread

Serves 10 to 12

½ pound sweet butter, softened
½ pound cream cheese, softened
1 teaspoon prepared mustard
½ small onion, finely minced
garlic powder, to taste
paprika

pumpernickel rounds or crackers

Blend butter, cheese, mustard, onion and garlic powder until smooth. Place in serving dish and sprinkle heavily with paprika. Cover and refrigerate. Serve with pumpernickel rounds or crackers.

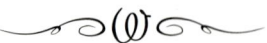

Liptoi Cheese Spread

Serves 12

½ pound Liptoi or cream cheese
¼ pound blue cheese
¼ pound butter
½ teaspoon caraway seeds
1 teaspoon capers, chopped

dark bread, thinly sliced, or crackers

Blend cheeses and butter. Mix in seasonings. Spread on thinly-sliced dark bread or crackers.

Italian Cheese Dip

Yield: 1½ cups

1   cup mayonnaise
½   cup Italian cheese, Provolone or Gorgonzola, grated
1   teaspoon Worcestershire sauce
¼   teaspoon garlic salt
2   tablespoons lemon juice

assorted raw vegetables, cut

Mix all ingredients, chill. Serve with cut vegetables.

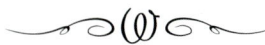

Emergency Cheese Things

Yield: 2 cups

1   cup sharp cheddar cheese, shredded
½ to ¾-cup onion, finely chopped
mayonnaise, enough to bind mixture together

party rye

Mix cheese and onion together. Add enough mayonnaise to bind it together, but not so much that it is sloppy. Spread on party rye and broil until cheese is thoroughly melted.

Note: This also makes a good open-faced sandwich.

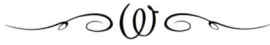

Marlene's Basil Pâté

Serves 10 to 12

4   full cups fresh basil
1   garlic clove
⅓   cup olive oil
1   pound Ricotta cheese
⅓   cup Parmesan cheese, grated
½   cup pine nuts, toasted
salt and pepper, to taste

cocktail rye or crackers

Mix all ingredients in food processor. Mold into mound on cold plate. Chill until set. Top with toasted pine nuts. Serve with cocktail rye or crackers.

Shrimp Mold

Serves 4 to 6

Also works well as a light lunch!

⅓ cup tomato soup
1 3-ounce package cream cheese
⅓ cup celery, chopped
⅓ cup onion, chopped
⅓ cup green pepper, chopped
1 small can medium shrimp
⅓ cup mayonnaise
3 tablespoons boiling water
½ package Knox gelatin
cocktail rye or crackers

Mix soup with cream cheese in a double boiler on top of stove until soft. In a separate bowl mix celery, onion, green pepper, shrimp and mayonnaise. Add that to soup mixture. Combine boiling water with Knox gelatin, blend well and add to rest of ingredients. Put in a small mold and jell at least 3 hours or more in refrigerator. Unmold and serve with cocktail rye or crackers.

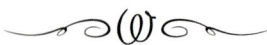

Shrimp, Cheese & Bacon Delight

Serves 8

16 jumbo shrimp (10 to 15 per pound), cleaned, peeled and deveined
4 ounces Monterey Jack cheese
8 slices bacon, cut in half
½ cup bread crumbs
vegetable oil
cocktail sauce

Cut a pocket about ¾-inch deep and 1½-inches long in each shrimp; in center of slit, make a small cut through shrimp. Cut cheese in a small triangle, about ½-inch thick. Tuck point of triangle into slit in shrimp, and tightly wrap a piece of bacon around shrimp, enclosing cheese. Place a wooden skewer through tail-end of shrimp, and then through bacon and cheese. If made ahead, cover and chill. In a 3 to 4-quart pan, heat 2 inches of oil to about 350 degrees. Cook shrimp 3 or 4 at a time, turning if needed until golden and cheese begins to melt, about 1½ minutes. Drain shrimp, keep warm; serve with cocktail sauce.

Shrimp in Cocktail Sauce

Serves 6

1 pound shrimp, cleaned, deveined, cooked and chilled

Cocktail sauce:
2 tablespoons capers, chopped
¼ teaspoon onion, grated
½ cup heavy mayonnaise
1 teaspoon dry dill, steeped in scalding water and drained dry
2 hard-boiled eggs, chopped
½ cup grapefruit sections, cut into pieces
1 teaspoon orange rind

To make sauce, combine all ingredients. To serve, pour over shrimp.

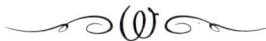

Bacon~Wrapped Shrimp

Serves 10

1½ pounds (30 to 40) shrimp, cleaned, deveined and cooked
1 16-ounce package lean bacon
¾ cup Teriyaki sauce

Preheat oven to 400 degrees. Cut bacon slices in half. Wrap bacon around shrimp and secure with wooden picks. Place in 9x13-inch baking dish. Pour Teriyaki sauce over shrimp. Cover and refrigerate one hour. Bake, uncovered, for 20 to 25 minutes.

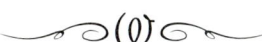

Louisiana Mustard Sauce Shrimp

Serves 6 to 8

3 pounds shrimp, cleaned, peeled, deveined and cooked

Mustard sauce:
¼ cup celery, coarsely chopped
¼ cup onion, coarsely chopped
¼ cup parsley, coarsely chopped
½ cup Dijon mustard
½ cup vinegar
½ cup olive oil
½ teaspoon paprika
1 tablespoon salt

Combine all sauce ingredients in food processor or blender; mix until smooth. Chill and serve over shrimp, or use as a dipping sauce.

Crab Meat Dip

Serves 6

- 1 6-ounce (4½-ounce drained) can crab meat, cleaned and drained
- 1 8-ounce package cream cheese, softened
- 2 tablespoons onion, grated
- 1 tablespoon milk
- ½ teaspoon prepared horseradish
- ¼ teaspoon salt
- ¼ teaspoon pepper

⅓ cup slivered almonds
rye crackers or cocktail rye bread

Preheat oven to 350 degrees. Mix together all ingredients, except almonds. Put mixture in small casserole dish. Top with almonds. Bake for 15 minutes. Serve with rye crackers or cocktail rye bread.

Hot Crab Fondue

Serves 6 to 8

- 1 6-ounce (4½-ounce drained) can crab meat, cleaned and drained
- 1 5-ounce jar Kraft sharp American cheese spread
- 1 8-ounce package Philadelphia cream cheese
- ¼ cup half-and-half
- ¼ teaspoon garlic salt
- ½ teaspoon Worcestershire sauce
- ¼ teaspoon cayenne pepper

melba toast, crackers or breadsticks

Combine all ingredients in a fondue pot or saucepan. Heat on medium until melted, then stir to mix flavors. Serve with melba toast or other full-bodied crackers. Sesame or regular breadsticks also work well with this fondue.

Note: Tastes best when you keep the mixture warm in a fondue pot. You can prepare this recipe in advance, refrigerate it and warm it up at the last minute.

Crab Meat Spread

Serves 12

1   6-ounce (4½-ounce drained) can crab meat, cleaned and drained
2   8-ounce packages cream cheese, softened

shrimp cocktail sauce

crackers

Flake the crab meat and stir into cream cheese. Form mixture into a ball. Chill. Before serving, pour shrimp cocktail sauce over crab meat mixture. Serve with crackers.

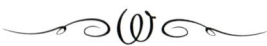

Salmon Spread

Serves 6

1   16-ounce can salmon, drained and flaked
1   8-ounce package light cream cheese, softened
½   tablespoon lemon juice
¼   teaspoon salt
2   teaspoons onion, grated
½   teaspoon liquid smoke
½   teaspoon horseradish

crackers or taco chips

Mix together all ingredients, taste and re-season if desired. Refrigerate. Serve on crackers or with taco chips.

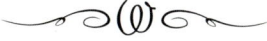

Chris' Clam Dip

Serves 6 to 8

2   6½-ounce cans minced clams, drained, reserve clam juice
1   8-ounce package cream cheese, softened
1   teaspoon lemon juice
1   tablespoon scallions (green onions), chopped
½   teaspoon Worcestershire sauce
½   teaspoon Tabasco sauce
1   dash pepper and seasoned salt, to taste

Mix together all ingredients, except the clams. Fold in clams. Thin with clam juice for desired consistency; use as a dip or spread.

Guacamole

Yield: 1 cup

In Spanish aguacate *(avocado) means alligator pear. When served as a spread or dip, aguacate is called guacamole!*

1 garlic clove
1 large avocado, peeled
¼ teaspoon salt
¼ teaspoon chili powder
1 teaspoon lemon juice
2 teaspoons onion, finely minced
mayonnaise

Rub wooden bowl with cut garlic clove. Place avocado in bowl and mash with silver fork. Add salt, chili powder, lemon juice and minced onion. Mix well and taste for seasoning. Put the guacamole in a serving bowl and cover with thin layer of mayonnaise, to prevent avocado from blackening. Stir well just before serving.

Note: This may be used as a canapé spread or a raw vegetable dip. Also very good as dressing for head-of-lettuce salad.

Nacho Dip

Yield: 2 quarts

2 8-ounce containers sour cream
2 8-ounce packages cream cheese, softened
1 package taco seasoning mix
1 cup picante sauce
1 cup scallions (green onions), chopped
½ cup black olives
1 cup Monterey Jack or cheddar cheese, shredded
nacho chips

Put sour cream, cream cheese and taco seasoning in blender or food processor, and blend until creamy. Pour into flat serving dish. Layer evenly on top: picante sauce, chopped scallions, black olives and shredded cheese. Serve with nacho chips.

Mexican Dip

Serves 6

- 1 8-ounce package cream cheese, softened
- 1 15-ounce can Hormel no-beans chili
- 8 ounces Monterey Jack cheese with jalapeño peppers, shredded
- 2 green onions, chopped
- 1 medium tomato, chopped

nacho chips

Preheat oven to 350 degrees. Spread cream cheese on serving dish. Spread chili on top. Place shredded Monterey Jack cheese on top of chili layer. Add chopped green onion and chopped tomato. Bake for 20 minutes. Surround the platter with nacho chips and enjoy.

Hot Chili Dip

Serves 8

- 2 8-ounce packages cream cheese
- 4 green onions, chopped
- ¼ teaspoon garlic salt
- 1 15-ounce can no-beans chili
- 2 cups cheddar cheese, grated

dip-size corn chips

Preheat oven to 250 degrees. Spread cream cheese in 9x13-inch baking dish. Cover with onions, garlic salt and chili. Top with cheese. Bake until cheese melts, about 30 minutes. Serve hot with corn chips.

"Girls' Day Out" Dip

Serves 8 to 10

- 2¼ cups sharp cheddar cheese, shredded
- 6 scallions (green onions), finely chopped
- 1 6-ounce can pitted black olives, chopped
- 6 tablespoons Hellmann's mayonnaise
- 1 pound bacon, fried, drained and crumbled

tortilla chips

In a mixing bowl, combine cheese, scallions and olives; mix. Stir in 4 tablespoons of mayonnaise, adding more until mixture pastes together. Prior to serving, blend in crumbled bacon. Serve with tortilla chips.

Note: Best made the night before.

Bruschetta

Serves 10

4 large tomatoes, chopped
1 small onion, chopped
2 garlic cloves, chopped
2 teaspoons balsamic vinegar
2 tablespoons Italian flat-leaf parsley
1 teaspoon oregano
salt and pepper, to taste
1 loaf crusty French bread
¼ cup olive oil
½ cup basil, chopped
½ cup Romano cheese, grated

Combine tomatoes, onion, garlic, vinegar, parsley and oregano. Add salt and pepper to taste. Add ⅛-cup olive oil. Mix well. Allow to rest while preparing bread. Cut bread into 2-inch slices. Place on cookie sheet. Brush with ⅛-cup olive oil and broil until golden; turn, brush other side and broil. Spoon mixture evenly onto bread. Top each with 1 teaspoon basil and 1 teaspoon Romano cheese. Warm in 350 degree oven, 1 to 2 minutes, and serve.

Caviar Cream Cheese Spread

Serves 10 to 12

2 8-ounce packages cream cheese, softened
1 3-ounce package cream cheese, softened
1 cup mayonnaise
1 small onion, grated
1 tablespoon Worcestershire sauce
1 tablespoon lemon juice
1 dash Tabasco sauce
1 3½-ounce jar black caviar, drained
4 eggs, hard boiled and finely chopped
1 cup fresh parsley, chopped
assorted crackers

Beat cream cheese in blender or food processor until smooth. Add mayonnaise, onion, Worcestershire sauce, lemon juice and Tabasco sauce; blend until creamy. Fold into serving dish. Top with caviar, eggs and parsley. Serve with assorted crackers.

Sausage & Sauerkraut Bites

Yield: 36 balls

8 ounces pork sausage, crumbled
¼ cup onion, finely chopped
vegetable oil
1 14-ounce can sauerkraut, drained, pressed dry and finely chopped
¾ cup plus 2 tablespoons dry bread crumbs, finely crushed
1 3-ounce package cream cheese, at room temperature
¼ teaspoon garlic powder
¼ teaspoon pepper
¼ cup all-purpose flour
1 egg, beaten with ¼-cup milk
1 cup bread crumbs
gourmet mustard, one or two kinds

In medium-size skillet, sauté sausage and onion in vegetable oil over medium heat, until lightly browned. Remove from heat. Drain off fat. Stir in sauerkraut, bread crumbs, cream cheese, garlic powder and pepper until thoroughly blended. Transfer to bowl; cover and chill until firm, at least 2 hours, or overnight. Shape mixture into ¾-inch balls. Roll in flour, then egg mixture and bread crumbs. Heat 2 inches oil in heavy 3-quart saucepan to 350 degrees. Fry 6 balls at a time, turning once, 2 to 3 minutes until lightly browned. Drain on paper towels. Serve hot, with one or two kinds of gourmet mustard.

Note: *Sausage & Sauerkraut Bites* may be fried ahead, then reheated on a jelly roll pan. Bake at 350 degrees for 10 to 15 minutes.

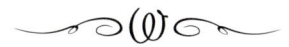

Curry Spread or Dip

Yield: 2 cups

1 8-ounce package cream cheese
1 cup cheddar cheese, grated
4 tablespoons cream sherry
1 teaspoon curry powder
chutney
green onions, snipped
crackers

Bring cream cheese, cheddar cheese and sherry to room temperature. Combine with curry powder, and shape into a ball. Pour chutney over top and garnish with green onions. Serve with crackers.

Kentucky Hot Brown Sandwiches

Yield: 4 sandwiches

Also works well as a light lunch!

- 8 slices bacon, cooked, drained and reserved
- 4 slices bread, toasted
- 4 to 6 slices turkey breast
- 4 to 6 thin slices baked ham
- 1 medium onion, chopped
- 2 tablespoons butter or margarine
- 5 tablespoons flour
- 3 cups milk
- 1 dash hot pepper sauce
- ¼ cup Swiss cheese, grated
- ¼ cup Parmesan cheese, grated

Butter a cookie sheet. Place toast on greased cookie sheet. Arrange ham and turkey slices on toast. Sauté onion in butter until soft and translucent. Add flour and stir 3 minutes over medium heat. Add milk, stirring constantly with whisk, until thick. Add pepper sauce and cheeses. Mix until dissolved and pour over meat and toast. Place sandwiches under broiler for about 5 minutes or until lightly brown. Put 2 slices bacon on top and serve.

Water Chestnuts in Bacon

Serves 12

- 2 8-ounce cans whole water chestnuts
- 1½ pounds bacon, cut strips into thirds
- 1 20-ounce bottle of catsup
- 8 heaping tablespoons brown sugar
- ¼ teaspoon Tabasco sauce

Preheat oven to 350 degrees. Drain water chestnuts and wrap each chestnut in a third of a slice of bacon. Place each in baking dish, wrapped end down. Bake for 40 minutes. Drain on paper towels. Mix brown sugar with catsup and Tabasco sauce. Pour over baked water chestnuts in baking dish. Cover and marinate overnight. Before serving; bake, uncovered, at 350 degrees for about 30 minutes.

Jean's Artichoke Dip

Serves 6 to 8

1 8-ounce can artichoke hearts, drained and mashed
½ cup Parmesan cheese, grated
4 drops Tabasco sauce
4 drops Worcestershire sauce
1 cup Hellmann's mayonnaise
paprika and parsley, chopped
crackers

Preheat oven to 350 degrees. Mix together artichoke hearts, Parmesan cheese, Tabasco, Worcestershire sauce and mayonnaise. Put in buttered casserole. Top with paprika and parsley. Bake for 20 minutes. Serve with crackers.

Artichoke Dip Bucaro

Serves 6 to 8

1 8-ounce can artichoke hearts, drained and chopped
1 cup mayonnaise
1 package Good Seasons Italian dressing mix
¼ cup parsley, chopped
½ cup Romano cheese, grated
crackers

Mix together artichoke hearts, mayonnaise, dressing mix and parsley; and spread in a shallow dish. Sprinkle with Romano cheese and heat in microwave for 3 minutes. Serve with favorite crackers.

Artichoke Balls

Yield: 48 balls

2 garlic cloves
2 tablespoons olive oil
1 8-ounce can artichoke hearts, drained and mashed
2 eggs, beaten
½ cup Parmesan cheese, grated
½ cup Italian bread crumbs

In a saucepan, cook garlic in olive oil. Add artichoke hearts and egg. Warm-through for 5 minutes on low heat. Add half the cheese and crumbs. Make balls. Roll in the remainder of cheese and crumbs.

Mushroom Turnovers

Yield: 3½ dozen

Also works well as a side dish!

Dough:
- 1   8-ounce package cream cheese, softened
- 1½ cups flour
- ½ cup butter or margarine

Mushroom filling:
- ½ pound mushrooms, minced
- 1 large onion, minced
- 3 tablespoons butter or margarine
- ¼ cup sour cream
- 1 teaspoon salt
- ¼ teaspoon thyme leaves
- 2 tablespoons flour
- 1 egg, beaten

In a large bowl, with mixer at medium speed, beat the cream cheese, adding flour and ½-cup butter or margarine. Mix until smooth. Shape into ball. Wrap and refrigerate one hour. Cook mushrooms and onions in 3 tablespoons of butter or margarine in skillet. Stir in cream, salt, thyme and 2 tablespoons flour. Set aside. Roll half the dough, on floured surface, to ⅛-inch thickness. Cut circles with floured 2½-inch cookie cutter. Preheat oven to 400 degrees. Place a scant teaspoon of mushroom mixture on half a circle. Brush edges of circles with egg. Fold dough over filling. Firmly press edges together with fork. Prick tops. Place turnovers on cookie sheet which has not been greased. Brush with remaining egg. Bake about 12 minutes, until golden.

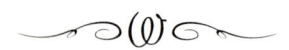

Crisp, Golden Mushrooms

Serves 4

Also works well as a side dish!

- 6 ounces fresh mushrooms
- ⅓ cup cornflakes, crushed into crumbs
- ½ teaspoon Italian seasoning
- ¼ teaspoon salt
- 1 dash ground red pepper, to taste
- ¼ cup cream or half-and-half

Preheat oven to 350 degrees. Wipe mushrooms with damp cloth. Place cornflake crumbs, seasoning, salt and red pepper into small paper or plastic bag. Dip mushrooms into cream, then shake with seasoned cornflakes. Place mushrooms on greased cookie sheet and bake for 15 minutes.

Stuffed Mushrooms

Yield: 12 to 16 caps

Also works well as a side dish!

1	pound fresh mushrooms
3	green onions, bulbs and stems thinly sliced
¼	cup butter
¼	cup fresh bread crumbs
3	tablespoons blue cheese, crumbled
1	tablespoon parsley, minced
1	tablespoon lemon juice
½	teaspoon salt

paprika, to taste

Preheat oven to 450 degrees. Remove the stems from mushrooms and mince; set aside caps. To make the filling, sauté the minced stems in butter with green onions until soft. Add bread crumbs, blue cheese, parsley, lemon juice and salt. Thoroughly blend the filling ingredients. Place the filling in the mushroom caps and sprinkle with paprika. Bake for 8 minutes.

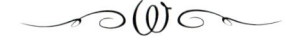

TV Party Mix

Yield: 4 quarts

4	cups Cheerios
6	cups Kix
3	cups Wheat Chex
3	cups slim pretzel sticks
1	pound mixed, salted nuts
½	cup butter or margarine
¼	cup bacon drippings
1	teaspoon Worcestershire sauce
1½	teaspoons seasoned salt
1	teaspoon garlic salt
1	teaspoon summer savory (optional)

Preheat oven to 250 degrees. Combine cereals, pretzels and nuts in large roaster pan. Melt butter and bacon drippings in saucepan. Add Worcestershire sauce and mix well. Pour over cereal mixture and mix. Combine seasonings. Put seasonings into an unused salt shaker and sprinkle over mixture, mixing well. Toast in oven for 1 hour, stirring every 15 minutes. Store in Tupperware containers.

Note: Recipe may be cut in half for smaller amount. *TV Party Mix* also makes nice gifts ~ just put Mix in baggies with bows, decorative jars or tins.

Spinach Appetizer Balls

Yield: 24 to 30 balls

2 10-ounce packages frozen, chopped spinach, cooked and well-drained
2 cups herb stuffing mix
1 cup Parmesan cheese, grated
6 eggs, beaten
¼ cup soft butter or margarine
salt and pepper, to taste

Preheat oven to 350 degrees. Combine ingredients and form small balls. Place balls on cookie sheet, cover with foil and freeze. To serve, bake frozen spinach balls on cookie sheet for 10 minutes, or until done.

Note: After frozen, *Spinach Appetizer Balls* may be put in a freezer container and stored for future use.

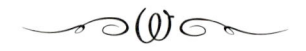

Spinach Strudel

Yield: 24 to 30 slices

2 10-ounce packages frozen, chopped spinach
    (place in refrigerator the night before using to thaw)
1 6-ounce package shredded mozzarella cheese
½ cup green onions, chopped
1 cup Parmesan cheese, grated
2 dashes ground cinnamon
salt and pepper, to taste
½ stick butter, cut into small pieces
phyllo dough (in sheets or leaves), thawed per package directions
1½ sticks of butter, melted
½ cup bread crumbs

Preheat oven to 350 degrees. Drain frozen spinach and squeeze to remove excess liquid. Mix together spinach, mozzarella, onions, Parmesan, cinnamon, salt, pepper and small pieces of butter; set aside. Place one phyllo sheet on a damp tea towel and brush with melted butter and sprinkle lightly with bread crumbs. Place another sheet on top and repeat butter and bread crumb routine, follow with third sheet. Place a third of spinach mixture along long end of phyllo sheet and roll as for jelly roll. Tuck ends in and with a sharp knife make diagonal cuts about three-quarters thru for serving portions. Repeat, for a total of 3 rolls. Bake for 45 minutes.

Note: This may be made the day before and refrigerated overnight. Leftovers reheat very well.

Deviled Ham Cornucopias

Serves 24

1 loaf white bread, cut into 24 thin slices
3 tablespoons mayonnaise
1 4½-ounce can deviled ham
2 hard-boiled eggs, finely chopped
1 tablespoon prepared mustard
1 tablespoon parsley
paprika (optional)

Preheat oven to 350 degrees. Cut bread with cookie cutter or glass. Flatten with rolling pin. Spread both sides with mayonnaise. Roll to form cornucopia. Fasten with toothpick. Place small ball of foil in center to prevent cornucopias from falling while baking. Bake on cookie sheet for 12 to 15 minutes. Remove toothpick and foil. To make filling, combine ham, eggs, mustard and parsley. Fill each cornucopia with a teaspoon of filling. Garnish with paprika

Spicy Broccoli Spread

Yield: ¾ cup

2½ cups broccoli florets
½ cup onion, chopped
1 small garlic clove, chopped
¼ teaspoon crushed red pepper
2 tablespoons olive oil
3 tablespoons Parmesan cheese, grated
toasted bread or crackers

In a small, covered saucepan, cook broccoli in a small amount of boiling, salted water for about 12 minutes, or until tender. Drain well. In a small skillet, cook onions, garlic and red pepper in hot olive oil until onions are soft; about 10 minutes. Combine broccoli, onion mixture and Parmesan cheese in a food processor. Cover and blend until smooth. Transfer to a small serving bowl. Serve at room temperature or cover and chill, for up to 24 hours. If chilled, let stand at room temperature 30 minutes before serving. Serve with toasted bread or crackers.

Becky's Bacon Breadsticks

Serves 4 to 6

1 cup brown sugar
cayenne pepper, to taste
1 pound bacon
1 package plain, Italian Stella D'ora breadsticks

Preheat oven to 350 degrees. Place a large piece of aluminum foil on the counter and spread brown sugar flat on surface. Sprinkle with cayenne pepper, to taste. With a fork, mix cayenne pepper into the brown sugar. Wrap a piece of bacon around each breadstick, leaving 1-inch on the end of each breadstick uncovered (for picking up). Roll bacon-wrapped breadsticks in brown sugar mixture and place on broiler pan (so bacon grease drips through it). Bake for 20 minutes. Turn breadsticks after 10 minutes, and continue baking. Move to cookie rack to cool. (Breadsticks will be limp until cool.) Serve when completely cooled.

Beefy Meatballs

Serves 10 to 12

Also works well as the main course!

2 pounds ground beef
2 cups stale bread, crumbled
2 eggs, slightly-beaten (or ½-cup Egg Beaters)
1 small onion, minced
1 garlic clove, minced
½ teaspoon pepper
2 teaspoons salt
½ teaspoon allspice
¼ cup milk
2 to 4 tablespoons butter or olive oil
¼ cup drippings, from the ground beef
1½ tablespoons flour
½ cup water
1 cup Burgundy or dry red wine
3 tablespoons dry beef and mushroom soup mix

Combine meat, bread, eggs, onion, garlic, seasonings and milk. Mix well. Form meatballs, about 1-inch in diameter. In a skillet, brown meatballs on all sides in butter or olive oil. Remove from pan. Retain drippings in pan and blend in flour, water, wine and soup mix. Cook, stirring constantly, until thick and smooth. Return meatballs to pan, cover and simmer 20 minutes. Transfer to chafing dish and keep hot on buffet table.

Meatballs Bourguignon

Serves 4 to 6

Also works well as the main course!

2 eggs
1 teaspoon garlic salt
¾ cup Burgundy ~ ¼-cup for meatballs, ½-cup for gravy
1½ pounds lean ground beef
½ cup bread crumbs, fine
1 to 2 tablespoons vegetable oil
2 packages onion gravy mix
½ cup water
1 teaspoon herb seasoning
1 pound noodles, cooked per package directions

Combine eggs, garlic salt and ¼-cup Burgundy. Add ground beef and bread crumbs. Mix lightly, and shape into small meatballs, using a round teaspoon for each. Brown in oil in a large skillet. Pour off fat. Combine the gravy mix with water, ½-cup Burgundy and the herb seasoning. Pour over the meat balls. Simmer, uncovered, for 15 minutes. Serve over noodles.

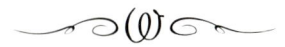

Crazy Meatballs

Yield: 70 meatballs

Also works well as the main course!

2 pounds ground beef
¼ cup bread crumbs
3 eggs, beaten
1 package onion soup mix
1 cup drained sauerkraut
1 16-ounce can cranberry sauce
1 10-ounce jar chili sauce
1 bottle of water (use chili sauce jar)
1 cup brown sugar

Preheat oven to 350 degrees. Combine ground beef, bread crumbs, eggs and onion soup mix. Shape into meatballs (around 70); set aside. In separate bowl; mix sauerkraut, cranberry sauce, chili sauce and water. Add brown sugar, mix well. Pour mixture over meatballs. Bake, uncovered, for 2 hours.

Swedish Meatballs

Serves 4 to 6

Also works well as the main course!

- ½ cup fresh white bread crumbs
- ½ cup milk
- ¼ pound ground beef
- ¼ pound ground pork
- 1 egg, slightly beaten
- 3 tablespoons onion, chopped
- 1½ teaspoons salt
- ¼ teaspoon white pepper
- ¼ teaspoon allspice
- 2 tablespoons butter
- 2 tablespoons flour
- 1 can beef broth
- ½ to 1 cup boiling water
- ½ cup light cream
- ½ cup milk
- 2 teaspoons dried dill weed
- 1 pound noodles, cooked per package directions

In a small bowl, soak bread crumbs in milk for 5 minutes. In a large bowl, combine meats, egg, onion, salt, pepper, allspice and bread mixture. Shape into meatballs. In a large skillet, in hot butter, sauté meatballs until they are browned and cooked-through. Remove meatballs to a 9x12-inch baking dish as they are cooked. Add flour to drippings in skillet and stir until smooth. Add beef broth and boiling water; whisk until smooth. Add cream, milk and dill weed; simmer gently for 3 minutes. Pour the sauce over the meatballs, coating them well. Bake, covered, for 1 hour. Serve over noodles.

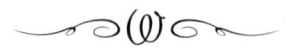

Quesadillas

Serves 4 to 6

- 6 flour tortillas
- ¾ cup Monterey Jack and/or cheddar cheese, shredded
- 6 tablespoons canned, diced chili peppers
- 6 tablespoons pimento, diced

Preheat oven to 350 degrees. Lay tortilla on baking sheet. Sprinkle layer of cheese over half. Dot with 1 tablespoon chilies and 1 tablespoon pimento, and fold. Repeat with remaining tortillas. Bake until cheese is melted, about 10 to 15 minutes. Cut folded tortillas into wedges and serve.

Sweet Brie

Serves 24

1   8-inch (24-ounce) round of Brie,
      not fully ripened, with top rind removed
1   cup pecans, chopped
2   cups brown sugar, firmly packed
crackers

Place Brie in 10-inch pie plate and sprinkle with nuts. Cover top and sides with brown sugar, patting gently. In preheated oven, broil on lowest rack until sugar bubbles and melts, about 3 minutes. Place Brie on serving plate, surround with crackers, and serve immediately.

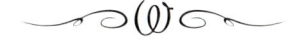

Steak Tartare

Serves 6

½   pound ground sirloin
1   egg yolk, beaten
½   tablespoon hot mustard
salt, to taste
pepper, freshly ground, to taste
1   dash Worcestershire sauce
1   dash Tabasco sauce
1   cup sour cream
caviar (optional)
½   cup sweet onion, finely chopped
rye bread sticks

Mix meat with yolk. Blend mustard with water and add seasonings. Mix with meat. Adjust seasonings to taste. Shape meat into mound on chilled plate. Cover mound with a layer of sour cream and top with caviar. Place onion and rye bread on the side of plate and serve.

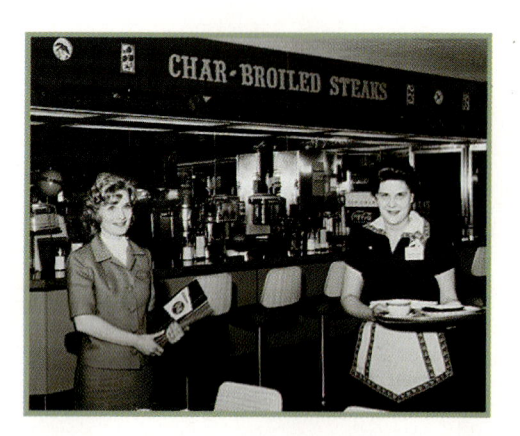

The in-store grills made their debut in the early 1960's, featuring pleasing decor, table seating and a wait staff.

Facing Page: *Salmon Chowder*
Photo: Scott Lanza, 1995
Stylist: F. Lynn Nelson

SOUPS & SALADS

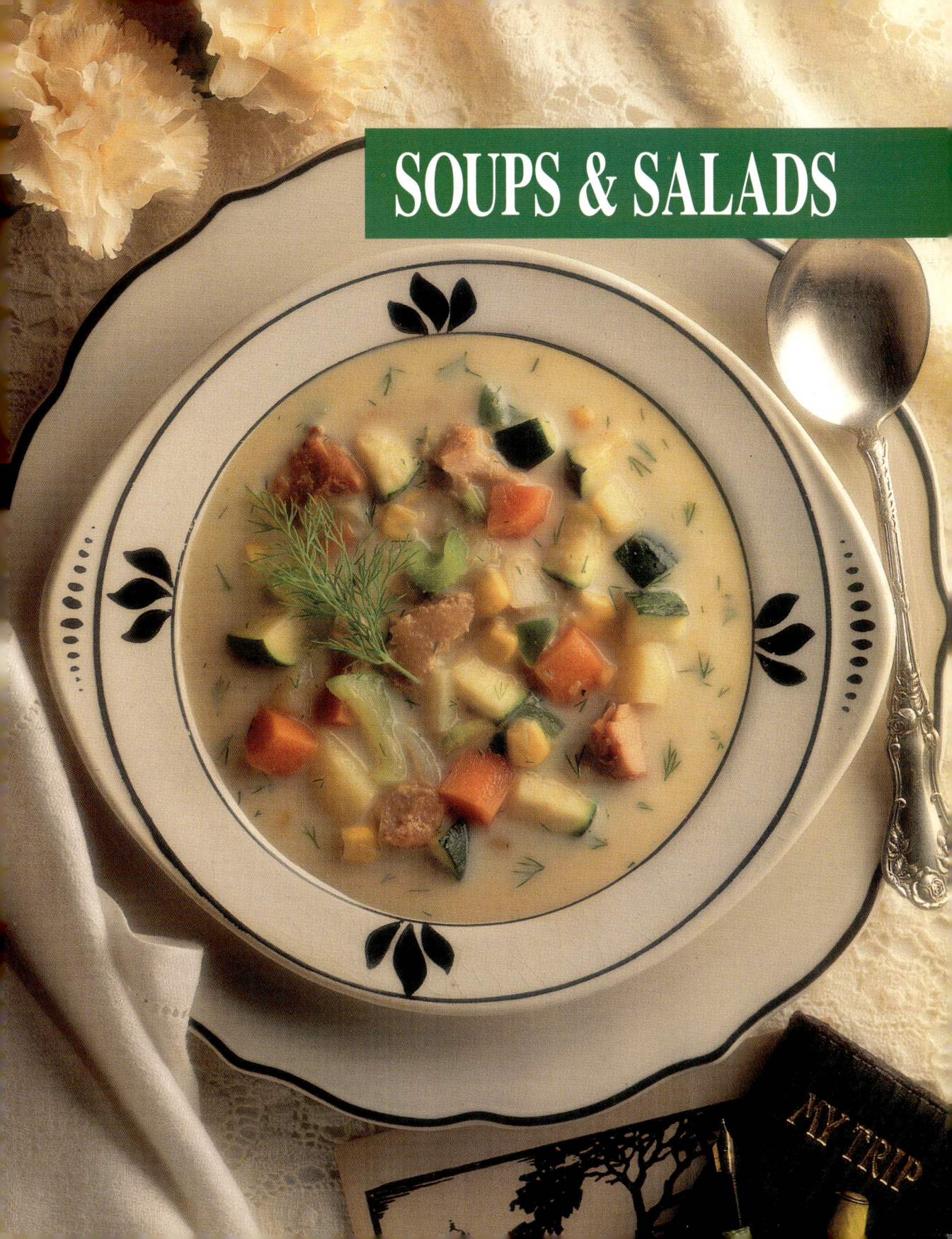

The In-Store Grills
Marvelous Food at Modest Prices

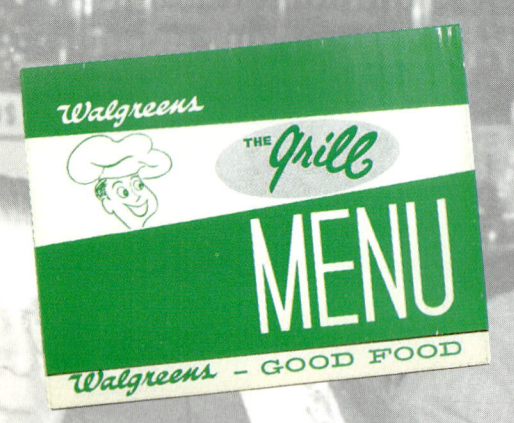

The "new" Pattie Melt was added to the menu in 1969 to appeal to the 27-and-under crowd...who made up 50 percent of the population!

Forming the greater share of Walgreens food service in the 1960's and 1970's were the in-store grills. Much more elegant than the old fry-cook counters, these grills featured soft lighting, thoughtfully-planned decor and table seating ~ plus, nearly every food item imaginable, all served by a wait staff! The carefully-prepared menus were complete and offered a medley of basic-to-fancy fare, from the newly-created Pattie Melt burger to the French-dipped roast beef sandwich, and appetizers galore! The food was affordable, the service, quick, and perhaps the most popular order on the menu was a sandwich with delicious homemade soup, like *French Onion*, *Vegetable Beef*, and *Bean & Bacon*.

Schwemm House Peanut Soup

Serves 8 to 10

- ½ cup celery, chopped
- 2 medium onions, diced
- ¼ pound butter
- 2 tablespoons flour
- 2 quarts chicken stock (bouillon)
- 8 ounces creamy peanut butter
- ¼ cup half-and-half
- ½ cup peanuts, finely chopped

Sauté celery and onions in butter. Thicken with flour, blending until smooth. Add chicken stock and blend until smooth. Reduce heat, add peanut butter and half-and-half. Heat through. Do not boil! Garnish with chopped peanuts.

Italian Sausage Soup

Serves 8

- 1 pound Italian sausage, removed from casing
- 1 cup onions, chopped
- 2 garlic cloves, minced
- 5 cups beef broth
- ½ cup dry red wine or water
- 1 28-ounce can tomatoes, drained and chopped
- 1 cup carrots, chopped
- ½ teaspoon basil
- ½ teaspoon oregano
- 1 8-ounce can tomato sauce
- 1½ cups chopped zucchini
- 8 ounces cheese tortellini
- 3 tablespoons fresh parsley, chopped
- 1 green pepper, chopped

Parmesan cheese, grated

Brown and drain sausage. Reserve 1 tablespoon drippings. Sauté onion and garlic with drippings. Add beef broth, wine or water, tomatoes, carrots, basil, oregano, tomato sauce and sausage. Bring to a boil. Reduce heat and simmer 30 minutes, uncovered. Skim fat. Stir in zucchini, tortellini, parsley and green pepper. Simmer uncovered 35 to 40 minutes or until tortellini is tender. Sprinkle with Parmesan cheese before serving.

Note: If using fresh or frozen tortellini, shorten cooking length.

Good's Gazpacho

Serves 8

- 3 cucumbers, chopped
- 3 green peppers, chopped
- 3 onions, chopped
- 8 radishes, chopped
- 4 ripe tomatoes, chopped
- 2 8-ounce cans chopped Italian tomatoes
- 2 tablespoons olive oil
- 2 teaspoons salt
- ½ teaspoon pepper
- 3 sprigs fresh dill

juice of 2 lemons

Combine cucumbers, green peppers, onions, radishes, tomatoes and Italian tomatoes. Add remaining ingredients, mix well and chill. Serve cold.

Clamato Gazpacho

Serves 8

- 3 fresh tomatoes, finely chopped
- 4 to 6 green onions and tops, finely chopped
- ½ green pepper, finely chopped
- 2 avocados, finely chopped
- 1 cup celery, finely chopped
- 1 tablespoon horseradish or Tabasco sauce, to taste
- ¼ cup Worcestershire sauce
- ½ cup catsup (optional)
- 2 tablespoons lemon juice
- 2 bottles Clamato juice
- 3 6½-ounce cans minced clams (optional)

salt and pepper, to taste

Mix ingredients together and chill. Serve cold.

Creamy Clam Chowder

Serves 4

- 2 medium potatoes, peeled and diced
- 1 large carrot, grated
- 2 cups water
- 1 teaspoon salt
- 2 6½-ounce cans minced clams, drained
- ¼ cup butter
- 2 tablespoons flour
- 1 cup canned evaporated milk
- 2 teaspoons sugar
- 1 tablespoon vinegar

Cook potatoes and carrot in salted boiling water until tender, about 8 minutes. Drain. Stir in minced clams. In separate saucepan, melt butter; stir in flour. Add milk, stirring constantly; cook until thickened. Stir in sugar and vinegar. Stir in vegetables and heat through. Serve immediately.

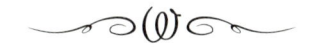

Mike's Clam Chowder

Serves 6

An original Hazelwood recipe!

- 2 slices bacon, finely cut
- ¼ cup onions, minced
- 2 tablespoons celery, chopped
- 3 6½-ounce cans minced clams, reserve liquid
- 2 cups raw potatoes, diced
- ½ cup hot water
- ¼ cup dry vermouth
- 1½ cups milk
- 2 tablespoons butter
- ½ teaspoon salt
- ⅛ teaspoon cayenne pepper
- ¼ teaspoon white pepper

Combine bacon, onions and celery in a hot skillet. Sauté until golden brown. Add clam liquid, potatoes, water and vermouth. Cook in covered saucepan until potatoes are tender, but still firm, about 10 minutes. Add clams, milk, butter, salt, cayenne pepper and white pepper. Bring to a boil, stirring occasionally. Serve hot.

Note: To make Manhattan-style clam chowder, omit milk and add 1½ cups of canned tomatoes.

Nova Scotia Seafood Chowder

Serves 6 to 8

- 1 pound shellfish ~ lobster, scallops, shrimp, crab, oysters, clams or mussels ~ in any combination
- 1 pound fish ~ halibut, turbot, haddock or salmon ~ in any combination
- ¼ cup butter
- ¼ cup chicken bouillon powder
- ¼ teaspoon white pepper
- 1 cup water
- 4 cups half-and-half or milk, or combination
- 1 cup onion, diced
- 2 tablespoons butter
- ½ cup celery, diced
- ½ cup green and red peppers, diced
- ½ cup flour
- 2 cups milk

If using fresh lobster, cook, prepare and reserve ¼-cup of cooking liquid. Cube fish into bite-size chunks. Melt ¼-cup butter in large, heavy saucepan. Stir in bouillon and white pepper. Add water and half-and-half, and mix. Keep warm over low heat; do not boil. Melt 2 tablespoons of butter in large skillet and sauté celery, onion and peppers; until just tender. Add fish and seafood (and reserved liquid, if any) and sauté until barely-cooked. Transfer mixture to the saucepan. Put flour in bowl, slowly whisk in milk, and beat until smooth. Pour mixture through strainer into saucepan. Heat soup until thickened and steamy; do not boil. Serve hot.

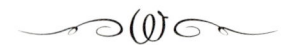

Northumberland White Fish Chowder

Serves 4 to 6

- 1 pound turbot, halibut or haddock ~ or your favorite white fish
- ¼ cup butter
- 1 small onion, finely chopped
- 3 to 4 medium potatoes, cooked and chopped
- ½ teaspoon salt
- ½ teaspoon white pepper
- 3 cups milk

Lightly sauté fresh or frozen fish in 1 tablespoon of the butter, or use canned. Brown onion and potatoes in butter, in a large skillet. Stir in salt and pepper. Transfer to a large saucepan and mix in milk. Heat, without boiling, stirring constantly. Add fish and heat again. Serve when nice and hot.

Salmon Chowder

Serves 6

- ½ cup onion, chopped
- ½ cup green pepper, chopped
- ½ cup celery, chopped
- 3 tablespoons butter
- 1½ cups potatoes, peeled and diced
- 1 cup carrots, diced
- ½ teaspoon pepper
- 1 teaspoon salt
- ½ teaspoon dill weed
- 1 14½-ounce can chicken broth
- 1 14¾-ounce can cream-style corn
- 1 12-ounce can evaporated milk
- 1 6½-ounce can flaked salmon, cleaned
- 1 cup zucchini, diced

Sauté first three ingredients in 3 tablespoons of butter. Add potatoes, carrots, spices and chicken broth. Cook until tender 30 to 40 minutes. When all vegetables are tender, add creamed corn, milk, salmon and zucchini. Heat thoroughly. Cooking time: 45 minutes.

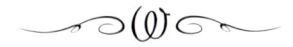

Halifax Vegetable Chowder

Serves 6

- ½ cup onion, chopped
- 1 cup carrots, chopped
- 1¼ cups potatoes, cubed
- 1 garlic clove, minced
- ¼ teaspoon nutmeg (optional)
- salt and pepper, to taste
- 2 tablespoons chicken bouillon powder
- 2 tablespoons butter or margarine
- ¾ cup broccoli (or asparagus, or other green vegetable), chopped
- 1 cup water
- 1 tablespoon cornstarch
- 2 cups milk
- 2 tablespoons sour cream or plain yogurt (optional)

Sauté onions, carrots, potato, garlic, seasonings and bouillon powder in a heavy saucepan with butter. Simmer, covered, for 10 minutes. Add broccoli; cook 5 minutes more. Place sautéed vegetables into blender. Add water; chop vegetables ~ do *not* purée. Return vegetables to saucepan. Mix in cornstarch and milk; cook for 2 minutes. Garnish with sour cream; serve hot.

Gourmet Potato Soup

Serves 4

- 2 chicken bouillon cubes
- ½ cup hot water
- 4 large potatoes, peeled and diced
- ½ cup onion, diced
- ½ cup celery, diced
- 2 cups milk
- 1 8-ounce container sour cream dip with chives
- 1 teaspoon flour

Dissolve bouillon cubes in hot water; add potatoes, onion, celery and milk. Cover and cook until vegetables are tender, about 15 minutes. Do not boil. Blend in sour cream dip and flour; heat until thickened and bubbly. Garnish with parsley or chives. Serve immediately.

Portuguese Potato Soup

Serves 10

- 1 stick margarine
- 1 very large Spanish onion, finely chopped
- 5 chicken bouillon cubes
- 2 bay leaves
- 2 teaspoons white pepper
- 2 pounds chorizos (Portuguese) or Polish sausage
- 3 pounds Idaho potatoes, peeled
- 1 very large head of cabbage, diced
- 3 tablespoons sugar
- 1 carrot, shredded

Sauté onions in margarine with sliced chorizo, chicken bouillon cubes, and bay leaves. When onions are transparent, add potatoes (diced very small) and cover with water. Cook until almost falling apart (about an hour). Add diced cabbage and cover again with water. Cook until cabbage is fully cooked and potatoes are almost all dissolved; about one hour. To serve, sprinkle shredded carrot over soup before serving.

German Potato Soup

Serves 2 to 3

1½ cups potatoes, diced
1½ cups boiling water
¼ cup green onion, chopped
¾ teaspoon salt
1 tablespoon butter or margarine
⅛ teaspoon white pepper
1 dash garlic powder
½ cup milk
1 egg yolk (optional)
fresh or dried parsley flakes, as garnish
croutons, as garnish

Combine potatoes, water, onions and salt in 2-quart saucepan. Cover, simmer until tender, about 15 to 20 minutes. Mash potatoes in pot until smooth, add butter, garlic powder and pepper, return to heat. Just before serving, blend milk into well beaten egg yolk. Blend slowly into soup, stirring constantly; cook just until heated through. Garnish with parsley and croutons.

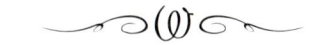

Janet Ann's Best Potato Soup

Serves 6

6 potatoes, peeled and diced
1 small onion, diced
3 or 4 celery stalks, diced
1 to 2 teaspoons parsley flakes
3 or 4 carrots, sliced
1½ teaspoons sugar
salt and pepper, to taste
3½ cups water
¼ stick butter or margarine
3 cups milk
2 tablespoons cornstarch or flour

Combine all ingredients, except last four (water, butter, milk and cornstarch), in large pan. Add water. Cover and cook until done, about 40 minutes. Add butter and milk. Heat to near-boiling. Add cornstarch or flour to thicken. Stir, and serve.

Swiss Broccoli Soup

Serves 4

5½ cups whole milk
1 10-ounce box frozen, chopped broccoli
2 tablespoons onion, chopped
2 tablespoons butter
1 tablespoon flour
1 8-ounce package shredded Swiss cheese
salt and pepper, to taste

Heat milk in large saucepan to simmering. Cook broccoli and onions in milk until tender. Melt butter in separate saucepan; stir in flour. Add this mixture to milk. Cook and stir 3 minutes. Remove from heat. Add shredded cheese and salt and pepper. Stir until cheese is melted. Serve immediately.

Cheesy Corn Soup

Serves 6

½ medium onion, chopped
¼ cup butter
3 10-ounce packages frozen, cream-style corn
chili peppers, to taste (optional)
1 large tomato, chopped
2 teaspoons salt
6 cups water
¾ cup Monterey Jack cheese, cubed
½ cup evaporated milk

In medium kettle, sauté onion in butter until soft, not browned. Add corn and chilies, and continue cooking for 2 minutes. Add tomato, salt and water; stir lightly. Simmer for 1 hour. Stir in Monterey Jack cheese and milk and continue heating until cheese starts to melt. Serve with tortillas.

Note: Chilies are optional, but may be used for a more spicy taste.

Hearty Tomato~Rice Soup

Serves 4

- 1 cup onion, chopped
- ½ cup celery, chopped
- 1 tablespoon butter
- 1 14½-ounce can stewed tomatoes
- 2 beef bouillon cubes
- ¾ cup uncooked rice
- 1 teaspoon salt
- ½ teaspoon chili powder
- 3 cups water

Sauté onion and celery in butter; add rest of ingredients and bring to a boil. Reduce heat and simmer for 20 minutes or until rice is tender. Serve immediately.

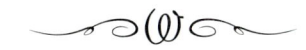

Ten~Minute Tomato Soup

Serves 4

- 1 cup onion, chopped
- 1 garlic clove, minced
- 2 tablespoons butter
- 4 cups tomatoes, chopped
- 4 cups water
- 1 or 2 bouillon cubes
- 1 tablespoon parsley, chopped
- 4 slices white toast
- 1 4-ounce package shredded mozzarella, or other soft cheese

Sauté the onions and garlic in butter in a large saucepan until lightly browned. Add the tomatoes, water and bouillon cubes and allow soup to boil for 5 minutes. Add parsley. Place a slice of toast into each of four soup bowls and ladle the tomato soup over the toast. Garnish with cheese, and serve piping hot.

Sweet & Sour Cabbage Soup

Serves 6

Adapted for your kitchen... from the original Walgreens recipe!

Corporate Cafeteria, Walgreen Company Headquarters

1 large onion, finely chopped
2 celery stalks, finely chopped
2 carrots, pared and finely chopped
1½ tablespoons butter or margarine
1 head green cabbage
6 cups canned beef broth
½ to 1 teaspoon salt
¼ teaspoon pepper
1 14½-ounce can tomatoes, drained and chopped
1 6-ounce can tomato paste
1 tablespoon white vinegar
1½ tablespoons sugar
salt and pepper, to taste

In a soup kettle, sauté chopped onion, celery, and carrots in butter until tender. Add beef broth, cabbage and remaining ingredients. Simmer until cabbage is tender, approximately 20 to 30 minutes. Adjust seasonings and add more beef broth if too thick. Serve immediately.

Polish Cabbage Soup

Serves 6 to 8

8 slices bacon, diced
1 pound cabbage, chopped
2 carrots, sliced
2 potatoes, sliced
1 celery stalk, sliced
1½ quarts water
2 tablespoons flour
2 tablespoons butter or margarine (room temperature)
salt and pepper, to taste
dumplings or pirogi (optional)

Fry bacon until golden, but not crisp in 3-quart saucepan. Add vegetables and water. Simmer 30 minutes, or until vegetables are tender. Blend flour into butter. Stir into soup. Bring soup to boiling, stirring. Season to taste with salt and pepper. If desired, serve with dumplings or pirogi.

Cream of Asparagus Soup

Serves 6

An original Hazelwood recipe!

2   tablespoons butter
2   cups leeks or green onions, sliced
6   cups asparagus stems, diced (reserve 1-cup asparagus tops)
1   quart chicken broth
1   cup light cream
2   tablespoons Parmesan cheese, grated
¼   teaspoon white pepper
salt, to taste
nutmeg, to taste

Melt butter in large soup pot and sauté leeks until limp, 3 to 5 minutes. Add asparagus stems and chicken broth. Simmer until asparagus is tender, 10 to 15 minutes. Cool the soup slightly, purée in a blender and reheat. Add the cream, Parmesan, pepper, salt and nutmeg. Garnish with steamed asparagus tops. Serve hot.

Cream of Celery Soup

Serves 6 to 8

Adapted for your kitchen... from the original Walgreens recipe!

Robin Hood & Briargate Restaurants, 1970's ~ 1980's

4   cups chicken broth
4   tablespoons margarine
2   cups celery with leaves, chopped
2   medium onions, coarsely chopped
3   cups milk, heated to boiling
2   tablespoons flour
¼   teaspoon white pepper
nutmeg, grated, to taste
2   tablespoons parsley, chopped

Bring chicken broth to boil. Sauté celery and onion in 2 tablespoons margarine. Add chicken broth and white pepper and simmer 10 minutes. Strain soup. Add strained soup to 3 cups boiling milk. Mix well. Combine 2 tablespoons margarine and flour to make a roux. Remove 1 cup soup mixture; blend with roux. Return to soup pot. Add white pepper. Stir until thickened. Serve hot, topped with a grating of nutmeg and chopped parsley.

Scotch Barley Soup

Serves 6 to 8

**Adapted for your kitchen...
from the original Walgreens recipe!**

Robin Hood & Briargate Restaurants, 1970's ~ 1980's

2½ pounds shoulder and neck of lamb
2 quarts water
½ cup barley
1 onion, julienne
2 carrots, pared and julienne
1 rib celery, julienne
1 medium turnip, julienne
3 tablespoons parsley, chopped
1 tablespoon salt
1 tablespoon margarine
1 tablespoon flour
¼ teaspoon Tabasco sauce (optional)

Preheat oven to 350 degrees. Cut meat away from bones; break bones. Put in small roasting pan; brown beef and bones in 350-degree oven. Remove; put water, bones, barley, onion, carrots, celery, turnip, 1 tablespoon parsley, and salt into soup pot. Bring to boil; skimming top of soup frequently. Remove bones, but leave meat. Reduce heat; simmer for 2 hours, adding more water if necessary. Blend butter with flour to make roux. Remove 1 cup soup and blend in roux. Return to soup pot. Add Tabasco sauce and stir soup until thickened slightly. Serve in soup plates, garnished with remaining parsley.

Low~Fat Cucumber Soup

Serves 4 to 6

3 medium cucumbers, peeled, seeded and cut into chunks
3 scallions with tops, cut into 2-inch pieces
¼ cup no-fat sour cream
¼ cup low-fat mayonnaise
1 cup low-fat canned chicken broth
1½ teaspoons dried dill weed
1 teaspoon salt
¼ teaspoon ground white pepper
½ cup skim milk
dill weed sprigs or thinly sliced cucumbers, as garnish

In food processor or blender, combine cucumber and scallions. Process until finely chopped and transfer to a large bowl. Add sour cream, mayonnaise, chicken broth, dill, salt and pepper. Mix well. Blend in milk, and chill for several hours. To serve, garnish with dill weed or cucumber.

Diet Vegetable Soup

Serves 2 to 3

½ head of cabbage, chopped in large pieces
2 or 3 onions, sliced lengthwise
1 green pepper, chopped in large pieces
6 celery stalks, chopped
1 14½-ounce can tomatoes, or fresh
1 package dry onion soup mix
Parmesan cheese, optional

Put all ingredients in pot and cover with water. Simmer until vegetables are cooked. Sprinkle with Parmesan cheese before serving.

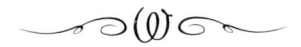

Lima Bean & Bacon Soup

Serves 8 to 10

Adapted for your kitchen... from the original Walgreens recipe!

Corporate Cafeteria, Walgreen Company Headquarters

1 pound lima beans, dry
1 gallon cold water
¼ pound bacon, diced
2 medium onions, coarsely chopped
3 carrots, pared and coarsely chopped
2 celery stalks, coarsely chopped
1 green pepper, coarsely chopped
2 garlic cloves, peeled and minced
3 tablespoons catsup
¼ teaspoon pepper
1 teaspoon marjoram
1 dash chili powder (optional)
2 tablespoons butter or margarine
2 tablespoons flour

Soak lima beans in water overnight. Drain beans. Sauté onions, carrots, celery, green pepper, garlic and bacon in soup pot until vegetables are tender. Add beans, water, catsup, pepper, marjoram and chili powder; cover and simmer approximately 1½ hours, or until beans are tender. Combine margarine and flour to make a roux. Remove 1 cup hot soup and blend in with roux. Return mixture to soup pot. Heat through and adjust seasonings.

French Onion Soup

Serves 6 to 8

*Adapted for your kitchen...
from the original Walgreens recipe!*

*Robin Hood
& Briargate
Restaurants,
1970's ~ 1980's*

- 3 large Bermuda onions, thinly sliced
- 5 tablespoons margarine
- 1 garlic clove, finely minced
- 2 tablespoons flour
- 1½ teaspoons salt
- ¼ teaspoon pepper
- 8 cups beef broth, brought to a boil
- 1 tablespoon Worcestershire sauce
- 8 slices crusty French bread
- 1 cup Parmesan cheese, grated
- 8 1-ounce slices Swiss cheese

Preheat oven to 350 degrees. In soup pot, sauté onions and garlic in margarine, over medium heat, until soft. Add flour; cook until bubbly. Add boiling broth; blend over medium heat. Bring to a boil, reduce heat; add Worcestershire sauce, salt and pepper. Stir and heat through. Pour into heated bowls; top with crusty French bread. Sprinkle Parmesan cheese on bread; top with Swiss cheese slice. Bake at 350 degrees for about 10 minutes, until cheese melts.

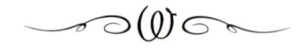

Split Pea Soup

Serves 6 to 8

*Adapted for your kitchen...
from the original Walgreens recipe!*

*Robin Hood
& Briargate
Restaurants,
1970's ~ 1980's*

- 1 pound split peas, well washed
- 1 meaty ham bone
- 10 cups water
- 1 onion, coarsely chopped
- 3 ribs celery, coarsely chopped
- 2 carrots, pared and coarsely chopped
- 2 garlic cloves
- 1 bay leaf
- 1 teaspoon sugar
- ¼ teaspoon thyme
- 1 dash cayenne pepper
- 2 tablespoons margarine
- 2 tablespoons flour

Cover peas with cold water overnight. Drain. Put peas, ham bone, and water in soup pot; simmer, covered, for 2½ to 3 hours. Add onion, celery, carrots, garlic, bay leaf, sugar, thyme, and cayenne; simmer 30 minutes longer. Remove ham bone. Put soup through a sieve. Combine flour and margarine to form a roux. Mix with 1 cup of soup. Return to soup pot and heat through until thickened. Serve soup hot.

Puerto Rican Beef Soup with Pigeon Peas

Serves 6 to 8

Adapted for your kitchen...
from the original Walgreens recipe!

Walgreen Grills in Puerto Rico, 1960's ~ 1980's

Originally called: Asopao de Gandules y Carne de Res

1 pound pigeon peas (or 1-pound can LaPreferida gandules*)
1 pound beef top round, cut into 1-inch cubes
1 tablespoon olive oil
1 garlic clove, peeled and chopped
½ cup tomato sauce
4 tablespoons Goya sofrito* (12-ounce bottle)
  (also see recipe in the RxCetera ~ Sauces & Garnishes chapter)
1 cup uncooked long-grain rice
1 pound fresh pumpkin, cooked, peeled and cut into 1-inch cubes
1 pound potatoes, cut into 1-inch cubes
3 packages Goya Sazan* (1.41-ounce box) with coriander and achiote
1½ quarts water

Cover peas with water overnight. Drain. Cover peas with water in large soup pot and simmer for 1½ hours. Drain and set aside. Heat olive oil; sauté beef with garlic until lightly browned. Add tomato sauce and Soffrito and simmer. Add the rice, pumpkin, potatoes, Sazon packets and 1½ quarts water. Stir and simmer 45 minutes or until rice is done. Add more water, if necessary.

Note: *Available in the ethnic or specialty sections of grocery stores.

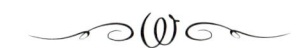

Swiss Mushroom Consommé

Serves 6

1 pound fresh mushrooms
4 tablespoons butter
2 10½-ounce cans Campbell's beef broth
2 soup cans water
¼ teaspoon nutmeg
¼ teaspoon black pepper
¼ cup green onions, sliced (use some tops, too)
2 tablespoons dry sherry

Clean and slice fresh mushrooms. In a large saucepan, melt butter. Add mushrooms and sauté 5 minutes. Add beef broth, water, nutmeg and black pepper. Bring to a boil, lower heat and simmer, uncovered, for 5 minutes. Stir in green onions and sherry. Simmer, uncovered, for 1 minute.

Petite Marmite Soup

Serves 6 to 8

**Adapted for your kitchen...
from the original Walgreens recipe!**

Corporate Cafeteria, Walgreen Company Headquarters

1 pound beef top round, cubed
1 3½-pound chicken, cut into serving pieces
2 large leeks, cut into match-like strips
1 large onion, coarsely chopped
3 ribs celery, cut into match-like strips
2 carrots, pared, cut into match-like strips
1 white turnip, cut into cubes
4 cups canned chicken broth
4 cups canned beef broth
1 teaspoon thyme
1 bay leaf
salt and pepper, to taste
¼ cup fresh parsley, chopped
¼ cup sherry wine

Cube beef, cut chicken into serving pieces, cutting legs and wings at joints and cutting each breast into 4 pieces. Cover with water; bring to boil and simmer 5 minutes. Remove from heat and run cold water over meats. Drain. Now combine all vegetables. Cover with cold water, bring to boil and simmer 15 minutes. Drain. Now combine meats and vegetables in soup pot. Cover with chicken and beef broths. Bring to boil. Add spices, seasonings and sherry. Simmer for 1 more hour; skim surface to remove any foam or fat. Serve hot in soup bowls, sprinkled with parsley.

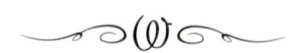

U.S. Senate Bean Soup

Serves 8

2 pounds Michigan navy beans
4 quarts water
1½ pounds ham hocks, smoked
1 onion, chopped
1 tablespoon butter
2 medium potatoes, cubed, boiled until soft and mashed
salt and pepper, to taste

Place beans in colander and rinse with hot water until water runs clean. Place rinsed beans in soup pot. Add 4 quarts of water. Add ham hocks. Brown onion in butter, and add to soup. Add mashed potatoes to soup. Bring soup to a boil, lower heat and simmer 3 hours. Remove 2 cups of beans, purée in blender and return to soup. Remove ham hocks, let soup cool. Dice meat; add to soup. Serve hot.

French Market Soup

Serves 6 to 8

Adapted for your kitchen... from the original Walgreens recipe!

Corporate Cafeteria, Walgreen Company Headquarters

- 1 pound navy beans
- 1 beef shin bone
- 2 quarts water
- 2 teaspoons salt
- 1 tablespoon margarine
- 3 carrots, pared and sliced
- 3 large potatoes, peeled and diced
- 1 turnip, peeled and diced
- 3 celery stalks, diced
- 2 medium onions, peeled and chopped
- ¼ pound green beans, sliced
- 1 cup frozen corn
- 1 cup kidney beans
- ½ cup lentils
- 1 teaspoon oregano
- 1 bay leaf
- ¼ teaspoon white pepper
- 3 sprigs fresh parsley, chopped

Pistou:
- 4 garlic cloves
- ¼ cup fresh basil, chopped or 2 teaspoons dried basil
- 4 large tomatoes, peeled, seeded, and chopped
- ¼ cup olive oil

Soak navy beans in water overnight. Drain. Return beans, beef shin bone, water, and salt to soup pot. Simmer 1¼ hours or until beans are tender. Remove beef bone. Sauté all vegetables in margarine in fry pan until soft, but not brown. Add to soup pot along with kidney beans, lentils, and all spices and seasonings. Heat through another 20 to 30 minutes. Make pistou. Crush garlic, basil, tomatoes in a mortar or blender to make a paste. Add olive oil slowly until mixture is consistency of mayonnaise. Add pistou to soup mixture. Bring back to boil and serve immediately.

Cuban Black Bean Soup

Serves 6 to 8

**Adapted for your kitchen...
from the original Walgreens recipe!**

Corporate Cafeteria, Walgreen Company Headquarters

- 1 1-pound package dried black beans
- 9 cups water
- 1 ham bone
- 2 garlic cloves, finely minced
- 2 tablespoons margarine
- 1 medium onion, chopped
- 1 rib celery, chopped
- 1½ tablespoons lemon juice
- salt and pepper, to taste
- 1 dash cayenne pepper
- 1 teaspoon cumin
- 1 teaspoon oregano
- 6 to 8 slices lemon
- 1 hard-boiled egg, chopped

Soak beans in cold water overnight. Drain. Return beans to pot with ham bone and 9 cups water. Simmer beans for 2-2½ hours or until beans are tender. Blend garlic, cumin, cayenne, and oregano to a paste. In saucepan, sauté onion and celery in margarine. Add vegetables, garlic paste, and lemon juice to soup pot and simmer 15-20 more minutes. Remove 2 cups of beans with liquid and purée in electric blender until smooth. Return to soup pot, mix thoroughly to thicken and heat through. Serve in soup bowls, garnished with a lemon slice and chopped hard-boiled egg.

Spanish Bean Soup

Serves 4

- ½ pound garbanzo beans (chickpeas)
- 1 tablespoon salt
- 1 beef bone
- 1 ham bone
- 2 quarts water
- 4 ounces white bacon
- 1 onion, chopped
- ¼ teaspoon paprika
- 1 pound potatoes, quartered
- 1 pinch saffron
- salt, to taste
- 1 Spanish sausage (*chorizo*), cooked and thinly sliced

Spanish Bean Soup, *continued on next page.*

Spanish Bean Soup, continued.

Soak garbanzo beans overnight with salt, in sufficient water to cover them. Drain salted water from beans. In soup pot, add 2 quarts water, ham bone and beef bone. Cook 45 minutes on low heat. Fry white bacon; drain. Fry onion with paprika in bacon fat. Add bacon, onions, beans, potatoes, saffron and salt to soup. When potatoes are done, add Chorizo slices. Serve hot.

Bavarian Lentil Soup

Serves 6-8

Adapted for your kitchen... from the original Walgreens recipe!

Corporate Cafeteria, Walgreen Company Headquarters

2	cups dried lentils
10	cups water
1	ham bone
1	bay leaf
3	tablespoons margarine
1	medium onion, finely chopped
3	celery stalks, finely chopped
3	carrots, pared and finely chopped
2	tablespoons white vinegar
1	tablespoon Worcestershire sauce
¼	teaspoon pepper
1	teaspoon thyme
2	tablespoons butter
2	tablespoons flour
1	pound sausage, cooked and sliced

Cover lentils with cold water overnight and drain. Put lentils in soup pot with ham bone and bay leaf. Cover with the 10 cups water and simmer 3 hours. Remove bay leaf and ham bone. Melt margarine in small frying pan; sauté onions, celery, and carrots. Add to soup pot along with vinegar and Worcestershire sauce. Combine butter and flour to make a roux. Put soup through a sieve; add roux to a small portion of the strained soup. Return soup to heat and cook until soup boils. Add soup-roux mixture to rest of soup pot. Heat through. Serve piping hot, garnished with sausage slices.

Bonsignore's Italian Chicken Soup with Meatballs

Serves 10 to 12

Soup:
- 1 whole stewing chicken, washed
- 1 bay leaf
- 2 tablespoons parsley flakes
- 1 tablespoon salt
- 1 teaspoon pepper
- 4 celery stalks, diced
- 4 large carrots, peeled and diced
- 4 medium onions, peeled and diced
- 2 cups rice
- Romano or Parmesan cheese, as garnish

Meatballs:
- 3 pounds meat loaf mix (ground beef, pork and veal)
- 1 medium onion, diced
- 1 egg
- 1 cup Italian seasoned bread crumbs
- ½ cup Romano or Parmesan cheese
- 2 tablespoons parsley flakes
- salt and pepper, to taste

To make soup, put chicken in very large pot and cover with water. Add bay leaf, parsley flakes, salt and pepper. Boil for 2 hours, making sure that chicken is covered with water at all times. Remove chicken and put in bowl. Cover with wet paper towels to make sure chicken does not dry out. Add celery, carrots and onions to pot. Bring to boil, then simmer while making meatballs.

To make meatballs, mix all ingredients well. Mixture should be of meat loaf consistency. If it is too dry, add another egg. Shape into quarter-size meatballs, and add to soup. Cook for several hours, until meatballs are tender.

One hour before serving, cook rice according to directions on box, then add to soup. Remove chicken from the bones and cut into serving-size pieces. Add chicken to soup and continue cooking for another 5 minutes.

Serve with shredded Romano or Parmesan cheese.

Note: This recipe makes several quarts of soup; the extra soup may be frozen for future use.

Dad's Homemade Chicken Soup

Serves 6 to 8

An original Hazelwood recipe!

2   2 to 3-pound fryers or stewing hens
2   bay leaves
1   teaspoon peppercorns
2   tablespoons parsley, chopped
1   teaspoon salt
4   celery stalks, sliced
5   carrots, sliced
4   parsnips, sliced
5   medium onions, quartered
1   1-pound package noodles, cooked per package directions, and drained
salt and pepper, to taste

Cut chickens in half. Place in large stockpot. Cover with water to top of chickens. Add bay leaves, peppercorns, chopped parsley, and salt. Bring to boil. Boil for 3 hours. Let soup cool overnight then remove top layer of fat. Heat chickens, when warm, remove from pot. Strain soup into another stockpot. Add vegetables and cook until tender. Meanwhile, bone and cut into small pieces. Add to soup. Bring to boil. Add noodles; serve hot. Season with salt and pepper.

Mofongo Dumpling Soup

Serves 6 to 8

Adapted for your kitchen… from the original Walgreens recipe!

Walgreen Grills in Puerto Rico, 1960's ~ 1980's

4   green plantains (*platanos*), cut into ½-inch pieces
vegetable oil
1   1-pound bag crispy pork rinds
1   teaspoon salt
7   cups canned chicken broth or homemade chicken stock

Deep-fry plantains in 360-degree oil in an electric skillet or frying pan until tender. Cool. In food processor, combine plantains, pork rinds and salt to make a paste or pudding. Shape mixture into balls or dumplings. Heat chicken broth and drop the mofongo dumplings into the hot soup.

Strega Nana's Pasta & Fagioli Soup

Serves 6 to 8

- 1 cup onion, chopped
- ½ cup celery, chopped
- 4 garlic cloves, minced
- ½ teaspoon crushed red pepper flakes
- 3 tablespoons olive oil
- 2 tablespoons butter
- 1 16-ounce can Italian plum tomatoes, drained and chopped
- 1 tablespoon salt
- 1 teaspoon pepper
- 1 teaspoon thyme
- 1 64-ounce (4-pound) can white cannellini beans
- 10 cups water
- 2 tablespoons parsley, chopped
- 1 tablespoon Parmesan cheese, grated
- 2 cups small pasta, cooked separately (ditalini, tabetti, elbow, etc.)
- 2 tablespoons basil, chopped

Sauté onions, celery, garlic and red pepper flakes in oil and butter. Cook until translucent. Add tomatoes, salt, pepper, and thyme; and simmer for 20 minutes. Add beans and water; simmer until heated through. Add parsley, grated cheese and cooked pasta. Pour into serving dishes and garnish with chopped basil. Serve immediately.

Tortellini Soup

Serves 6

- 2 garlic cloves
- 1 tablespoon butter or margarine
- 1 12-ounce package tortellini
- 6 cups canned chicken broth
- 1 10-ounce package frozen, chopped spinach, thawed
- 1 tablespoon oregano
- 1 14½-ounce can tomatoes, chopped and undrained
- 1 tablespoon sugar

Parmesan cheese, grated

Cook garlic in margarine for 2 to 3 minutes. Add broth and tortellini, heat to a boil. Reduce heat and simmer 10 minutes. Add spinach, oregano, tomatoes and sugar. Simmer 5 more minutes. Serve topped with cheese.

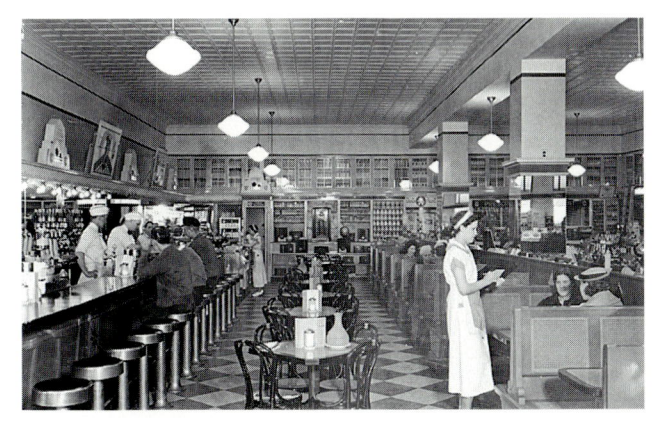

A spacious 1940's soda fountain in Clinton, Iowa.

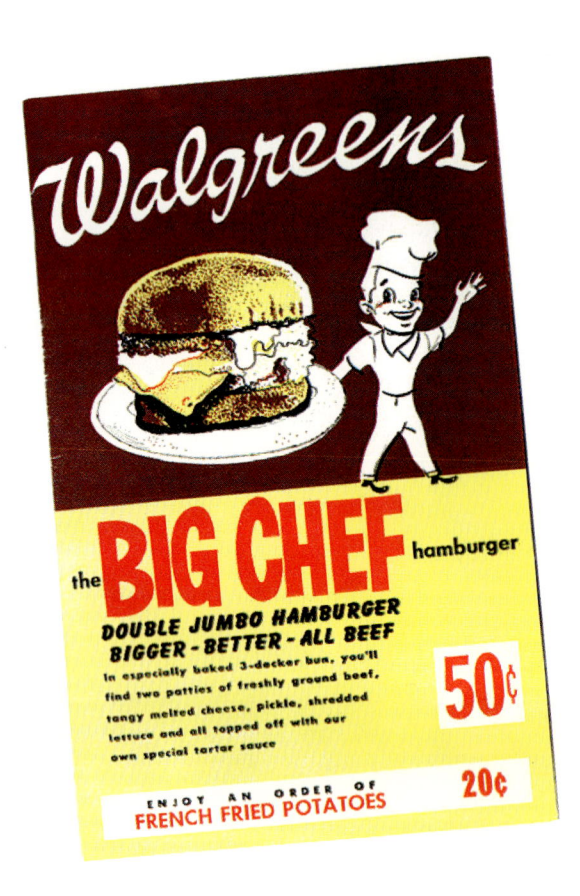

A 1957 Walgreens grill menu featuring the 50¢ "double jumbo" Big Chef hamburger with a triple-decker bun…and French-fried potatoes for 20¢!

Insalata La Famillia

Serves 8 to 10

Salad:
- ½ head iceberg lettuce
- 1 head Boston or Bibb lettuce
- 1 head red-tipped lettuce
- 1 cup seasoned croutons
- 1 green pepper, chopped
- ½ large, red onion, thinly sliced
- 6 large radishes, sliced
- 1 large tomato, diced
- 1 cucumber, sliced
- 1 can artichoke hearts, chopped
- 1 cup black olives, pitted
- 1 cup Fontinella cheese, chopped into small pieces

Red wine vinaigrette:
- ¼ cup virgin olive oil
- 2 teaspoons balsamic vinegar
- ⅛ cup red wine
- ½ teaspoon garlic salt
- ¼ teaspoon oregano

salt and pepper, to taste

Wash, dry and tear lettuce into medium-size pieces. Add croutons, vegetables and cheese. To make dressing, whisk together all ingredients. Just before serving, pour dressing lightly over salad and toss.

Cran~Apple Salad Mold

Serves 10 to 12

- 2 3.6-ounce boxes strawberry Jello
- 2 cups boiling water
- 1 16-ounce can whole-cranberry sauce
- 1 cup applesauce
- ½ cup port wine or fruit juice
- ¼ cup walnuts, chopped

Dissolve Jello in boiling water. Stir well and cool slightly. Add cranberry sauce, applesauce, wine and chopped nuts. Pour into a greased, 6½-cup mold. Stir when partially thickened so fruit will be well mixed. Do not cover. Place in refrigerator overnight. Unmold when ready to serve.

Blackstone Caesar Salad

Serves 4, generously

An authentic recipe from the maître d' at the Blackstone Hotel ~ Chicago, 1957

1½ pounds romaine lettuce
1   6-ounce box caesar salad croutons

Caesar dressing:
1   garlic clove
1   2-ounce can flat anchovies
8   tablespoons olive oil
4   tablespoons red wine vinegar
4   eggs
¼   teaspoon celery salt
1   teaspoon black pepper, freshly ground
1   tablespoon Worcestershire sauce
4   ounces Parmesan cheese, grated

Clean romaine lettuce. Remove center vein from large leaves. Cut leaves in small pieces. Set aside. Crush garlic in salted wooden bowl and rub around. Add anchovies, mash with fork. Add olive oil and wine vinegar. Stir for a few minutes. Add celery salt, eggs, and black pepper. Grind black pepper on the yolks of each egg until covered. Add Worcestershire sauce and Parmesan cheese. Add romaine lettuce and salad croutons. Toss salad and dressing until very little dressing is left in bottom of bowl.

Greek Tomato Salad

Serves 10

6   medium tomatoes, sliced
¼   pound feta cheese, crumbled
1   small onion, thinly sliced
1   7-ounce can sliced, ripe olives

Red wine vinaigrette:
½   cup olive or salad oil
⅓   cup red wine vinegar
2   tablespoons parsley
4   teaspoons sugar
½   teaspoon basil
¼   teaspoon salt
¼   teaspoon cracked pepper

Place tomatoes, feta, onions and olives in salad bowl. Mix together ingredients for marinade. Pour dressing over salad, toss and marinate in refrigerator for at least 2 hours.

Salad Niçoise

Serves 2

1½ heads lettuce (Boston, green leaf, endive or combination)
½ pound new potatoes, steamed and sliced
1 small tomato, sliced
2 hard-boiled eggs, sliced
1 6-ounce can tuna or 5-ounce can chicken, drained
½ pound fresh green beans
1 small red onion, thinly sliced
1 2¼-ounce can sliced black olives
1 8-ounce can artichoke hearts, halved (optional)
1 small red pepper, thinly sliced (optional)
1 small cucumber, sliced (optional)
capers

Apple cider vinaigrette:
6 tablespoons olive oil
2 tablespoons apple cider vinegar
1 teaspoon salt
¼ tablespoon pepper

Wash and dry lettuce. Make vinaigrette and toss gently with tomatoes and potatoes. Place lettuce on plates. Arrange potatoes, tomatoes and all remaining ingredients on top. Garnish with parsley or capers. Serve with extra dressing on side.

Sliced Tomatoes with Blue Cheese Dressing

Serves 6

4 firm, ripe tomatoes, thinly sliced
1 bermuda onion, very thinly sliced
¼ cup parsley, minced
salad greens

Blue cheese dressing:
¼ cup blue cheese, crumbled
½ cup olive oil
2 tablespoons lemon juice
1 teaspoon salt
¼ teaspoon sugar

Peel tomatoes by dropping briefly in boiling water; slice. Place on greens arranged on a large, round platter. Place an onion slice on each tomato. Sprinkle with parsley. Blend blue cheese, olive oil, lemon juice, salt and sugar. Pour over tomatoes. Chill at least 20 minutes before serving.

Honey~Pear Tossed Salad

Serves 6 to 8

Honey-mustard vinaigrette:
- 1 large shallot, minced
- ½ cup safflower oil
- 2 tablespoons red wine vinegar
- 2 tablespoons honey
- 1 tablespoon mustard
- 1 tablespoon water
- ¼ teaspoon coarse pepper
- ⅛ teaspoon salt

Salad:
- 2 large, firm pears, peeled and diced
- 6 cups mixed greens, torn (red leaf lettuce, Boston lettuce, Romaine lettuce, curly endive and arugula)
- ⅓ cup feta cheese, crumbled
- ¼ cup pine nuts, toasted
- salt and pepper, freshly ground, to taste

To make dressing, put ingredients into jar and shake vigorously to mix. For salad, toss diced pears with ¼-cup dressing, and refrigerate for an hour. Toss greens with remaining dressing. Add cheese, pine nuts, salt and pepper.

Calico Vegetable Salad

Serves 8 to 10

- 1 15-ounce can tiny green peas
- 1 14½-ounce can diced carrots
- 1 12-ounce can tiny white corn
- 1 14½-ounce can French-cut green beans
- 1 2-ounce jar pimentos, diced
- 1 cup celery, diced
- 1 cup onions, chopped
- 1 medium green pepper, chopped

Cider marinade:
- ¾ cup cider vinegar
- 1 cup sugar
- ¼ cup oil
- salt, to taste

Drain all vegetables before adding marinade. Boil marinade ingredients. Pour marinade over vegetables while hot. Refrigerate overnight.

Hot Chicken Salad

Serves 16

Salad:
- 4 cups chicken, cooked and cubed
- 8 hard-boiled eggs, diced
- 1½ cups Hellmann's mayonnaise (no substitute)
- 1½ cups cream of chicken soup, undiluted
- 4 cups celery, diced
- 2 tablespoons onion, finely chopped
- 2 teaspoons salt
- 4 tablespoons lemon juice

Topping:
- 2 cups cheddar cheese, grated
- 1 tablespoon butter or margarine
- 3 cups potato chips, crushed
- 1⅓ cups slivered almonds

Mix all salad ingredients together. Put into greased 9x13-inch casserole dish. Place cheese on top. Lightly-sauté almonds in butter, mix with chips. Place on cheese. Refrigerate overnight. Let stand at room temperature before baking. Bake, uncovered, at 400 degrees for 30 minutes.

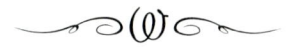

Summer Chicken Salad

Serves 12 to 15

- 4 pounds boneless, skinless chicken breasts
- 2 pounds asparagus, cut into 1-inch pieces
- ½ cup red pepper, chopped
- 2 green onions, chopped
- 2 celery stalks, chopped
- 3 teaspoons dried tarragon
- 3 tablespoons lemon juice
- 2 cups Miracle Whip salad dressing

red or green grapes, cut (optional)

Cover chicken breasts in a small amount of water and steam for 20 to 30 minutes, or until done. Set aside to cool, then cut into bite-size pieces. Add asparagus, red pepper, green onions, celery stalks to chicken. Mix in tarragon. Blend lemon juice with Miracle Whip, and add to chicken mixture. Chill well before serving. Garnish with red or green grapes.

Hawthorn Club Chinese Vegetable Salad

Serves 10 to 12

1 head iceberg lettuce, washed and shredded
1 head Romaine lettuce, washed and shredded
1 head Boston lettuce, washed and shredded
2 cups celery, thinly sliced on diagonal
1 bunch radishes, thinly sliced
1 Chinese cabbage (bok choy), thinly sliced
1 bunch scallions (green onions), finely chopped
1 package crispy rice or won ton noodles, crushed
2 cups peanuts, chopped

Sesame vinaigrette:

¼ cup vinegar
4 teaspoons salt
2 teaspoons Accent
¼ cup sesame seed oil
1 tablespoon sesame seeds, toasted and ground
½ cup sugar

Mix dressing ingredients together. Combine and lightly toss salad ingredients. Serve salad on individual plates and garnish with dressing. (Or toss dressing in with salad before serving.)

Chinese Chicken Salad

Serves 6

4 chicken breasts, skinless and boneless
1 head Romaine lettuce, washed and shredded
1 bunch scallions (green onions), chopped

Sesame vinaigrette:

½ cup sesame seeds, baked
½ cup olive oil
½ cup vinegar
2 tablespoons soy sauce
2 tablespoons honey
1 garlic clove, crushed

Steam chicken breasts in water, covered, until tender, about 10 to 20 minutes. Meanwhile, make dressing. Bake sesame seeds at 350 degrees for 5 minutes, or until golden. Mix sesame seeds, olive oil, vinegar, soy sauce, garlic and honey; whisk well. Shred chicken and marinate in dressing. Right before serving, toss chicken with lettuce and garnish with chopped scallions.

Spicy Szechwan Noodle Salad

Serves 4 to 6

- 4 cups linguini, cooked per package directions and chilled
- 1 cup cooked chicken, slivered
- 1 cup green onions, slivered
- 2 red sweet peppers, slivered
- 1 green pepper, slivered
- 1 cup pea pods, blanched

rice noodles

Sesame vinaigrette:

- 2 tablespoons soy sauce
- 3 tablespoons red wine vinegar
- 2 tablespoons fresh ginger, minced
- 1½ tablespoons sugar
- 1 to 2 tablespoons sesame oil
- 1 teaspoon chili paste with garlic
- ¼ teaspoon salt

Prepare pasta. Toss with small amount of oil to prevent sticking. Prepare chicken and vegetables. Toss all ingredients except dressing. Set aside or refrigerate until ready to serve. Prepare dressing; combine all ingredients, blending well. Toss with salad just prior to serving. Garnish with toasted sesame seeds or rice noodles. Serve at room temperature.

Endive & Escarole Salad with Raspberry Vinaigrette

Serves 6 to 8

Salad:

- 1 small head escarole, torn in pieces
- 2 heads Belgium endive, cut in 1-inch pieces
- 1 fennel bulb, thinly sliced
- 1 cup hazelnuts, cracked, roasted and chopped
- 1 cup Granny Smith apples, peeled and chopped

Raspberry vinaigrette:

- ⅓ cup raspberry vinegar
- ⅔ cup light olive oil
- 1 tablespoon honey

Mix together all salad ingredients, then mix all dressing ingredients. Pour dressing over salad and toss lightly.

Korean Spinach Salad

Serves 6 to 8

1 10-ounce bag fresh spinach
2 hard-boiled eggs, chopped
6 strips bacon, crumbled

Vinaigrette:

½ cup sugar
¼ cup white vinegar
1 cup salad oil
1 onion, grated
2 tablespoons Worcestershire sauce
¼ cup catsup

Wash spinach. Drain on paper towel. Hard boil eggs. Fry bacon. Set aside to cool while making dressing. Heat sugar and vinegar until sugar dissolves. Add oil, onion, Worcestershire sauce and catsup. Arrange spinach leaves, add chopped eggs and crumbled bacon. Add dressing and toss.

Spinach Salad with Cranberry and Orange

Serves 6 to 8

2 cups fresh cranberries
½ cup water
¼ cup sugar
½ pound spinach
3 oranges, peeled and thinly sliced
8 ounces jicama, peeled and grated
¼ cup walnuts, toasted

White wine-honey vinaigrette:

¼ cup white wine vinegar
2 tablespoons salad oil
2 tablespoons honey
1 tablespoon cranberry liquid

Combine cranberries, water and sugar. Bring to a boil. Stir to dissolve sugar; gently boil 2 minutes. Drain, reserving 1 tablespoon of cranberry liquid. Transfer cooked and drained cranberries to a bowl, cover and chill. Combine dressing ingredients by shaking well. Toss spinach with dressing. Arrange spinach on salad plate. Top with orange slices, jicama, cranberries and walnuts.

Spinach Crunch Salad

Serves 4

1 pound spinach, washed and stems removed
1 bunch green onions, finely chopped

Crunch Mixture:
2 3-ounce packages Ramen noodles, without seasoning packet
1 tablespoon sesame seeds
1 ounce slivered almonds
1 tablespoon butter or margarine, melted

Dressing:
½ cup vegetable oil (preferably canola oil)
¼ cup sugar
2 tablespoons soy sauce

After cleaning spinach, use salad spinner to remove as much water as possible. Carefully cut or tear into bite-size pieces and place in large bowl with chopped green onions. Leave Ramen noodles in package and crush with hands to uniform consistency. In small bowl, mix noodles (without seasoning packet) with the sesame seeds and slivered almonds. Coat mixture with melted butter. Place evenly on cookie sheet and bake at 375 degrees about 3 minutes to toast lightly. Watch carefully. Let cool. Add to spinach and onions. Stir vegetable oil, sugar and soy sauce in bowl until mixture thickens. Pour dressing over salad and toss.

Grace's Red Raspberry~Cranberry Relish Salad

Serves 10 to 12

2 3.6-ounce packages raspberry Jello
1½ cups water, boiling
½ cup ginger ale
1 10-ounce box frozen red raspberries, thawed
1 10-ounce container frozen cranberry relish, thawed
juice of 1 lemon
rind of 1 lemon, grated
lettuce leaves

Prepare Jello in boiling water. Quickly stir in ginger ale, frozen raspberries, cranberries, lemon juice and rind. Pour into flat, oblong Pyrex or glass dish. Allow to set in refrigerator. Cut and serve on salad plates over lettuce.

Note: May also be molded in individual serving-size glass dishes.

Mom's Potato Salad

Serves 8 to 12

4 pounds unpeeled red potatoes, cooked in boiling, salted water
1½ cups celery, chopped
4 large green onions with tops, chopped
2 green peppers, chopped
salt and pepper, to taste
3 tablespoons oil
1 tablespoon vinegar
⅛ tablespoon dry mustard
3 hard-boiled eggs, chopped

For the following day:
1½ cups Hellmann's mayonnaise
1½ teaspoons French's mustard
1 hard-boiled egg, sliced
paprika, to taste

Chop everything in advance, because potatoes must still be warm when mixed with the other ingredients! Cook potatoes and, while warm, remove skins. Slice potatoes and start layering them with the chopped vegetables. Use salt and pepper in each layer. Mix oil, vinegar and dry mustard. Pour mixture over layered potatoes and vegetables, and mix. Add 3 chopped eggs and mix. Cover with plastic and let sit overnight. The next day, mix in mayonnaise and mustard; season to taste. Garnish with sliced egg and paprika.

Summer Pasta Salad

Serves 10 to 12

1 pound box thin spaghetti noodles, cooked
½ jar McCormick Vegetable Supreme (spice)
2 packages Good Seasons Italian dressing, prepared as directed
1 green pepper, finely chopped
1 cucumber, finely chopped
3 large tomatoes, finely chopped
3 celery stalks, finely chopped
2 4½-ounce cans chopped black olives

Mix all ingredients together. Store overnight in refrigerator, stirring occasionally.

Sour Cream Potato Salad

Serves 6 to 8

3 to 5 pounds potatoes, peeled and cubed
1½ cups mayonnaise
½ cup sour cream
¼ cup mustard
1 cup celery, chopped
1 medium onion, chopped or grated
1 dash salt
1 dash pepper
1 dash garlic powder

Cook potatoes. Mix mayonnaise, sour cream and mustard. Add celery, onions, salt, pepper and garlic powder.

Note: Prepare a day in advance for better flavor.

Artichoke & Shrimp Pasta Salad

Serves 6

1 16-ounce packages frozen artichoke hearts
1½ pounds medium shrimp, cooked, peeled and deveined
1 pound medium pasta shells, cooked and cooled

Red wine-mustard vinaigrette:
½ cup red wine vinegar
¼ cup Dijon mustard
¼ cup fresh chives, snipped
2 egg yolks
2 tablespoons shallots, minced
1 cup olive oil
½ cup vegetable oil
salt and pepper, to taste

Cook artichoke hearts according to package directions. Drain and place in large bowl. Add shrimp. Combine vinegar, mustard, chives, yolks and shallots in blender or processor. With machine running, gradually add both oils in thin stream. Season with salt and pepper. Pour over artichoke hearts and shrimp. Cover and refrigerate for 2 to 4 hours, stirring occasionally. Add cooked and slightly cooled pasta shells, and toss thoroughly. Cover and refrigerate until well chilled. Serve cold.

Note: May be prepared a day ahead.

Mexican Corn Chip Salad

Serves 4

- 1 pound ground chuck
- 1 small garlic clove, crushed
- 1 14½-ounce can tomatoes, drained
- 1 cup onion, finely chopped
- 1 4-ounce can green chilies, chopped
- salt and pepper, to taste
- 2 heads crisp lettuce, chopped
- 1 6-ounce package corn chips
- 1 cup green peppers, diced
- 2 cups cheddar cheese, grated
- 1 cup tomatoes, diced
- 1 cup avocados, diced
- ½ cup pitted black olives, sliced
- 1 cup sour cream

Sauté chuck and garlic in medium skillet, breaking up meat with fork until browned. Drain. Add tomatoes, onions, green chilies, salt and pepper. Cook over low heat for 30 minutes. Line glass bowl with chopped lettuce. Layer corn chips and meat mixture. Garnish with spoonfuls of green pepper, cheese, tomatoes, avocados, olives and a dollop of sour cream.

Red~Bean Taco Salad

Serves 4

- 1 onion, chopped
- 4 tomatoes, chopped
- 1 head iceberg lettuce, chopped
- ½ cup cheddar cheese, grated
- 1 8-ounce jar French dressing
- Tabasco sauce, to taste
- 1 bag taco-flavored Doritos
- 1 large avocado, sliced
- 1 pound ground beef
- 1 15½-ounce can red beans, with juice
- ¼ teaspoon salt

Chop onion, tomatoes, head of lettuce. Toss with grated Cheddar cheese, French dressing and hot sauce. Crush and add taco-flavored Doritos. Slice and add avocado. Set aside. Brown ground beef. Drain. Add red beans and salt. Cook 10 minutes. Add cooked mixture to salad ingredients.

Three~Bean Salad with White Wine Vinaigrette

Serves 8 to 10

- 1   14½-ounce can green beans
- 1   14½-ounce can yellow wax beans
- 1   15½-ounce can red kidney beans
- 1   medium onion, chopped
- 1   medium green pepper, chopped
- ½   cup celery, diced

White wine vinaigrette:
- ¾   cup sugar
- ½   cup white wine vinegar
- ½   cup salad oil
- ½   teaspoon salt
- ½   teaspoon pepper

Drain beans. Add onion, green pepper and celery. In a small bowl, whisk together sugar, vinegar, oil, salt and pepper. Pour mixture over beans and mix well. Refrigerate overnight.

Jean's Mustard Three~Bean Salad

Serves 8 to 10

- 1   14½-ounce can green beans
- 1   14½-ounce can wax beans
- 1   15½-ounce can kidney beans
- 1   medium green pepper, sliced
- 1   medium onion, chopped

Mustard vinaigrette:
- ½   cup sugar
- ½   cup vinegar
- 1   teaspoon salt
- ½   cup salad oil
- ½   teaspoon dry mustard

Drain beans. Place beans, green pepper and onion in large bowl. Mix all dressing ingredients together and pour over bean mixture. Cover. Let marinate in refrigerator several hours or overnight. Stir once or twice. Serve with slotted spoon.

Madge's Kidney Bean Salad

Serves 6 to 8

- 3 15½-ounce cans kidney beans, drained and washed
- 2 cups celery, finely chopped
- 1 cup green onions, finely chopped
- ¼ cup sweet pickle relish
- 1 tablespoon pepper, freshly ground
- 1 teaspoon celery salt
- 1 16-ounce jar Hellmann's mayonnaise
- 2 hard-boiled eggs, cut into slices

paprika

Mix all ingredients well, except eggs and paprika. Garnish with egg slices and paprika.

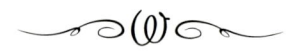

"Dressed-Up" Coleslaw

Serves 6

- 1 cup mayonnaise
- 2 tablespoons fresh lime juice
- ½ teaspoon lime rind, minced
- ½ head green cabbage, shredded
- ½ head red cabbage, shredded
- 1 cup seedless red or green grapes, cut in half
- 4 green onions, cut into thin rings
- 4 green onion tops, minced
- ½ cup walnuts, finely chopped

Combine mayonnaise, lime juice and rind in large bowl. Add remaining ingredients and mix well. Chill and serve.

Note: May be prepared a day ahead.

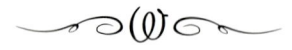

Yacht Club Coleslaw

Serves 8

- 1 head cabbage, shredded
- 1 cup raisins
- 1 large apple, cored and chopped
- 1 cup salted peanuts, halved
- 1 8-ounce bottle coleslaw dressing

Mix above ingredients and chill.

"Sis W" Coleslaw

Serves 16 to 18

- 1 large head white cabbage, shredded
- 1 large head red cabbage, shredded
- 2 large onions, minced
- 1 large green pepper, minced
- 1 large red pepper, minced
- 2 cups mayonnaise
- 1 teaspoon Worcestershire sauce
- 1 tablespoon dry mustard
- 1 tablespoon celery seed
- 1 teaspoon sugar
- ½ cup olive oil
- 1 tablespoon lemon juice
- ⅓ cup balsamic vinegar
- 1 teaspoon salt
- 1 teaspoon pepper
- 1 teaspoon Tabasco sauce

Combine all ingredients; mix well. Refrigerate until serving.

Note: Keeps several days in covered container in refrigerator.

Sweet & Sour Cucumbers

Serves 12

- 7 to 8 medium unpeeled cucumbers, washed and thinly sliced
- 1 teaspoon salt

Sweet-sour vinaigrette:
- 1 cup white or cider vinegar
- ¼ cup dry sherry (optional)
- 2 cups sugar
- 1 cup onion, chopped
- 1 cup green pepper, chopped (optional)
- ¼ teaspoon celery salt
- 1 teaspoon dill weed
- ¼ teaspoon black pepper

Sprinkle unpeeled cucumber slices with 1 teaspoon salt, and let stand for one hour. Mix ingredients for vinaigrette. Heat until warm, but not hot. Pour over cucumbers. Serve warm or cold.

Note: Keeps in refrigerator for two weeks.

Cranberry Waldorf Salad

Serves 6

1 8-ounce package cranberries
2 cups miniature marshmallows
1 cup sugar
2 cups tart apples, diced
½ cup seedless grapes
½ cup walnuts
¼ teaspoon salt
1 cup whipping cream, whipped
lettuce (optional)

Grind cranberries in food processor. Combine with marshmallows and sugar. Cover and refrigerate overnight. The next day, add all other ingredients. Fold in whipped cream. Serve in large bowl or on individual salad plates, on lettuce.

Fruit & Nut Tossed Salad

Serves 8

1 pound spinach, torn
1 head romaine lettuce, torn
1 cup green seedless grapes, halved
½ cup slivered almonds, toasted
1 11-ounce can mandarin oranges, chilled and drained
1 small avocado, peeled and sliced

Vinaigrette:

½ cup oil
¼ cup vinegar
¼ cup sugar
½ teaspoon salt

In large bowl combine spinach, lettuce, grapes, almonds and oranges. In screw-top jar combine dressing ingredients. Shake well. Just before serving, toss some dressing with salad and garnish with avocado.

Waldorf Raisin Salad

Serves 8

6 Red Delicious apples, diced
2 tablespoons lemon juice
1 cup raisins
2 tablespoons sherry
1 cup pecans or walnuts, halved
1 cup celery, diced
1 cup miniature marshmallows
¼ to ½-cup mayonnaise
lettuce leaves

Soak apples in lemon juice. Heat raisins in sherry until plump. Cool. Mix all ingredients, adding mayonnaise to moisten. Serve on lettuce leaves.

German Cottage Cheese

Serves 4 to 6

1½ 8-ounce containers cottage cheese
2 tablespoons green onions or chives, finely chopped
½ teaspoon Beau Monde seasoning
¾ teaspoon caraway seeds
1 pinch black pepper, freshly ground

Mix all ingredients together. Cover tightly and refrigerate overnight.

Note: Will keep for several days.

Pineapple~Mandarin Fruit Salad

Serves 8 to 10

Also works as a dessert!

1 8-ounce container Cool Whip
1 14-ounce can Eagle Brand condensed milk
1 8-ounce can crushed pineapple
1 21-ounce can cherry pie filling
½ cup nuts, chopped
½ cup coconut
2 cups miniature marshmallows
1 11-ounce can mandarin oranges, drained

Mix Cool Whip and Eagle Brand milk. Fold in remaining ingredients, chill until served.

Bing~Banana Salad

Serves 8 to 10

Also works as a dessert!

- 2 cups miniature marshmallows
- 1 20-ounce can bing cherries, undrained
- 1 8-ounce container Cool Whip
- 1 3.6-ounce package instant banana pudding
- 2 bananas, sliced

Mix all ingredients and pour into mold or 8x10-inch Pyrex dish. Refrigerate overnight.

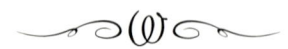

Pistachio Salad with Sherbet

Serves 10

Also works as a dessert!

- 1 20-ounce can crushed pineapple
- 1 3.6-ounce package instant pistachio pudding
- 1 pint lime sherbet
- 1 8-ounce container Cool Whip

Drain pineapple and add juice to pudding. Stir in sherbet and mix well. Add pineapple and Cool Whip to pudding mixture. Pour into a greased jello mold, and freeze. Unmold onto platter and serve.

Note: Keeps well in freezer for a few days.

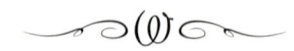

Layered Jello Salad

Serves 10 to 12

Also works as a dessert!

- 1 3.6-ounce package raspberry Jello
- 1 15-ounce can frozen raspberries, thawed and drained
- 1 3.6-ounce package lemon-lime Jello
- 1 16-ounce can fruit cocktail, drained
- 1 3.6-ounce package strawberry-banana Jello
- 1 large banana, sliced
- 1 15-ounce can frozen strawberries, thawed and drained

Cool Whip (optional)

Prepare raspberry Jello as directed. Add drained raspberries. Put in decorative clear bowl large enough for all Jello flavors. Let chill until thickened. Prepare lemon-lime Jello and add drained fruit cocktail. Add to top of chilled raspberry Jello. Let chill until firm. Prepare strawberry Jello and add banana and strawberries. Serve as a dessert with Cool Whip, or as a side salad without.

Pretzel Pie Salad

Serves 8 to 12

Also works as a dessert!

Crust:
- 2½ cups pretzels, crushed (not too fine)
- ¾ cup butter or margarine, softened
- 3 tablespoons sugar

Pie:
- 1 8-ounce package cream cheese, softened
- 1 cup sugar
- 1 package Dream Whip
- 2 3.6-ounce packages strawberry Jello
- 2 cups boiling water
- 2 10-ounce boxes frozen strawberries

Preheat oven to 375 degrees. Mix pretzels, butter or margarine and 3 tablespoons sugar, and press in 10x13-inch pan (do not grease pan). Bake 10 minutes. Cool. Mix softened cream cheese with 1-cup sugar. Whip Dream Whip according to directions. Fold into cream cheese mixture. Spread over pretzel crust. Dissolve 2 packages Jello into 2 cups boiling water. Add two 10-ounce packages frozen strawberries. Stir until strawberries are melted. When almost set, spread over cheese mixture. Chill.

Taffy Apple Salad

Serves 6 to 8

Also works as a dessert!

- 1 20-ounce can pineapple tidbits
- 4 cups miniature marshmallows
- ½ cup sugar
- 1 tablespoon flour
- 1 egg, well beaten
- 1½ tablespoons white vinegar
- 1 12-ounce container Cool Whip
- 3 large, unpeeled apples, diced
- 1 cup Spanish peanuts, chopped (save some for topping)

Drain pineapple, reserving juice. Mix pineapple with marshmallows (set aside). In small saucepan, combine juice, flour, sugar, egg and vinegar. Cook until slightly thickened. Cool. When mixture is cold, combine with Cool Whip. Fold in marshmallow mixture. Add apples and peanuts, mix well. Sprinkle extra peanuts on top.

Creamy Garlic House Dressing

Yield: 1 quart

Adapted for your kitchen... from the original Walgreens recipe!

Robin Hood & Briargate Restaurants, 1970's ~ 1980's

- 2 egg yolks
- ¾ teaspoon salt
- ½ teaspoon dry mustard
- ¼ teaspoon sugar
- 1 pinch cayenne pepper
- 4 to 5 teaspoons lemon juice
- 1 garlic clove, minced
- 2 tablespoons onion, finely chopped
- 1½ cups salad or olive oil
- 4 teaspoons hot water
- ½ cup sour cream

In blender, combine egg yolks, salt, mustard, sugar, cayenne pepper, lemon juice, onion and garlic. Mix at low speed for 15 seconds. Increase speed, open blender and slowly drizzle in ¼-cup oil in a fine, steady stream. As mixture thickens, continue adding oil, alternating with hot water, until all the oil and hot water have been added. Scrape down the sides of blender. Pour mixture into bowl and fold in sour cream with a wire whip. Refrigerate.

Creamy Pepper Dressing

Yield: 3 cups

- 2 cups mayonnaise
- ½ cup milk
- ¼ cup water
- 4 tablespoons Parmesan cheese
- 1 tablespoon pepper, freshly ground
- 1 tablespoon cider vinegar
- 1 teaspoon fresh lemon juice
- 1 teaspoon onion, finely chopped
- 1 teaspoon garlic salt
- 1 dash of Tabasco sauce
- 1 dash of Worcestershire sauce

Combine ingredients in blender. Refrigerate for several hours before serving.

Honey Dressing for Fruit Salad

Serves 4 to 6

½ cup vegetable oil
¼ cup fresh lemon juice
¼ cup fresh lime juice
½ teaspoon salt
cayenne pepper, to taste
¼ cup honey

Combine oil, juices and seasonings. Add honey and beat well. Chill and serve over fruit salad.

Mustard~Wine Vinaigrette with Pecans

Serves 6 to 8

¼ cup sherry wine vinegar
1 shallot, minced
1 teaspoon Pommery or any Dijon-style mustard
1 tablespoon fresh lemon juice
¾ cup vegetable oil
4 tablespoons pecans, chopped and toasted
salt and pepper, to taste

Combine vinegar, shallot, mustard and lemon juice in bowl (metal, if possible). Gradually whisk in oil. Add toasted pecans, while they are hot, to vinaigrette. Season with salt and pepper. Serve over fruit salad.

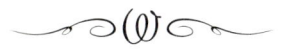

Raspberry~Poppy Seed Dressing

Yield: 3 cups

1½ cups sugar
2 tablespoons onion juice
⅔ cup raspberry vinegar
1 tablespoon Coleman's English or any Dijon-style mustard
1 teaspoon salt
2 cups vegetable oil
3 tablespoons poppy seeds

Mix all ingredients together in a blender, except oil and poppy seeds. Blend well. Slowly add oil until dressing is thick. Add poppy seeds and blend. To serve, chill and spoon over fresh fruit or salad.

KBW's World~Famous Blue Cheese Dressing

Serves 8 to 10

- ½ pound blue cheese
- ½ cup milk
- 1 cup mayonnaise
- 1 teaspoon Worcestershire sauce
- ¼ teaspoon Tabasco sauce
- 2 teaspoons balsamic vinegar
- ¼ cup olive oil
- 1 garlic clove, minced (optional)

salt and pepper, to taste

Reserve ¼ of the blue cheese hunk; grate the rest with a large hand grater. With a whisk, combine remaining ingredients. Crumble the rest of the blue cheese and combine with the other ingredients. Serve over salad.

Note: May be stored in air-tight container in refrigerator for up to 7 days.

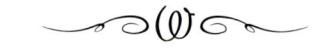

Blue Cheese~Yogurt Dressing

Yield: 1½ cups

- 1 16-ounce container plain, low-fat yogurt
- ¾ cup non-fat buttermilk
- ½ cup blue cheese, crumbled
- 1 teaspoon cider vinegar
- ¼ teaspoon pepper
- ⅛ teaspoon salt
- 1 small garlic clove, pressed

Spoon yogurt onto several layers heavy-duty paper towels. Spread to ½-inch thickness. Cover with additional paper towels. Let stand 5 minutes. Scrape into small bowl, using a rubber spatula. Add buttermilk and remaining ingredients, stir well. Cover and chill. Serve over mixed greens.

Tara's Western Dressing

Yield: 1½ cups

- 1 10¾-ounce can tomato soup
- ¾ cup cider vinegar (or white tarragon, or mixture)
- ½ cup salad oil
- ¼ cup sugar
- 1 tablespoon Worcestershire sauce
- ¼ teaspoon onion powder (or 1 tablespoon onion, grated)
- 1 teaspoon salt
- 1 teaspoon dry mustard
- 1 teaspoon paprika

Combine ingredients in blender and mix well. Chill to serve. Keeps well refrigerated.

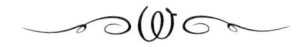

A~1 French Dressing

Yield: 1½ cups

- ½ cup Mazola oil
- ½ cup catsup
- ¼ cup vinegar
- ½ cup sugar
- 1 teaspoon paprika
- 1 small onion, chopped
- 1 teaspoon A-1 sauce

Combine all ingredients in blender and mix well. Chill to serve.

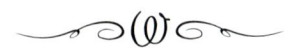

Spicy Dill Dressing

Yield: 1½ cups

- 1 cup mayonnaise
- ⅓ cup sour cream
- ½ teaspoon garlic salt
- 1 dash tabasco
- 1 tablespoon dill pickle juice
- 1 tablespoon dill weed, fresh or dried

salt and pepper, to taste

Mix mayonnaise and sour cream in food processor or blender. Add remaining ingredients and blend well. Refrigerate for at least 3 hours before serving.

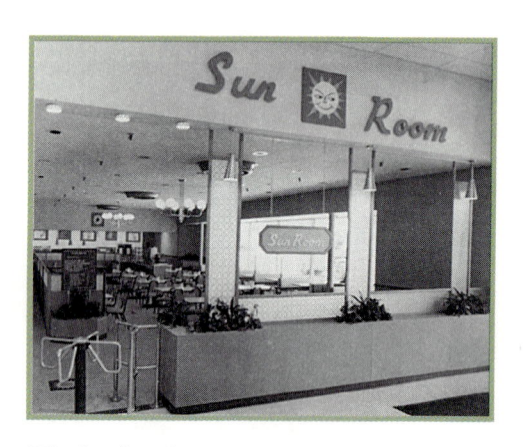

The bright, cheery Sun Rooms were a part of the Walgreen-owned Globe Discount Cities chain.

Facing Page: *Salmon & Shrimp Terrine*
Photo: Scott Lanza, 1995
Stylist: F. Lynn Nelson

FISH & SEAFOOD

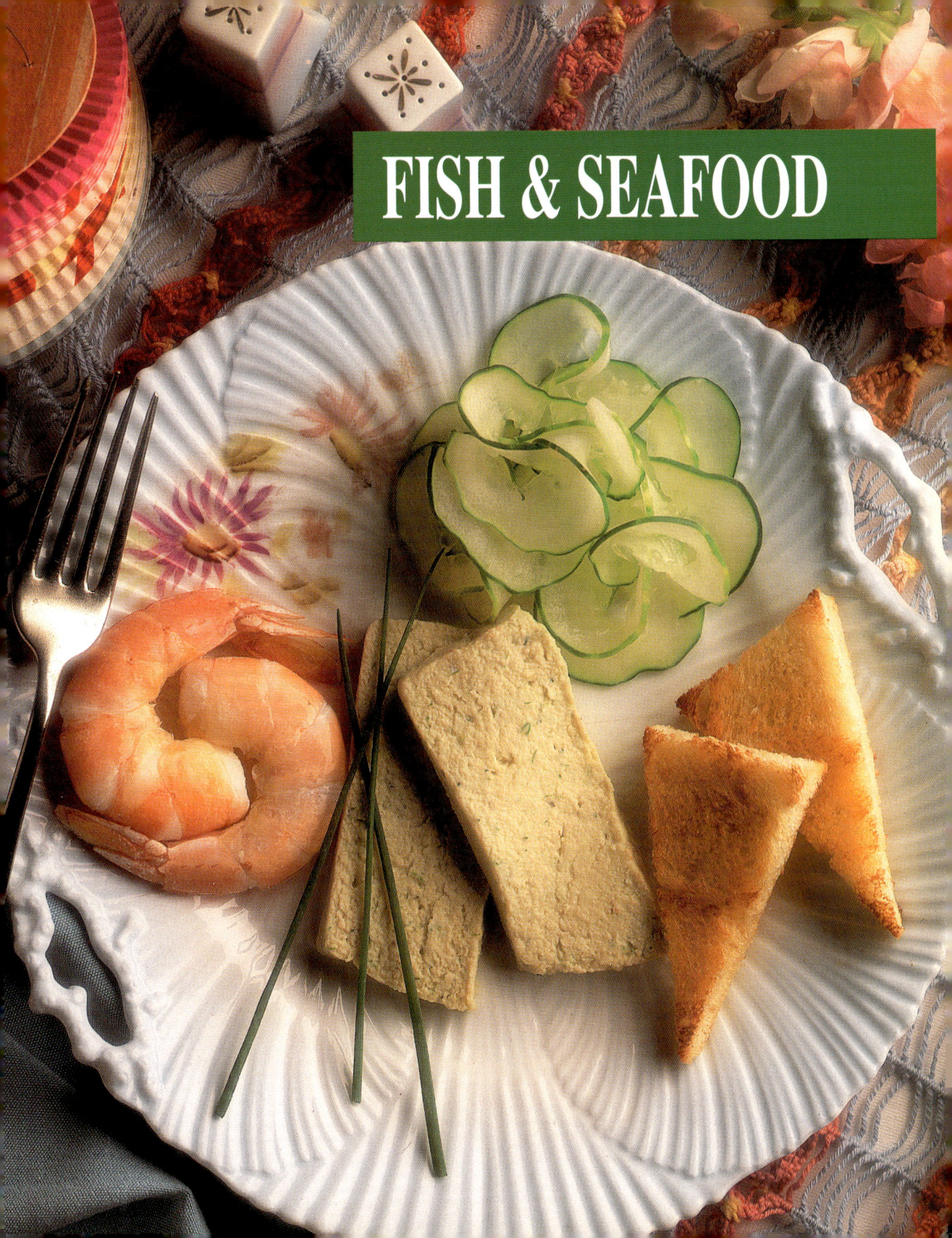

The Villager Room & The Globe Stores
Favorite In-Shop Dining Stops

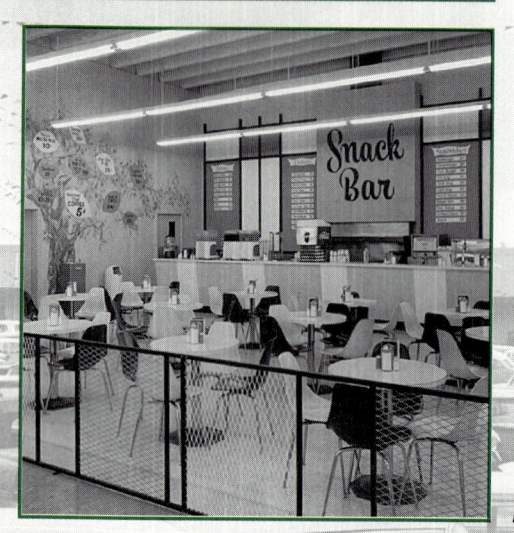

1962 proved to be a big year for Walgreens, which opened its first full-scale restaurant, The Villager Grill Room. That same year the company purchased the first Globe Department Store.

The Villager Room in Oak Park, Illinois opened in 1962 and was Walgreens first full-scale restaurant and grill room. Tastefully decorated and carpeted, it was hard to believe the restaurant was part of a Walgreens drug store! The Villager Room became well-known throughout the town with its second-to-none seafood bar, carving bar and salad bar, plus quick breakfasts, luscious luncheons and a scrumptious weekend buffet.

Walgreens bought the first *Globe Discount Cities* department store in 1962, and soon expanded, opening 30 stores. The Globe stores were spacious, around 100,000 square feet, and with them came the opportunity to build the first comprehensive in-store dining centers. Among these were the popular short-line cafeterias or *Sun Rooms* (named so because many had sunrooms in front). The "bigger is better" idea was prevalent with these huge stores, and one of the largest, in San Antonio, had a snack bar and bakery running the length of its front lobby and adjacent cafeteria!

Vermouth White Sauce Fish

Serves 4 to 6

8 fish fillets
1 teaspoon parsley, chopped

Vermouth white sauce:
4 tablespoons butter
¼ cup flour
¼ teaspoon salt
¼ teaspoon Tabasco sauce
¼ teaspoon garlic powder
½ teaspoon sugar
¾ cup dry vermouth
¼ cup milk

To make sauce, combine butter, flour and salt in a saucepan and cook over low heat, stirring constantly, for 5 minutes. Be careful not to brown! Add Tabasco, garlic powder, sugar and dry vermouth. Continue cooking over low heat until sauce starts to bubble. Then, slowly whisk in milk. Whisk sauce until it thickens. Meanwhile, heat oven to 325 degrees. Put fish fillets on greased baking sheet and bake for 10 to 15 minutes, or until fish is flaky. Remove fish from oven to serving platter and spoon sauce over fish. Garnish with parsley and serve with leftover sauce.

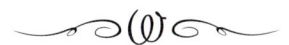

Swordfish in Citrus~Ginger Marinade

Serves 4

2 swordfish steaks, boneless, ¼-inch thick each

Ginger marinade:
2 tablespoons soy sauce
2 tablespoons orange juice
1 tablespoon lemon juice
½ teaspoon catsup
½ teaspoon ginger root, minced
1 garlic clove, minced

Combine all ingredient to make marinade. Marinate swordfish for 1 hour. Remove swordfish from marinade and charcoal grill or broil until done, approximately 10 to 15 minutes.

Halibut with Crumb~Nut Topping

Serves 4 to 6

4 pounds halibut steak, filleted

Crumb-nut topping:
2 cups bread crumbs
½ cup butter or margarine, melted
½ teaspoon salt
½ cup Parmesan cheese, grated
1 tablespoon lemon peel, grated
¾ cup fresh parsley, chopped
2 tablespoons fresh basil, chopped
1 cup pine nuts or pecans, coarsely chopped

Preheat oven to 350 degrees. To make topping, place bread crumbs, butter, salt, Parmesan cheese, lemon peel, parsley and basil in mixing bowl. Add nuts, and stir. Place fish in buttered baking dish. Top with crumb-nut mixture. Bake at 350 degrees for 20 minutes, or until done.

Baked Halibut, Greek Style ~ Plaki

Serves 6

2 pounds boneless halibut fillets
⅛ cup olive oil

Greek tomato sauce:
⅛ cup olive oil
4 onions, thinly sliced
1 garlic clove, pressed
2 cups tomatoes or 1 cup tomato pureé, diluted with 2 cups water
½ cup parsley, chopped
1 teaspoon oregano
⅛ teaspoon cinnamon
½ teaspoon salt
½ cup red or port wine
pepper, to taste

Preheat oven to 350 degrees. Cut fish in pieces and rinse with cold water. Grease baking dish (sauce will run off in oven if put on a flat pan) with ⅛-cup oil. Place slices of fish in dish. To make sauce, heat ⅛-cup oil in frying pan, and sauté onions and garlic on medium heat for 5 minutes. Add remaining sauce ingredients and cover. Cook 10 minutes. Pour sauce over fish. Bake at 350 degrees for 45 minutes.

Halibut Creole

Serves 4

2 pounds halibut steaks, filleted

Creole sauce:
2 tablespoons butter or margarine
1 tablespoon flour
1 tablespoon green onion, finely chopped
1 green pepper, chopped
2 cups tomatoes, diced and cooked
1 teaspoon white pepper
salt and pepper, to taste
1 cup rice, cooked per package directions

Preheat oven to 400 degrees. To make creole sauce, melt butter and blend in flour. Add green onion and green pepper. Cook 3 minutes. Add tomatoes and white pepper. Cook until thickened. Stir constantly. Simmer 10 minutes longer. Place fish in lightly-greased baking dish and pour creole sauce over fish. Bake at 400 degrees for 30 minutes. Add salt and pepper to taste. Serve with rice.

Flounder Fillet with Onions

Serves 4

2 pound flounder fillets
salt, pepper and paprika, to taste
4 tablespoons butter
1 large onion, thinly sliced
2 lemon wedges
2 dashes Worcestershire sauce

Wipe flounder with a damp paper towel. Season lightly with salt, pepper and paprika. Heat butter in a large skillet and sauté onions until lightly browned. Set onions aside. Add a little more butter if needed, and sauté fish fillets over medium heat until done, about 5 minutes for thin fillets. Return onions to pan. Squeeze lemon juice, from wedges, over fish and onions. Add generous dashes of Worcestershire sauce. Serve immediately.

Sole with Lemon and Capers

Serves 4

Fish:
4 6-ounce sole fillets
salt and pepper, to taste
½ cup all-purpose flour
4 tablespoons vegetable oil
4 tablespoons salted butter or margarine

Garnishes:
2 slices day-old bread, crusts removed
2 tablespoons butter or margarine
1 lemon, peeled, with pith and seeds removed, and diced
2 tablespoons capers, drained
3 tablespoons unsalted butter or margarine, melted and seasoned with salt and pepper
2 tablespoons fresh parsley, chopped

Season fillets with salt and pepper. Dredge in flour, shaking off excess. In each of two medium skillets, heat 2 tablespoons oil and 2 tablespoons of salted butter over medium-high heat. Add fillets, lower heat and sauté for 4 to 5 minutes on each side until cooked through and golden. Lift each fillet onto warmed plate. To prepare garnishes, cut bread into ¼-inch cubes and brown in 2 tablespoons of butter to make croutons. Add croutons, lemon and capers to each fillet. Sprinkle with 3 tablespoons melted, seasoned, unsalted butter. Top with chopped parsley.

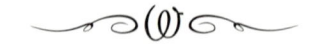

Singapore Steamed Fish

Serves 4

1 whole firm-bodied white fish, washed and towel dried
1½ tablespoons sesame oil
2 onions, diced
2 garlic cloves, minced
1½ tablespoons dark soy sauce
2 tablespoons oyster sauce
1 or 2 red hot chilies, very thinly sliced (optional)

Heat sesame oil in sauté pan; simmer the onions and garlic until cooked. Add soy sauce, oyster sauce and chilies until well-blended. Place fish in steaming basket or colander over boiling water; do not allow fish to touch the water. Pour sauce on top of uncooked fish. Cover tightly and steam 10 to 12 minutes per inch of thickness of fish. Serve immediately.

Granny Gunn's Finnan Haddie

Serves 6 to 8

2 pounds smoked haddock (finnan haddie)
1 tablespoon butter

White sauce (optional):
4 tablespoons butter
4 tablespoons flour
¾ teaspoon salt
¼ teaspoon white pepper
2½ cups milk, heated

6 potatoes, boiled

Preheat oven to 350 degrees. Put fish in covered dish with a very small amount of water. Add butter and bake at 350 degrees until heated through. For sauce, melt butter in saucepan, blend in flour; add salt and white pepper. On low heat, slowly whisk in milk, stirring constantly. Pour sauce over fish and serve with boiled potatoes.

Note: *Finnan haddie* (or *findhorn haddock*) originated in Scotland.

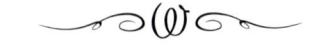

Beer Batter Fish

Serves 6

2 pounds fish fillets
3 to 4 tablespoons Bisquick
vegetable oil

Beer batter:
1 cup Bisquick
½ teaspoon salt
1 egg
½ cup beer

To make batter, combine Bisquick, salt, egg and beer. Mix well. Coat fish with 3 to 4 tablespoons of Bisquick, then in batter. In frying pan heat 1½-inches vegetable oil to 360 degrees. Deep-fry fish for about 2 minutes, or until golden brown. Drain on a brown paper bag.

Ceviche

Serves 6 to 8

Adapted for your kitchen... from the original Walgreens recipe!

Sanborns, Mexico, 1946 ~ 1984

Although this dish usually appears as an appetizer on Mexican restaurant menus, Ceviche *(pickled fish)* is frequently served as a main course in Mexico.

Also called **Seviche**.

3½ pounds fresh mackerel or kingfish, skinned and cut into cubes
juice of 3 fresh limes
salt, to taste
2 large tomatoes, skinned, seeded and cubed
1 onion, minced
1 tablespoon cilantro, coarsely chopped
½ cup green olives, minced
1 ripe avocado
2 canned chilies serranos, finely chopped
1 tablespoon vinegar
½ teaspoon oregano, dried

Garnishes:
8 lettuce leaves
8 slices avocado
8 whole olives
Chinese parsley (fresh cilantro), to taste
8 lemon slices (optional)
saltine crackers (optional)

Cover cubed fish with lime juice. Cover bowl and refrigerate for five hours. Add salt. Add tomatoes to fish. Add onion, olives, chilies serranos, vinegar, and oregano. To serve, place lettuce leaf on plate. Spoon a serving of ceviche on lettuce; top with sliced avocado and Chinese parsley. Ceviche may also be served on saltine crackers with lemon slices.

Mustard~Baked Fish Fillets

Serves 4 to 6

2 pounds white fish fillets, skin removed
1 egg white
¼ cup fat-free mayonnaise
1 tablespoon Dijon mustard
¼ teaspoon salt
¼ teaspoon pepper

Preheat oven to 400 degrees. Arrange fillets in a lightly-greased shallow baking dish and set aside. Beat egg white until stiff. Fold in remaining ingredients. Cover fillets with egg white mixture. Bake for 20 to 25 minutes or until puffed and golden.

Broiled Salmon with Grapes

Serves 4

- 2 pounds salmon fillets
- ½ cup lemon juice
- 1 tablespoon black pepper, freshly ground
- 2 tablespoons mayonnaise
- 4 teaspoons Dijon mustard
- 6 scallions (green onions), chopped
- 2 to 3 tablespoons Dip-idy Dill* mixture
- 2 cups green, seedless grapes, halved

Preheat broiler 10 minutes. Sprinkle fish with lemon juice and black pepper. Combine mayonnaise and mustard; brush fish with mixture. Sprinkle more pepper on fish. Sprinkle fish with Dip-idy Dill and chopped scallions. Place grapes in rows, covering fish completely. Broil fish for 10 minutes (grapes will be brown-black); cover fish with foil and broil 3 to 5 more minutes, depending on thickness, until fish flakes easily.

Note: *Dip-idy Dill may be found in the spice section of most grocery stores.

Honey Salmon Fillet

Serves 4

- 2 pounds salmon fillets
- 1 tablespoon olive oil

Honey sauce:
- ½ cup honey
- 1 teaspoon chili powder
- 2 garlic cloves, minced

lemon or lime wedges

To prepare honey sauce, mix together the honey, chili powder and garlic. Over medium-high heat, warm a heavy cast iron skillet until hot. Mask with olive oil. Cook salmon approximately 3 minutes per side until light pink throughout, but still firm. (Thicker fillets will take a little longer.) Just before fish is done, add honey mixture. Let mixture bubble vigorously. Remove fish to warm serving plates; pour sauce over fish. Garnish with lemon or lime wedges.

Salmon with Cilantro Oil & Mango Salsa

Serves 4

4 6 to 8-ounce salmon fillets, skin removed

Cilantro oil:
½ bunch cilantro, cleaned
4 ounces extra virgin olive oil
1 garlic clove, minced
salt and pepper, to taste

Mango salsa (may use papaya):
2 cups mango or papaya, peeled and cut into ¼-inch cubes
½ cup cucumber; peeled, seeded and cut into ¼-inch cubes
¼ cup cilantro, chopped
2 tablespoons green onion, finely chopped
½ jalapeño pepper, seeded and finely chopped
3 tablespoons fresh lime juice
1 teaspoon fresh ginger root, peeled and minced
1 dash pepper

To make salsa, combine all ingredients and refrigerate at least 1 hour to allow flavors to blend. (Add 1 teaspoon honey if papaya is used.) To make cilantro oil, place cilantro in a colander or strainer and immerse in a pot of boiling water for 2 seconds only. Remove and run cold water from tap over immediately. Purée cilantro and remaining ingredients in blender. Place in jar or squirt bottle. Cut salmon into ½-inch thick scallop, if desired. Heat cilantro oil in a non-stick pan and sauté salmon for about 5 minutes. Refrigerate extra oil and decorate serving plate with squiggles of chilled cilantro oil. Pass salsa to accompany salmon.

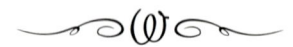

Salmon & Shrimp Terrine

Serves 8

1 8-ounce salmon, skinned and boned
8 ounces shrimp, shelled and deveined
3 egg whites
3 tablespoons fresh chives, chopped, or green onions, sliced
½ teaspoon dried dill weed
½ teaspoon salt
¼ teaspoon pepper
1½ cups whipping cream
whole shrimp, cooked (optional)

Salmon & Shrimp Terrine, *continued on next page.*

Salmon & Shrimp Terrine, continued.

Thaw salmon and shrimp, if frozen. Rinse the fish and pat dry with paper towels. Coarsely chop fish, then place in food processor. Process until smooth, stopping frequently to scrape sides of bowl. (Or, place half the fish in blender and blend until smooth; repeat with other half, then return all fish to blender.) Add egg whites, chives or green onions, dill weed, salt and pepper to fish in processor or blender. Process or blend until mixture resembles a thick paste, stopping to scrape sides as necessary. With processor or blender running, gradually add the cold whipping cream, stopping to scrape sides as necessary. Process 30 to 60 seconds more until mixture is thick.

Line an 8x4x2-inch loaf pan with foil, extending foil over edges. Grease foil. Spread fish mixture evenly in pan. Cover pan with foil. Place loaf pan in 13x9x2-inch baking pan. Pour hot tap water into the baking pan around the loaf pan to a depth of 1-inch. Bake at 350 degrees for 30 to 35 minutes, or until a knife inserted near center comes out clean. Remove loaf pan from baking pan. Cool to room temperature. Chill.

To serve, unmold the chilled terrine onto a serving platter. Garnish with additional cooked, whole shrimp, if desired.

Creamed Salmon with Peas

Serves 6

Adapted for your kitchen... from the original Walgreens recipe!

Walgreens Cafeterias 1940's ~ 1960's

1	1-pound can salmon
½	cup canned peas

White sauce:

2	tablespoons butter
2	tablespoons flour
⅛	teaspoon pepper
¼	teaspoon salt
1	cup milk

6 slices toast or patty shells, prepared per package directions

Drain salmon, remove bones and dark skin. Break into large pieces. Drain peas. To make sauce, bring milk to boil. In another pan melt butter or margarine; blend flour and seasoning, stirring constantly. Bring mixture to a boil. Remove from heat and add hot milk, stirring until smooth. Return to low heat, bring to a boil, stirring constantly. Add salmon and peas. Heat thoroughly. Season to taste. Serve on toast or in patty shells. May also be served over rice or with noodles in a casserole.

Alaskan Salmon Loaf with Creole Sauce

Serves 6 to 8

*Adapted for your kitchen...
from the original Walgreens recipe!*

Walgreens Cafeterias 1940's ~ 1960's

- 1 16-ounce can red Alaska salmon
- ¼ cup milk
- 1 cup dry bread crumbs
- ½ cup celery, finely chopped
- 2 eggs, beaten
- 1½ tablespoon butter or margarine, melted
- 1 teaspoon Worcestershire sauce
- ½ teaspoon white pepper

Creole sauce:
- 2 teaspoons vegetable oil
- ½ cup celery, chopped
- ½ cup green pepper, chopped
- ½ cup onion, chopped
- ½ cup mushroom, sliced (optional)
- ½ pound can chopped tomatoes
- 1 teaspoon salt
- ½ teaspoon pepper, freshly ground
- ¼ teaspoon Tabasco sauce

To make sauce, sauté celery, green pepper, onion, mushrooms in oil until lightly browned. Add tomatoes, salt, pepper, tabasco. Simmer 15 minutes. Drain salmon, remove dark skin and bones, and flake. Add remaining ingredients and mix thoroughly. Pack into a well-greased and foil-lined 9x5x3-inch loaf pan. Set loaf pan in a pan of hot water, cover with foil and bake at 350 degrees for 1 hour. Uncover and bake for 30 more minutes, or until top is lightly browned and firm to the touch. Remove from oven. Let stand before serving. Reheat creole sauce and serve hot over sliced loaf.

Broiled Salmon with Tarragon Butter

Serves 4

- 4 1-inch thick salmon fillets
- 6 tablespoons butter
- 3 tablespoons fresh lemon juice
- salt and pepper, to taste
- 3 tablespoons fresh tarragon, minced (or 2 teaspoons, dried)

Broiled Salmon with Tarragon Butter, *continued on next page.*

Broiled Salmon with Tarragon Butter, *continued.*

Preheat broiler. Melt butter with lemon juice in small saucepan over low heat. Remove from heat and add generous amount of pepper. Arrange salmon skin-side down on broiler pan. Brush with half of butter mixture. Season with salt. Broil, without turning, until just cooked through. Add tarragon to butter in saucepan; heat. To serve, spoon over salmon on plates.

Michigan Farmhouse Salmon Loaf

Serves 8

2	16-ounce cans of salmon, reserve liquid from can
2	eggs
1	cup milk
3	cups Saltine cracker crumbs
2	tablespoons lemon juice
2	teaspoons onions, chopped
¼	teaspoon salt
¼	teaspoon pepper

lemon wedges

Flake salmon, removing bones and skin. Reserve liquid from cans. Blend 2 eggs into salmon. Add milk to salmon, making 1½ cups of mixture. Stir reserved liquid into the salmon and egg mixture. Add cracker crumbs, lemon juice, onions, salt and pepper. Mix well. Spoon lightly into a greased 9x5x3-inch loaf pan. Bake at 350 degrees for 45 minutes. Serve with lemon wedges.

Scotch~Mustard Salmon

Serves 4

4	salmon fillets, about 6 ounces each

Scotch-mustard marinade:

½	cup safflower or canola oil
2	tablespoons soy sauce
2	tablespoons Scotch whiskey
2	tablespoons rice vinegar
1	tablespoon Dijon mustard
2	tablespoons green onion, finely chopped

To make marinade, combine ingredients. Pour over salmon and marinate for 1 to 2 hours. Broil or charcoal grill salmon for 6 to 8 minutes without turning. Brush with marinade while cooking. Heat remaining marinade just to the boiling point. Serve hot with cooked salmon.

Baked Walleye in Wine Sauce

Serves 2 to 4

2 to 4 walleye fillets or other white fish
2 tablespoons lime juice
5 tablespoons white wine
5 whole green onions, chopped
¼ pound butter or margarine
½ cup Parmesan cheese
½ cup bread crumbs

Preheat oven to 375 degrees. Place fish on rack in poacher. Pour lime juice and wine over fish. Poach in 375-degree oven for about 10 minutes. Remove rack with fish, set poached fish in bottom of broiling pan. Drain poaching liquid into a saucepan; reduce by half. In another saucepan, sauté onions in butter until soft or translucent. Top fish with cheese and bread crumbs, salt and pepper to taste. Pour reduced wine sauce over fish; top with sautéed onions. Broil until onions are lightly browned and fish is flaky.

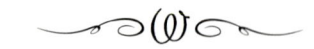

Broiled Brook Trout Amandine

Serves 4

**Adapted for your kitchen...
from the original Walgreens recipe!**

Robin Hood & Briargate Restaurants, 1970's ~ 1980's

4 8-ounce brook trout, boned
½ cup unsalted butter, melted
1 teaspoon salt
¼ teaspoon black pepper, freshly ground
¼ teaspoon paprika
2 tablespoons lemon juice

Amandine sauce:
4 tablespoons butter
½ to ¾ cup almonds, thinly sliced

Preheat oven to 450 degrees. Place foil on baking sheet, leaving an overhang to help in removal of fish. Brush foil with melted butter. Combine butter, salt, pepper, paprika and lemon juice. Arrange fish on baking sheet and brush with basting mixture. Bake in oven for 4 minutes, turn, brush other side with basting mixture; bake for 4 more minutes. Do not over-cook. To prepare amandine, heat butter in saucepan and sauté almonds until delicately golden. Do not over-cook. Remove fish to serving dishes and pour sauce over top. Serve immediately.

Baked Trout with Dill Sour Cream

Serves 4

- 4 8-ounce salmon or brown trout
- 3 tablespoons, plus 2 teaspoons butter at room temperature
- 1¼ teaspoons lemon pepper
- ½ teaspoon garlic powder
- 1 lemon, thinly sliced
- 4 green onions
- 4 fresh dill sprigs
- 1 tablespoon lemon juice

Dill sour cream sauce:

- 1 cup sour cream
- 2 tablespoons fresh dill, minced
- 1 teaspoon lemon juice

salt and pepper, to taste

Preheat oven to 350 degrees. Grease 8x12-inch baking dish with 1 tablespoon butter. Sprinkle with ¼-teaspoon lemon pepper. Rub cavity of each fish with 2 teaspoons butter. Sprinkle each cavity with ¼-teaspoon lemon pepper and ⅛-teaspoon garlic powder. Divide lemon slices among fish cavities. Place 1 green onion and 1 dill sprig in each cavity. Arrange trout in prepared dish. Sprinkle with 1 tablespoon lemon juice. Cover and bake until fish is no longer pink in center, about 15 minutes. Meanwhile, combine sour cream, minced dill and 1 teaspoon lemon juice. Season with salt and pepper. Remove lemon, green onion and dill sprig from fish and discard. Serve immediately with sour cream sauce.

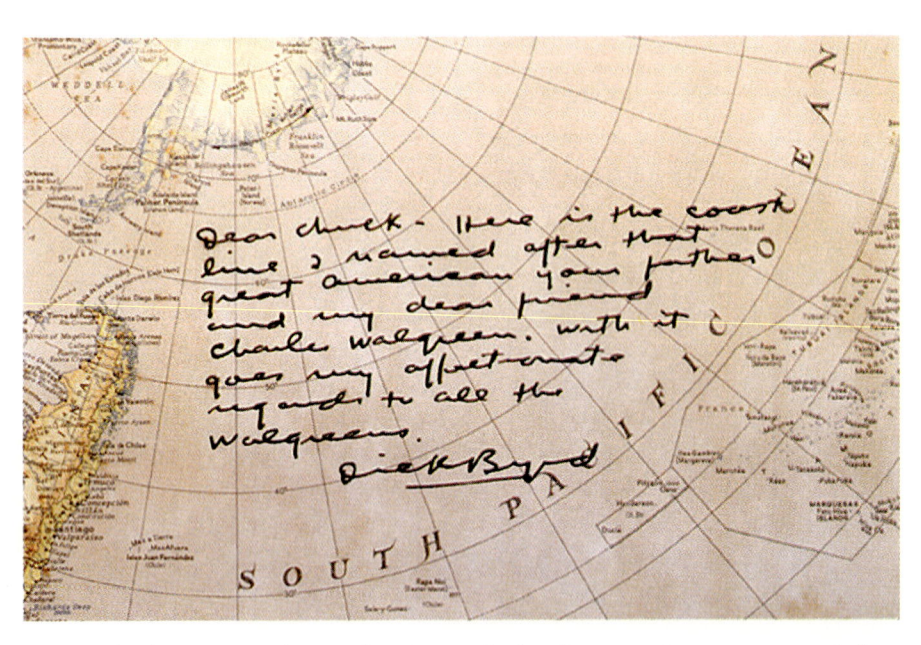

"Dear Chuck ~ Here is the coastline I named after that great American, your father, and my dear friend, Charles Walgreen. With it goes my affectionate regards to all the Walgreens." Dick Byrd

Upon returning from one of his exploratory trips to Antarctica, Admiral Richard E. Byrd presented Charles R. Walgreen, Jr. with a map of the continent. Byrd had named a 1,000-mile section of coastline *Walgreen Coast*, after Charles R. Walgreen, Sr., who was a close friend of his. Walgreen, Sr., donated supplies to Byrd for the expedition, including specially-made malt tablets, which could be easily stored on board the ship! The name can be found on atlases today.

Fresh, North Atlantic Lobster

Yield: 1 lobster per person

The authentic way to cook a fresh-from-the-sea lobster is in fresh, boiling seawater, over a bonfire, on a sandy beach!

live Maine or Nova Scotia lobsters ~ 1 per person
water
salt, 1 teaspoon per quart of water

butter, melted
lemon, cut into wedges

How to cook lobster:

Test lobster: straighten tail, if it springs back into curled position, lobster is okay (alive). (Watch out for those big claws!) Prepare a large stockpot of boiling, salted water. Plunge lobster headfirst into the boiling water. (Lobsters are always cooked alive!) Cover pot and return to a rolling boil. Begin timing: cook lobster 10 to 15 minutes for the first pound, and 3 to 5 minutes for each, additional pound. Lobster is cooked when bright red *and* legs pull easily away from the body.

How to serve lobster:

Flip lobster on its back and open by slitting shell (down center of lobster's front) from head to tail with a sharp knife or scissors. Remove dark green intestinal vein and organs, and discard. Crack claws with a nut cracker. Serve right-side-up on platter with lemon wedges, and melted butter in a dish, for dipping.

Nova Scotia~Style Lobster

Serves 4, 1 cup each

2 cups fresh lobster*, cooked and shelled
2 tablespoons butter
1 cup light or whipping cream
1 teaspoon cider vinegar
salt and pepper, to taste
paprika (optional)

your favorite side dish, or pastry shells

Cut, chop or shred freshly-cooked lobster into pieces. (Or, use frozen lobster meat.) Melt butter in large skillet. Add lobster meat and sauté for about 3 to 5 minutes (lobster will turn red). Stir in cream, vinegar, salt and pepper. Heat thoroughly over medium-low heat (being careful not to over-cook), about 3 to 5 more minutes. Garnish lightly with paprika, and serve with a favorite side dish (like rice, potatoes or pasta), or in puff pastry shells.

Note: *See above recipe for cooking lobster.

Cajun Crawfish Étouffée

Serves 4

12 to 16 ounces crawfish (crayfish) tails, fresh or frozen (may be ordered at specialty grocers)
- ¼ cup margarine
- 2 tablespoons salad oil
- 1 heaping tablespoon flour
- 1 tablespoon cornstarch
- 1 cup celery, chopped
- 1 cup onion, chopped
- 1 garlic clove, minced
- ⅛ teaspoon red cayenne pepper
- 1 teaspoon salt
- 1 cup water, boiling
- 2 tablespoons tomato paste (optional)
- 2 tablespoons fresh parsley, chopped
- 2 cups rice cooked per package directions

Melt margarine in a large skillet. Blend in oil. Stir in flour and cornstarch. When flour mixture starts to brown, add celery, onion, garlic, cayenne pepper and salt. Simmer until vegetables become transparent, about 3 to 5 minutes. Add crawfish and stir for 5 minutes. Then add hot water to make a thin gravy. Add tomato paste, if desired. Allow to simmer for 15 to 20 minutes until gravy thickens. Stir in parsley when ready to serve. Serve over rice.

Indian~Broiled Shrimp

Serves 6

- 3 pounds shrimp, cleaned and deveined

Indian marinade:
- 1½ cups oil
- 5 garlic cloves, crushed
- 2 tablespoons mint, chopped
- 2½ teaspoons chili powder
- 1 tablespoon turmeric, ground
- 1 tablespoon basil
- 2 tablespoons vinegar
- 1 teaspoon salt

pepper, freshly ground

To make marinade, combine ingredients. Add shrimp and refrigerate for at least 6 hours. Pour shrimp and marinade into shallow pan and broil under high heat for 6 to 10 minutes, turning once. Serve with the marinade.

Shrimp Tempura

Serves 4

Adapted for your kitchen... from the original Walgreens recipe!

Robin Hood & Briargate Restaurants, 1970's ~ 1980's

Tempura batter:
- 3 egg yolks (or 2 eggs)
- 1 cup ice water
- 1 cup flour
- ½ teaspoon salt
- 1 pinch paprika
- ½ teaspoon baking powder

Tempura sauce:
- ½ cup soy sauce
- ¼ teaspoon horseradish
- ¼ cup saki (sweet rice wine)
- 1 tablespoon sugar
- ¼ cup water
- ¼ cup clam juice

- 10 to 15 shrimp, boiled, peeled and deveined
- 2 cups rice, cooked per package directions

To prepare batter, blend egg yolks and ice water with wire whip. Mix flour, salt, and paprika into egg and water mixture. When mixture is smooth, blend in baking powder. Mixture should have consistency of whipping cream. Refrigerate for about 15 minutes.

To prepare sauce, combine all dipping sauce ingredients, blending well; refrigerate for about 15 minutes. To deep fry, pour oil 1½ inches deep in skillet or electric frying pan. Heat to 350 degrees.

To prepare shrimp, remove batter from refrigerator. Dip each shrimp into batter and gently slip into hot oil. Fry until golden brown. Drain fried shrimp on paper towel. Serve with bowls of dipping sauce and hot rice.

Shrimp Curry

Serves 6

4 pounds shrimp, cleaned and deveined
1 quart water
1 tablespoon salt
1 medium onion, sliced
1 lemon, sliced
6 whole peppercorns

Curry sauce:

3 tablespoons butter or margarine
1 cup onion, chopped
1 cup apple, pared and chopped
1 garlic clove, crushed
2 or 3 teaspoons curry powder
¼ cup all-purpose flour, unsifted
1 teaspoon salt
¼ teaspoon ginger
¼ teaspoon cardamom
¼ teaspoon pepper
2 10½-ounce cans condensed chicken broth
½ cup chutney
2 tablespoons lime juice
2 teaspoons lime peel, grated

2 cups rice cooked per package directions

Accompaniments:
chutney, chopped
pickled watermelon rind
green peppers, chopped
onion, chopped
avocado, diced
bacon, sliced
peanuts, chopped
raisins
pineapple chunks

Shrimp Curry, *continued on next page.*

Shrimp Curry, continued.

Prepare accompaniments and place in small serving dishes. To make curry sauce, melt butter and sauté onion, apple, garlic and curry powder in a large skillet for about 5 minutes, or until onion is tender. Remove from heat; blend in flour, 1 teaspoon salt, ginger, cardamom and pepper. Gradually, stir in chicken broth, chutney, lime juice and grated lime peel. Bring to boiling, stirring constantly. Reduce heat and simmer, uncovered, for 20 minutes. Meanwhile, rinse shrimp under cold, running water. In saucepan, combine water; 1 tablespoon salt; onion; lemon; and peppercorns. Bring to a boil, and add shrimp. Return to a boil, reduce heat and simmer shrimp 5 minutes. Drain, discarding liquid. Add shrimp to curry sauce and heat gently. Serve shrimp curry over rice with accompaniments.

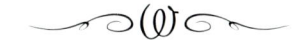

Shrimp de Jonghe

Serves 6 to 8

3 pounds shrimp, shelled and deveined
2 tablespoons boiled butter, for sauté
2¼ cups dry white wine, hot
1½ cups bread crumbs, toasted
¾ cup parsley, minced
1½ garlic cloves, minced
1¼ teaspoon salt
¼ teaspoon pepper
4 tablespoons butter, softened
6 tablespoons Parmesan cheese
2 tablespoons butter, melted

Preheat oven to 350 degrees. Sauté shrimp in 2 tablespoons of butter, over medium heat, for 2 minutes. Place in shallow 2-quart casserole. Pour hot wine over bread crumbs and mix well with fork. Let stand while absorbed. If too thick, add more wine. Add parsley, garlic, salt, pepper and 4 tablespoons softened butter. Mix thoroughly, and spread over shrimp. Sprinkle with Parmesan cheese. Drizzle 2 tablespoons melted butter on top. Bake at 350 degrees for 30 minutes. Turn oven heat to broil. Place shrimp under broiler to brown. Allow only a few minutes and watch carefully to prevent shrimp from burning.

Barbecued Shrimp

Serves 4

2 pounds fresh, unshelled jumbo shrimp

Sherry marinade:
1 cup olive or vegetable oil
1 cup dry sherry
1 cup soy sauce
2 garlic clove, minced

Butter sauce:
½ pound butter
½ teaspoon salt
1 tablespoon Worcestershire sauce
1 tablespoon soy sauce
3 to 4 dashes Tabasco sauce
juice of 1 lemon

To prepare shrimp, combine marinade ingredients and pour over shrimp. Refrigerate for 3 to 4 hours. Shell and devein shrimp. Grill shrimp over hot charcoal fire for 2 to 3 minutes per side; be careful not to over-cook. To prepare sauce, melt butter in small saucepan; add remaining ingredients for sauce and keep warm. Serve hot, cooked shrimp with butter sauce.

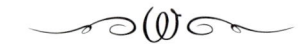

Shrimp Creole Allen

Serves 4

1 pound shrimp, cooked and cleaned
¼ cup butter
1 medium onion, chopped
1 garlic clove, minced
½ green pepper, diced
1 teaspoon salt
¼ teaspoon pepper
⅛ teaspoon rosemary, crushed
¼ teaspoon paprika
2 cups canned tomatoes
2 cups rice, cooked per package directions

Melt butter in skillet. Add onions, garlic, green pepper, salt, pepper, rosemary, paprika and tomatoes. Simmer 15 minutes. Add shrimp; heat only until shrimp are warm. Serve on hot rice.

Shrimp Kebabs with Curry Butter

Serves 4

- 6 tablespoons butter
- 4 tablespoons onion, minced
- 1 tablespoon curry powder
- 1 tablespoon chopped chutney
- 4 slices bacon
- 1½ pounds medium-size shrimp, peeled and deveined
- 4 wooden cooking skewers
- 1 cup rice, cooked per package directions

To make sauce, melt butter in small skillet or saucepan. Sauté onion until softened. Add curry powder, stir and cook a few minutes. Then, stir in chutney. Set aside until ready to use. To cook shrimp, start with bacon; if bacon is thick or extra-fatty, fry until about half-cooked. Cut slices into 6 to 8 pieces. Alternate with shrimp on 4 skewers. Grill 8 to 10 minutes, turning occasionally. Or place skewers on oiled broiler pan in center of 450-degree oven and cook until done, approximately 10 minutes. Reheat sauce. Spoon serving of rice onto serving plate, top with shrimp kebabs, and cover rice and shrimp with reheated sauce.

Gulf Coast Shrimp Casserole

Serves 4 to 6

- 1 pound fresh or frozen shrimp, deveined
- ¼ cup ripe olives, quartered
- 1 cup rice, uncooked
- 1 can condensed consommé *
- 1 cup water
- 2 teaspoons instant minced onion
- 1 tablespoon lemon juice
- ½ teaspoon Worcestershire sauce
- ¼ teaspoon salt
- ⅛ teaspoon garlic powder
- 1½ cups American cheese, diced into cubes
- 1 10-ounce package frozen peas, thawed

Preheat oven to 350 degrees. Combine shrimp, olives, rice and consommé in a 1½-quart casserole dish. Combine water, onion, lemon juice, Worcestershire sauce, salt and garlic powder, and stir into the casserole. Add ½-cup cheese cubes. Cover and bake at 350 degrees for 1 hour. Uncover and stir in remaining cheese and uncooked peas. Bake uncovered 10 minutes.

Crab Cakes in Tangy Mustard Sauce

Serves 2

- 8 ounces frozen or canned crab meat, cleaned and flaked
- 2 tablespoons parsley, chopped
- ½ cup cooked corn (optional)
- ½ to 1 teaspoon Dijon mustard
- 1 egg
- 2 tablespoons flour
- ¼ cup cracker crumbs, plus additional to coat cakes
- vegetable or olive oil and margarine, for frying

Mustard Sauce:
- ½ cup mayonnaise
- ½ tablespoon water
- 1 teaspoon Dijon mustard
- 1 teaspoon Coleman's dry mustard
- 1 teaspoon dry white wine
- 1 teaspoon fresh lemon juice
- 2 drops Tabasco sauce
- 2 teaspoons Worcestershire sauce
- salt and pepper, to taste

To prepare mustard sauce, mix all ingredients together; refrigerate. Prepare crab mixture; mix all ingredients, except oil and margarine, together. Form mixture into crab cakes; roll cakes in extra cracker crumbs. Heat oil and margarine in large skillet. Fry cakes, turning once, until browned. Serve hot crab cakes with mustard sauce.

Crab Custard Casserole

Serves 4

- 4 slices bread
- 2 tablespoons butter
- 1 6-ounce (4½-ounce drained) can crab meat, cleaned and flaked
- 1½ cup sharp cheddar cheese, grated
- 1 teaspoon mustard
- 3 eggs, beaten
- ½ teaspoon salt
- 1½ cup milk

Crab Custard Casserole, continued on next page.

Crab Custard Casserole, continued.

Preheat oven to 350 degrees. Butter bread on both sides and cut into cubes. Put buttered bread cubes, flaked crab meat, and grated cheddar cheese into well-greased casserole dish. Mix mustard, eggs, salt and milk; pour over crab combination in casserole. Cover and refrigerate all day or overnight. Bake at 350 degrees for 45 minutes. Serve immediately.

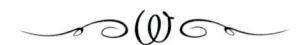

Kerstner's Fresh Crab Cakes

Serves 4

- 1 pound fresh, lump crab meat, cleaned and flaked
- ½ cup (lightly-packed) *fresh* bread crumbs
- 2 tablespoons fresh, flat-leaf parsley, chopped
- 2 tablespoons heavy cream
- 1 tablespoon fresh lemon juice
- 2 teaspoons fresh chives, snipped
- 1 teaspoon Dijon mustard
- ½ teaspoon lemon zest, grated
- ⅛ teaspoon cayenne pepper
- 1 large egg
- 1 large egg yolk

pepper, freshly ground, to taste

- ⅓ cup *dry* bread crumbs
- 2 tablespoons unsalted butter
- ¼ cup olive oil

Tartar Sauce, heated (see recipe in the *RxCetera ~ Sauces & Garnishes* chapter)

Place all ingredients, except last four (*dry* bread crumbs, butter, olive oil and tartar sauce), in mixing bowl and stir to combine. Shape into 2½-inch crab cakes, gently squeezing out excess liquid. Spread dry bread crumbs in shallow bowl and coat both sides of each cake with bread crumbs, gently shaking off excess. Heat half the butter and olive oil in large skillet, over medium heat. Add half the crab cakes and cook, turning once, until golden brown, about 4 to 6 minutes. Keep warm in oven. Repeat with remaining butter, olive oil and cakes. Serve crab cakes with hot *Tartar Sauce.*

Stuffed, Deviled Crab

Serves 6

Adapted for your kitchen... from the original Walgreens recipe!

Walgreens Cafeterias, 1940's ~ 1960's

1 pound fresh, lump or back-fin crab meat, cleaned and flaked
½ teaspoon salt
1 teaspoon paprika
½ teaspoon powdered mustard
juice of ½ lemon
¼ teaspoon Tabasco
⅛ teaspoon white pepper
1 tablespoon Worcestershire sauce
1 medium onion, finely chopped
½ green pepper, finely chopped

White sauce:
4 tablespoons butter or margarine
4 tablespoons flour
1¼ to 1½ cups milk

1 cup bread crumbs
butter

Preheat oven to 350 degrees. Combine all ingredients (except for the sauce ingredients, bread crumbs and butter). To prepare sauce, melt butter in a small saucepan over moderate heat; slowly blend in flour. Add milk and heat through, stirring until thickened. Mix sauce into crab meat mixture. Pour into a greased, 1½-quart casserole or individual ramekins. Top with bread crumbs and dot with butter. Bake at 350 degrees, uncovered, for 1 hour, until browned and bubbly. May serve in individual ramekins, crab shells or ceramic shell dishes.

Oven~Fried Scallops

Serves 2 to 3

1 pound raw scallops
1 egg
2 tablespoons water
½ teaspoon thyme
½ teaspoon dill weed
salt and pepper, to taste
1 cup cracker crumbs
2 tablespoons butter, melted

Oven-Fried Scallops, *continued on next page.*

Oven-Fried Scallops, continued.

Preheat oven to 450 degrees. Rinse scallops and dry on paper towel. Break egg into a mixing bowl and beat until foamy. Add water, thyme, dill weed, salt and pepper. Mix thoroughly. Dip scallops into egg mixture and then into cracker crumbs. Arrange in a shallow baking dish. Pour melted butter over scallops. Bake in pre-heated oven at 450 degrees for 20 minutes.

Scallops in Parchment

Serves 2 to 3

1 pound bay scallops
parchment paper
3 small, new red potatoes, sliced ¼-inch thick
1 cup asparagus, julienne, 2x¼-inch strips
½ large, red pepper, seeded, julienne
½ large, yellow pepper, seeded, julienne
2 scallions (green onions), thinly sliced
2 teaspoons fresh ginger, minced
1 teaspoon lemon zest, grated
¼ cup fresh lemon juice
1 tablespoon vegetable oil
2 teaspoons balsamic vinegar
¼ teaspoon pepper, freshly ground
salt

Preheat oven to 350 degrees. Cut parchment paper (or aluminum foil) into two 24x16-inch pieces. Fold each piece in half lengthwise, so each measures 16x12-inches. On fold of each piece, cut out half a heart (to form whole heart when unfolded).

In small saucepan, cover potatoes with cold water, add salt and heat to boiling. Cook over medium heat for 3 minutes. Drain thoroughly. Open hearts, and place potatoes in center of each, next to fold. Combine remaining ingredients in mixing bowl and spoon over potatoes. Fold paper or foil over and double-fold edges to seal tightly. Place packets on baking sheets and bake for 30 minutes. Transfer packets to plates and open.

Herb~Basted Bay Scallops

Serves 4

2 pounds bay scallops

Herb sauce:
4 tablespoons salad oil
4 tablespoons lemon juice
½ tablespoon paprika
½ tablespoon marjoram, basil or thyme leaves

Combine sauce ingredients in a small bowl. Place scallops on broiling pan. Using a basting brush, apply sauce to scallops during broiling. Broil 5 to 6 minutes, or until done.

Conch Fritters

Serves 6

2 eggs, beaten
1⅓ cups flour
¾ teaspoon salt
¼ teaspoon pepper
1 tablespoon butter, melted
2 teaspoons baking powder
½ teaspoon lime juice
¾ cup flat beer
2 teaspoons onion, minced
2 tablespoons parsley, minced
1 dash tabasco sauce
1 cup ground conch (about ½ pound)
hot pepper sauce
lime wedges

Mix beaten eggs, flour, salt, pepper, butter, baking powder, lime juice and beer together. Fold in onion, parsley, tabasco sauce, and conch. Pour oil 1½ inches deep in a frying pan or electric skillet. Heat to 375 degrees. Take 1 tablespoon of conch mixture and drop into deep fat. Fry until golden brown. Serve with hot pepper sauce and fresh lime wedges.

Scalloped Oysters

Serves 4 to 6

8 tablespoons butter
1 to 1½ cups cracker crumbs
1½ pints oysters, with ½-cup liquid reserved
salt and pepper, freshly ground, to taste
Tabasco sauce
½ cup heavy cream
½ cup bread crumbs, finely crushed

Preheat oven to 400 degrees. Melt 4 tablespoons butter in saucepan. Brush baking dish with some of the melted butter; reserve rest for bread crumbs. Cover bottom of baking dish with a layer of cracker crumbs. Put half of the oysters on the crumbs, then another layer of cracker crumbs. Break remaining 4 tablespoons butter into small pieces and dot the oyster-crumb layers with half the pieces. Sprinkle lightly with salt, pepper, and Tabasco. Layer again with oysters and cracker crumbs and dot with remaining butter. Sprinkle again with salt, pepper, and Tabasco. Pour liquid from oysters and heavy cream over top. Lightly sauté bread crumbs in remaining melted butter until golden, tossing well. Sprinkle over top of oyster mixture. Bake at 400 degrees for 25 minutes. Serve immediately.

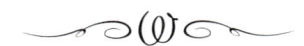

Mussels Marinere

Serves 4

½ cup yellow onion, minced
½ cup butter
3 dozen mussels in the shell, scrubbed and bearded
4 sprigs parsley
2 sprigs fresh thyme or ½-teaspoon dried thyme
1 bay leaf
2 cups dry white wine
2 tablespoons parsley, minced
salt, to taste

Sauté onion in butter 5 to 8 minutes in large, heavy kettle over moderate heat until golden. Add mussels, herbs, and wine; cover, bring to boil and simmer 3 minutes until mussels open. Discard any unopened or empty mussels. Transfer mussels to heated soup tureen. Strain cooking liquid through cheesecloth into saucepan; add remaining butter and minced parsley. Heat, stirring until butter melts. Salt to taste. Pour over mussels. Serve immediately with hot French bread.

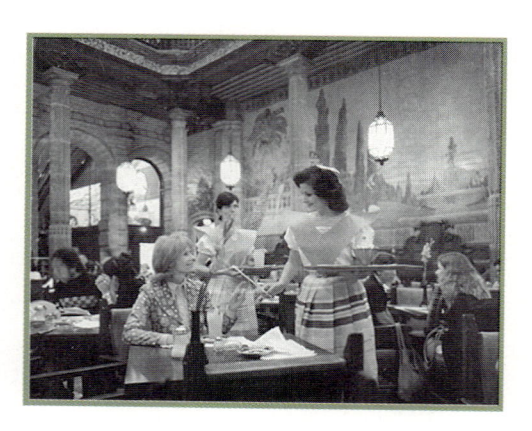

When Sanborns was purchased in 1946, Walgreens restored its historic House of Tiles (circa 1596), creating a beautiful and popular restaurant.

Facing Page: *Kathy's South-of-the-Border Pork Tenderloin*
Photo: Scott Lanza, 1995
Stylist: F. Lynn Nelson

MEAT & MORE

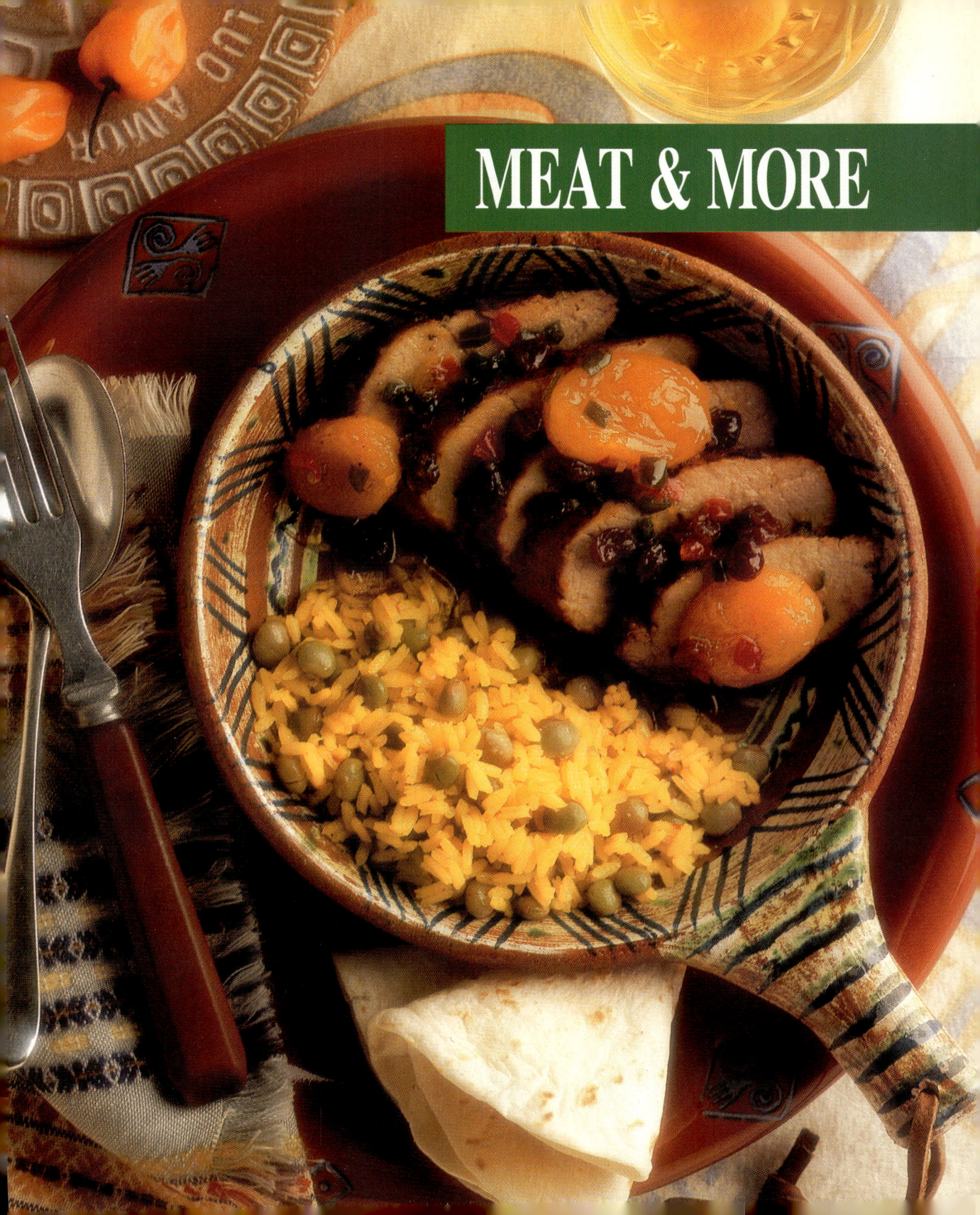

Sanborns House of Tiles
To Dine with the Spanish Conquistadors

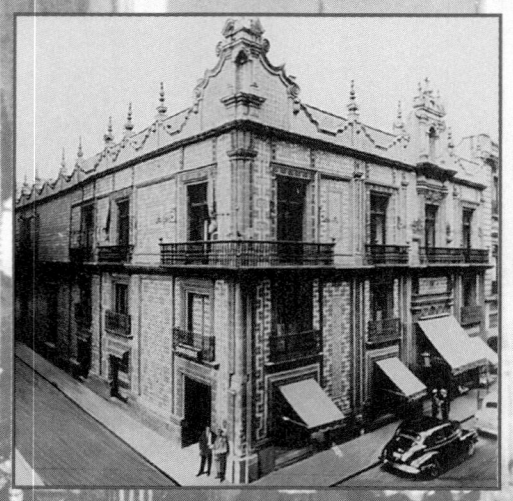

"Our Sanborns stores sold more silverware than Marshall Fields!"
Charles R. Walgreen, Jr., 1995

Imagine for a moment...sitting in 16th-century Mexico, encompassed by a mosaic of hundreds of hand-glazed blue tiles ~ a veritable palace, with gleaming bronze handrails, banisters and balconies. You drink from a crystal glass as you savor your freshly-cut steak, and then try a pastry, right out of the oven. Your meal is so delectably *fresh*, it could be fit for kings...but this is the *20th* century!

Such a vision was reality at the historic and famous *House of Tiles* (circa 1596) which, in 1903, housed a small drugstore and soda fountain. The drugstore became *Sanborns* (named for its founding brothers), a well-known silver shop and restaurant. Walgreens acquired Sanborns House of Tiles in 1946, and created within it, an immaculate and immensely-popular restaurant ~ and one of only a handful of Mexican diners to use fresh ingredients in its recipes! From this historic landmark, Walgreens went on to build Sanborns into Mexico's largest and finest chain of retail stores and restaurants.

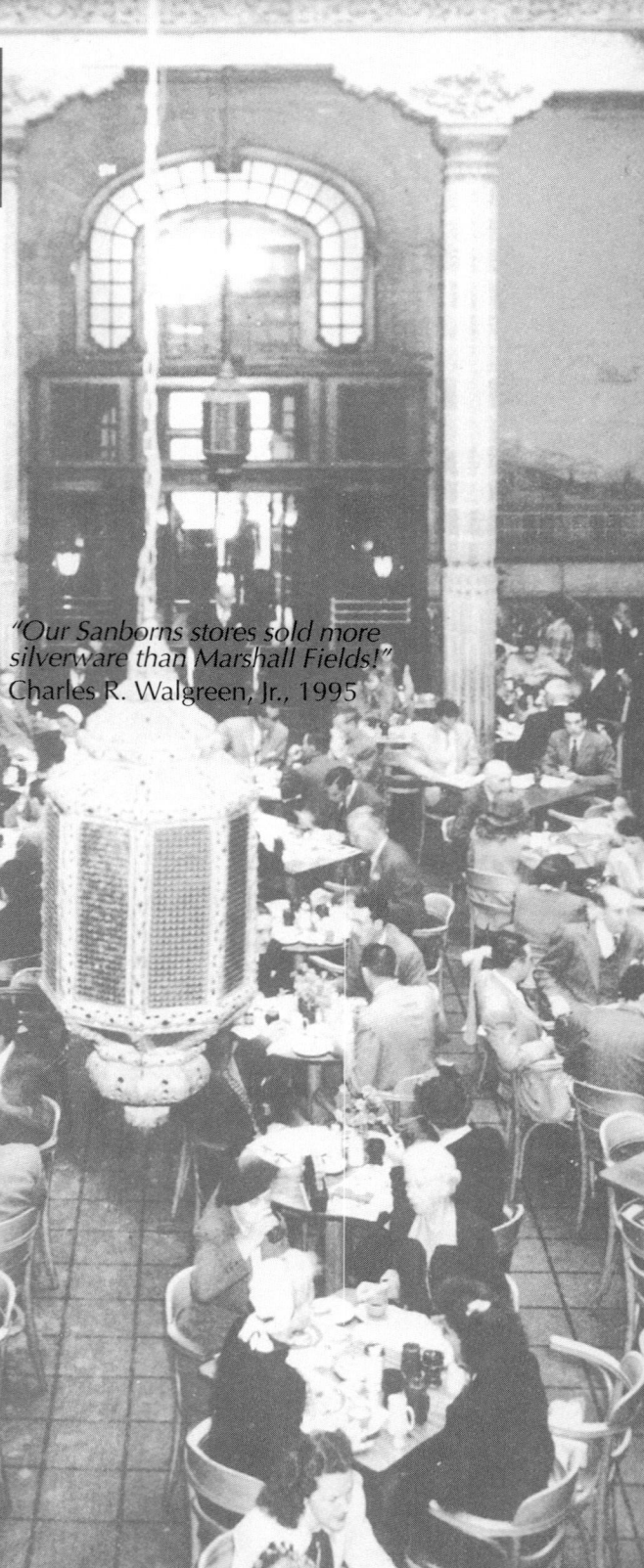

The Famous Patty Melt

Serves 1

The original recipe…invented at Walgreens!

Walgreens Cafeterias, 1960's; a mainstay at Wag's, 1970's ~ 1980's!

1   6-ounce hamburger patty
2   slices rye bread, spread on one side with butter
2   slices American cheese
1   tablespoon onion, finely chopped
2   pickle chips

Begin cooking hamburger patty on griddle or in frying pan. When patty is half-cooked, place bread on grill, buttered side down. Top each slice of bread with cheese, place onions on one side and place cooked patty on top of cheese. Close sandwich; cut in half diagonally. Serve with pickle chips.

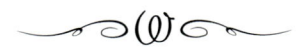

Roasted Short Ribs with Vegetables

Serves 4

3 to 4 pounds short ribs, cut into 3-inch pieces
2   tablespoons vegetable oil
4   medium potatoes, quartered
4   medium carrots, quartered
1   medium onion, sliced
1   tablespoon cider vinegar
1   tablespoon horseradish
1   tablespoon prepared mustard
1   tablespoon pepper
2   tablespoons sugar
2   tablespoons catsup
1   10½-ounce can Campbell's beef broth

Gravy (optional):
1   cup beef bouillon
2   cups cold water
¼   cup flour
salt and pepper, to taste

Preheat oven to 300 degrees. Brown short ribs in oil and pour off fat. Discard fat. Place ribs in roasting pan and arrange potatoes, onion and carrots around meat. Combine all other ingredients and pour on top of ribs. Simmer 6 to 8 hours in oven. Remove meat and set aside on warm serving platter. To make gravy, pour remaining fat from roasting pan into saucepan. Add 1 cup cold water; bring to boil while whisking and continually scraping sides. Slowly whisk in flour, 1 cup water, salt and pepper into pan drippings. Ladle a small amount of gravy on short ribs; serve with remaining gravy and vegetables.

Beef Roulades

Serves 6

- 6 slices raw bacon, diced
- ¾ cup onion, finely chopped
- 6 slices white bread, toasted and cubed
- 3 tablespoons fresh parsley, chopped
- ¼ teaspoon basil leaves, chopped
- ¼ teaspoon thyme leaves, chopped
- ¼ teaspoon marjoram leaves, chopped
- ¼ cup butter, melted
- ½ teaspoon salt
- 1¾ pounds round steak, cut in half-inch slices
- salt and pepper, to taste
- 6 to 12 toothpicks
- 1 10½-ounce can Campbell's beef broth
- ¾ cup water
- 1 15-ounce can herb tomato sauce
- 2 tablespoons butter
- ¾ pound mushrooms, thinly sliced

Sauté bacon and onion, until bacon is crisp and onion is tender. Toss bread, parsley, basil, thyme, marjoram and ½-teaspoon salt in a bowl. Stir in bacon mixture and ¼-cup melted butter. Reserve for meat stuffing. Pound meat until 1/16-inch thick, season on both sides with salt and pepper. Spread each piece of meat with a little stuffing mixture, roll meat and secure with toothpick. Place meat rolls in large skillet and add beef broth, water and herb tomato sauce. Cook slowly for 1 hour turning occasionally. When done, remove roulades to serving platter. Heat 2 tablespoons butter in second skillet, add mushrooms and cook until tender. Stir into the sauce and pour over the meat rolls.

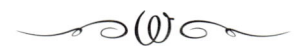

Beef Bourguignon

Serves 8 to 10

- 3 pounds sirloin tip, cubed
- ¾ cups Burgundy wine
- 2 cans golden mushroom soup
- ½ package Lipton onion soup mix
- ½ pound fresh or canned mushrooms, drained
- 1 1-pound package noodles, cooked per package directions

Preheat oven to 325 or 350 degrees. Mix all ingredients and pour into 4-quart casserole. Cover, and bake at 350 degrees for 3 hours, or 325 degrees for 4 hours. Serve over noodles.

Mexican Roast Beef a la Sanborns

Serves 6

Adapted for your kitchen... from the original Walgreens recipe!

Sanborns, Mexico, 1946 ~ 1984

Originally called: Carne Asada a la Sanborns

3	pounds beef fillet, trimmed
4	tablespoons olive oil
1	teaspoon salt
½	teaspoon pepper
1	cup refried beans (black or red)
2	tablespoons cotija cheese* or Parmesan cheese, grated
12	pieces totopos* (deep-fried tortillas) or tostados
6	tortillas, flour or corn
¾	11-ounce jar Señor Baca Ranchera Sauce*
½	pound chihuahua cheese*, grated
6	lettuce leaves
1	cup prepared guacamole
½	cup sour cream
1	4-ounce can poblano (green) chilies*, sliced
6	sprigs Chinese parsley (fresh cilantro)

Preheat oven to 400 degrees. To prepare meat, rub fillet with olive oil and pepper. Place on oiled rack in a roasting pan and bake for 30 minutes, or until meat thermometer registers 125 degrees. Salt roast when done and let stand 10 minutes. To serve, portion all ingredients among 6 plates. On each serving dish, spoon refried beans with the cotija or Parmesan cheese grated on top and 2 topopos or tostados on each side of the beans. Prepare tortillas by pouring ranchero sauce generously over tortilla and sprinkle chihuahua cheese over sauce. Broil or bake at 450 degrees, until cheese melts. Put 1 tortilla on each serving plate. Add 1 lettuce leaf to the plate, topped with guacamole and sour cream mixed with sliced poblano chilies. Slice beef fillet and place lengthwise on the plate surrounded by all the above condiments. Garnish each plate with a sprig of Chinese parsley.

Note: *Available in the ethnic or specialty sections of grocery stores.

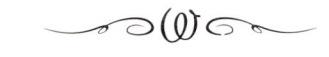

Roast Beef Louise

Serves 6

2	10⅛-ounce cans cream of mushroom soup, undiluted
1	envelope Lipton dry onion soup mix
1	cup red wine
1	3-pound chuck roast

Preheat oven to 325 degrees. Place beef in roasting pan. Mix together mushroom soup, onion soup mix and red wine in a small bowl. Pour over roast. Bake, covered, for 3 hours.

Roast Beef au Jus

Serves 8 to 10

¼ cup flour, lightly browned
1 tablespoon dry mustard
pepper, freshly ground, to taste
1 5 to 8-pound rib roast of beef
6 tablespoons beef drippings or butter
1 piece beef suet or fat, flattened
6 tablespoons red wine or water, warmed
salt and pepper, to taste

au jus:
roast beef juice and meat bits, fat removed
¼ to ½-cup red wine
2 to 4 tablespoons butter
1 to 2 teaspoons Worcestershire sauce

Lightly brown flour in 250-degree oven or frying pan. Preheat oven to 425 degrees. Mix dry mustard, pepper and lightly-browned flour. Spread beef with drippings or butter, and sprinkle with flour mixture. Tie flattened piece of suet or fat on top of roast. Place meat on rack in roasting pan. Brown in oven for 15 minutes. Reduce heat to 325 degrees. Add warmed red wine or water. Continue to roast, basting frequently. Allow 15 to 18 minutes per pound for rare, 20 to 24 minutes for medium and 25 to 30 minutes for well done meat. When done, season with salt and pepper. Move to serving platter. Let stand 15 to 20 minutes by oven door before carving.

Prepare au jus. Pour off fat from roasting pan. Use a suction tool to draw up pink juices from roast as it sets. Pour juices into saucepan. Scrape up all crusty bits of meat from pan and stir into the juices to make a clear sauce. Add red wine, butter and Worcestershire sauce. Bring to a boil and simmer 1 to 2 minutes. Strain. Serve in a sauceboat with the roast.

French Dip Beef au Jus

Serves 10

1 5 to 6-pound rump roast
red wine and water
1 tablespoon peppercorns, cracked
1 tablespoon rosemary
1 tablespoon summer savory
1 tablespoon oregano

French Dip Beef au Jus, continued on next page.

French Dip Beef au Jus, *continued.*

2 bay leaves
1 cube beef bouillon
1 teaspoon garlic powder
1 tablespoon thyme
10 French rolls or rye buns
gourmet mustard and horseradish sauce (optional)

Place roast in large pot, adding enough water and wine to just cover meat. Add seasonings. Cover and cook on top of stove on high until boiling. Reduce heat and simmer 8 to 10 hours. If necessary, add more water. Remove beef from pan and shred; reserve cooking water (au jus). To serve, place shredded meat on rolls with au jus on the side in individual crocks. May also serve with gourmet mustard and horseradish sauce.

Tenderloin Deluxe

Serves 8

1 3-pound whole tenderloin, trimmed of fat
2 tablespoons butter, softened
¼ cup scallions (green onions), chopped
2 tablespoons butter
2 tablespoons soy sauce
1 teaspoon Dijon wine mustard
1 dash ground pepper
¾ cup sherry
parsley

Béarnaise Sauce (see recipe in the *RxCetera ~ Sauces & Garnishes* chapter)
Mushrooms in Wine Sauce (see recipe in the *Vegetables* chapter)

The tenderloin should sit at room temperature for 2 to 3 hours before roasting. Preheat oven to 400 degrees. Spread tenderloin with the softened butter. Place on a rack in a shallow roasting pan and bake, uncovered, for 20 minutes. Meanwhile, sauté the scallions in the remaining butter until tender. Add the soy sauce, mustard and pepper. Stir in the sherry and heat until just boiling. When the meat has baked 20 minutes, pour the sauce over it and bake another 20 to 25 minutes, to serve medium-rare. Baste frequently. Remove from oven and let sit for 10 minutes. Carve into 1-inch slices. Overlap slices on a warm platter; garnish with parsley. Serve with *Béarnaise Sauce* and *Mushrooms in Wine Sauce* in separate, individual crocks or serving bowls.

Beef Stroganoff

Serves 6

- 2 pounds sirloin, trimmed and sliced into strips
- 4 tablespoons butter
- 1 cup onion, chopped
- 1 garlic clove, minced
- ½ pound fresh mushrooms, sliced
- 3 tablespoons flour
- 1 tablespoon catsup
- ½ teaspoon salt
- ⅛ teaspoon pepper
- 1 10½-ounce can Campbell's beef broth
- ¼ cup dry white wine
- ¼ teaspoon dill weed
- ½ to ¾-cup sour cream
- 1 1-pound package noodles, cooked per package directions

Trim meat and slice into thin strips. Melt 1 tablespoon butter in skillet. Sear meat and remove as browned. Add 3 tablespoons butter in same skillet and sauté onion, garlic and mushrooms until soft. Remove from heat and add flour, catsup, salt, pepper and stir until smooth. Gradually add beef broth, bring to a boil and simmer 5 minutes. Add wine, dill and meat. Cover and simmer 1 hour. Add sour cream, heat and serve over noodles.

Fruited Pot Roast

Serves 6

- 1 3 to 4-pound round, or blade bone roast
- 1½ teaspoons salt
- ¼ teaspoon pepper
- ¼ cup Burgundy wine
- 1 garlic clove, minced
- ⅓ cup carrots, finely chopped
- ½ cup onion, finely chopped
- 1½ cups hot water
- 1 11-ounce package mixed, dried fruit
- 3 tablespoons all-purpose flour
- ½ cup cold water

Fruited Pot Roast, *continued on next page.*

Fruited Pot Roast, *continued.*

Trim fat from meat. Cook in large skillet until there are about 2 tablespoons of melted fat. Remove trimmings. Brown meat in fat. Add salt, pepper, wine, vegetables and garlic. Cover and cook over low heat for 2 hours. Meanwhile, pour the hot water over the fruit and let stand one hour. Drain fruit, reserving liquid. Place fruit on meat. Cover and cook 45 minutes to one hour more, until meat is tender. Remove meat and fruit to platter. Skim fat from pan juices. Add reserved liquid to juices; makes about 1½ cups. Blend flour and cold water, and whisk into juices. Cook and stir until thickened and boiling. Pour juices over roast.

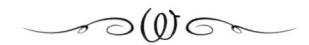

American Pot Roast with Noodles

Serves 6 to 8

Adapted for your kitchen…
from the original Walgreens recipe!

Walgreens Cafeterias 1940's ~ 1960's

1	4 to 5-pound rump, chuck or round roast
2½ to 3	teaspoons salt
½	teaspoon pepper
¼	cup flour
4	tablespoons vegetable oil
1	cup beef broth or water
1	small to medium yellow onion, coarsely chopped
2	carrots, scraped and coarsely chopped
2	celery stalks, coarsely chopped
1	8-ounce package broad noodles, cooked per package directions
1	tablespoon butter

Gravy (optional):
3   cups broth and water combined
6   tablespoons flour
1 to 2 tablespoons butter or margarine
salt and pepper, to taste

Rub meat with salt, pepper; dredge in flour. Heat the oil in a Dutch oven or roasting pan on top of stove. Brown meat in oil on all sides. Sprinkle chopped vegetables over roast; add broth or water. Bring to a simmer and place covered in a preheated 300-degree oven. Continue to cook for about 2 hours, or until tender. Prepare noodles; drain. Mix with butter. To make gravy, strain broth from cooking beef and add enough water to equal 3 cups. Blend broth and water with flour and stir all slowly back into the Dutch oven or roaster. Heat over medium heat, stirring until thickened. Reduce heat and simmer 2 to 3 minutes. Add the butter, salt and pepper. Slice pot roast. Add noodles and top both with gravy.

Brisket of Beef

Serves 6 to 8

Adapted for your kitchen... from the original Walgreens recipe!

Robin Hood & Briargate Restaurants, 1970's ~ 1980's

- 1 5-pound brisket, well-trimmed
- 4 celery stalks
- 1 onion, sliced
- 2 peppercorns
- 2 tablespoons beef bouillon granules
- 2 quarts cold water

Horseradish sauce:
- 1 cup brisket stock
- 1 cup béchamel (white sauce)
  (see recipe in the *RxCetera ~ Sauces & Garnishes* chapter)
- 2 to 3 tablespoons prepared horseradish
- 1 teaspoon sugar
- 1 teaspoon dry mustard
- 1 tablespoon vinegar

Place brisket in a heavy pot; cover with water, celery, onions, peppercorns and beef bouillon. Bring to a boil and reduce heat to simmer meat for 2½ to 3 hours or until meat is tender, occasionally skimming fat off the top of the water. Remove from heat and allow brisket to cool in its liquid. Skim fat from sauce. To prepare sauce, remove 1 cup skimmed brisket stock and heat in saucepan. Heat cream sauce in another saucepan. Combine the two when properly heated. Add horseradish, sugar, mustard and vinegar, and blend. To serve, slice meat across grain. Arrange on serving platter and pour sauce over brisket slices. Sliced brisket may also be heated (and reheated) with the sauce in a 350-degree oven.

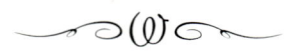

Corned Beef

Serves 6

Adapted for your kitchen... from the original Walgreens recipe!

Robin Hood & Briargate Restaurants, 1970's ~ 1980's

- 1 5-pound brisket
- 1½ quarts water
- 1 cup brown sugar
- ½ teaspoon dry mustard
- 6 cloves

Soak brisket overnight in refrigerator; discard water. Place brisket in Dutch oven or deep skillet; cover with water. Bring to boil and simmer on top of stove for approximately 4 hours, or until tender. Discard water. Preheat oven to 375 degrees. Score fat side of cooked brisket. Mix brown sugar and mustard; rub into brisket. Place in roasting pan and sprinkle cloves on top. Bake for about 30 minutes, or until beef is tender.

Corned Beef Hash

Serves 6 to 8

Adapted for your kitchen... from the original Walgreens recipe!

Robin Hood & Briargate Restaurants, 1970's ~ 1980's

2	medium yellow onions, finely chopped
3	tablespoons butter or margarine
3	cups corned beef scraps, diced (see *Corned Beef* recipe, previous page)
3	cups cold potatoes, cooked and diced
2	teaspoons Worcestershire sauce
1	cup beef broth
⅛	teaspoon pepper
½	teaspoon salt

Preheat oven to 350 degrees. Heat margarine in frying pan and sauté onions until brown. In a shallow baking pan, mix cooked onion, corned beef, potatoes, Worcestershire sauce, beef broth, salt and pepper. Bake for 30 to 45 minutes, or until liquid is absorbed and hash begins to brown. If desired, cook longer, mashing mixture down with spatula; bottom should begin to form a crust.

Braised Beef & Noodles

Serves 6 to 8

Adapted for your kitchen... from the original Walgreens recipe!

Walgreens Cafeterias 1940's ~ 1960's

3	pounds rump or chuck roast, cut into 1 to 1½-inch cubes
2	medium-size yellow onions, peeled and sliced thin
4	tablespoons vegetable oil
½	cup flour
1	14½-ounce can tomatoes, drained
4	cups canned beef broth, heated
2	teaspoons salt
¼	teaspoon pepper
1	teaspoon Kitchen Bouquet
1	8-ounce package broad noodles, cooked per package directions
1 to 2 tablespoons butter	

Heat oil in a Dutch oven or stew pot. Brown beef and onions in hot oil. Remove from heat; add flour and blend in with beef and onions. Add tomatoes and part of hot broth, stirring constantly. Return to heat, bring to boil. Add remaining broth and salt and pepper. Simmer until beef is tender, approximately 2½ hours. Add Kitchen Bouquet and season to taste. Prepare noodles; drain. Mix with butter. Serve braised beef over heated noodles.

Swiss Steaks in Pan Gravy

Serves 6 to 8

Adapted for your kitchen... from the original Walgreens recipe!!

Walgreens Cafeterias 1940's ~ 1960's

1	2-pound round steak, cut into 8 (4-ounce) steaks
½	cup flour
1	teaspoon salt
¼	teaspoon pepper
¼	cup vegetable oil or shortening
1	onion, finely diced
1	14½-ounce can tomatoes
1	16-ounce can brown gravy

Preheat oven to 350 degrees. Mix flour, salt and pepper and pound into steaks on both sides, using back of knife or meat mallet. Heat oil in heavy frying pan and brown steaks on both sides. Place in a baking pan, sprinkle onions on top of steaks, add tomatoes and brown gravy. Bake for about 1½ hours, or until tender.

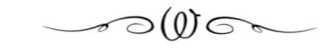

Mrs. B's Swiss Steak

Serves 6 to 8

¼	cup flour
1½	teaspoons salt
¼	teaspoon pepper
1	3-pound round steak, cut 2 inches thick
3	tablespoons vegetable oil
2	cups water
2	celery stalks, coarsely chopped
2	large onions, coarsely chopped
1	bay leaf
¼	teaspoon thyme
1	garlic clove, minced
2	whole cloves
1	15-ounce can tomato sauce
2	teaspoons dry mustard
1½	tablespoons catsup

Mix flour, salt and pepper. Sprinkle 2 tablespoons mixture on one side of steak; pound into steak with meat mallet. Turn and repeat on other side. Brown meat in heavy skillet or Dutch oven in 3 tablespoons oil; sear on both sides. Pour off fat. Add water, celery, onions, bay leaf, thyme, minced garlic and cloves. Simmer over medium-low heat for 1 hour, stirring occasionally. Add tomato sauce, dry mustard and catsup. Cook 1 more hour. To serve, cut meat into serving size pieces; cover with gravy.

Pepper Steak

Serves 4

- 1½ pounds round steak, cut into ¼-inch strips
- ½ cup Kikkoman soy sauce
- 4 garlic cloves, minced
- 3 medium tomatoes, quartered
- 1 medium onion, chopped
- ½ teaspoon black pepper
- 1 green pepper, sliced into ¼-inch strips
- 1 red pepper, sliced into ¼-inch strips
- 1 cup rice, cooked per package directions

Combine beef, soy sauce, garlic, tomatoes, onions and black pepper. Cook on medium heat for about 25 minutes. Add peppers, and cook 10 minutes more. Serve over rice.

Beef Chow Mein

Serves 4

- 1 pound round steak, cut into ¼-inch strips
- 1 tablespoon butter
- ½ cup onion, chopped
- ½ cup celery, chopped
- ½ cup green pepper, chopped
- ¾ cup rice, uncooked
- ¾ cup water
- 1 10¾-ounce can cream of chicken soup
- 1 10¾-ounce can cream of mushroom soup
- 1 7.3-ounce (4¼-ounce drained) jar sliced mushrooms
- ½ cup soy sauce
- 1 5-ounce can Chow Mein noodles

Preheat oven to 350 degrees. Brown round steak strips in butter. Add onions, celery and peppers; sauté until soft. Add rice, water, soups, mushrooms and soy sauce. Pour into a greased 9x13-inch baking dish. Bake for 1 hour and 15 minutes. Sprinkle Chow Mein noodles on top. Bake for 15 minutes. Remove from oven. Let stand for 5 minutes before serving.

Marie's Casserole Enchiladas

Serves 4 to 6

1½ dozen corn tortillas
2 tablespoons vegetable oil
½ lettuce head, chopped
½ onion, chopped
3 tomatoes, chopped
½ pound long horn cheese, grated
1 29-ounce can chili, heated

Preheat oven to 350 degrees. Heat oil in a skillet and fry the tortillas; remove to a plate with paper towels to absorb all of the oil. Layer half the tortillas in a casserole dish and spread half the ingredients on top. Repeat. When all tortillas and other ingredients have been layered, pour chili over the top. Bake for 20 minutes, or until cheese melts.

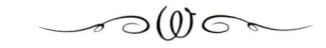

Southwestern Fajitas

Serves 6

2 medium sweet onions, quartered
2 green peppers, sliced
2 tablespoons vegetable oil
1 boneless strip steak, cut across the grain into 1¼-inch strips
1 16-ounce container sour cream
½ teaspoon salt
½ teaspoon pepper
½ teaspoon garlic salt
¼ teaspoon cayenne pepper
12 flour tortillas, warmed
1 16-ounce container fresh salsa

Stir-fry onions and peppers in small amount of oil until tender. Add steak, and sauté a few minutes. To sour cream, add salt, pepper, garlic salt and cayenne pepper. To serve, divide sour cream mixture among tortillas and spread evenly. Add even amounts of steak mixture and salsa. Roll up tortilla, enclosing filling.

Chipped Beef and Noodles au Gratin

Serves 6 to 8

Adapted for your kitchen... from the original Walgreens recipe!

Walgreens Cafeterias 1940's ~ 1960's

1   8-ounce package broad noodles, cooked per package directions
1   8-ounce package dried, chipped beef
boiling water

Cheese sauce:
½   cup butter or margarine
½   cup flour
4   cups milk, heated thoroughly
1   teaspoon salt
¼   teaspoon pepper
½   cup Kraft's grated American cheese

Crumb topping:
1   tablespoon butter or margarine
¼   cup cracker meal
¼   cup Kraft's grated American cheese

Preheat oven to 350 degrees. Prepare noodles. Cut beef into smaller pieces and cover with boiling water (blanch); drain meat. Make the cheese sauce: in a saucepan, heat butter, and blend in flour and seasonings. Cook over medium heat until mixture bubbles. Remove from heat and add heated milk, stirring until smooth. Return to heat, add the grated American cheese, and mix thoroughly. Combine cooked noodles, blanched chipped beef and sauce; mix. Pour into a 9x13-inch greased baking dish or a round, greased casserole dish. To make crumb topping, melt butter in a small frying pan. Add cracker meal; mix thoroughly. Add grated cheese and mix well. Top casserole with crumb mixture. Bake for about 20 minutes or until crumb topping is lightly browned.

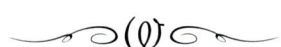

Hot~Mouth Salsa Burgers

Serves 4 to 6

1   pound lean ground beef
1   16-ounce jar hot or medium salsa
1   dash Tabasco sauce (or more, to taste)
salt and pepper, to taste
hamburger buns

In a large bowl, combine the beef with 8 ounces of salsa, Tabasco sauce, salt and pepper. Mix thoroughly, and form patties. Brown patties on both sides in skillet, or on barbecue grill. Serve on hamburger buns. Garnish (optional) with the rest of the salsa.

Texas Spiced Beef

Serves 12 to 14

2   4-ounce cans green chilies, diced
1½ to 3 tablespoons chili powder
1   teaspoon oregano
2   garlic cloves, minced
4   pounds beef chuck roast, bone in
½   14½-ounce can stewed tomatoes
salt, pepper and cayenne pepper, to taste
1   package tostados or nachos

Preheat oven to 300 degrees. Mix together green chilies, chili powder, oregano and garlic. Spread mixture on top of beef. Wrap beef in heavy foil and place in roasting pan. Bake in 300-degree oven for 4 to 4½ hours, or until tender. Remove beef from foil and shred with two forks. Discard bones, fat, and gristle. Add tomatoes, salt, pepper and cayenne to beef mixture. Serve with tostados or nachos.

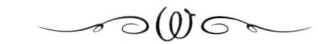

Emily's Barbecue Beef

Serves 6 to 8

2   pounds ground beef
2   tablespoons vegetable oil

Barbecue sauce:
2   cups catsup
2   tablespoons vinegar
1½ tablespoons brown sugar
¾   teaspoon yellow mustard
½   teaspoon cinnamon
¼   teaspoon cloves, ground
½   cup onion, chopped
½   cup green pepper, chopped
1   tablespoon salt
8   hamburger buns, or loaf of French bread

Heat oil and brown meat in skillet, then drain fat. Add remaining ingredients and blend well. Cook over low heat, stirring occasionally, for one hour. Serve over hamburger buns or French bread.

Crock-Pot Sloppy Joes

Serves 4 to 6

1 to 1½ pounds lean ground beef
1 small onion, minced
2 celery stalks, minced
3 tablespoons margarine or olive oil
1 10-ounce jar chili sauce
2 tablespoons brown sugar
1 tablespoon Worcestershire sauce
1 teaspoon salt
2 teaspoons sweet pickle relish
⅛ teaspoon pepper
hamburger buns or French rolls

In large skillet, cook beef with onion and celery until meat is browned. Pour off excess fat. In crock-pot; combine meat, onion and celery with remaining ingredients. Cover and cook on low for 3 to 4 hours. Spoon over toasted hamburger buns or French rolls.

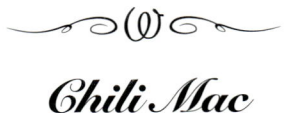

Chili Mac

Serves 6

1½ pounds ground beef
1 small onion, chopped
2 tablespoons butter
1 tablespoon chili powder
1 46-ounce can V-8 juice
2 15½-ounce cans kidney beans
1 cup macaroni, cooked per package directions

Sauté onion in butter until lightly browned. Add beef and cook until brown. Drain excess fat. Add chili powder, V-8 juice and kidney beans. Mix with macaroni and serve.

Firehouse Chili

Serves 20

- 6 medium onions, finely chopped
- 6 green peppers, finely chopped
- 3 garlic cloves, minced
- 6 tablespoons olive or vegetable oil
- 4 pounds ground round or chuck
- 4 16-ounce cans Italian-style tomatoes, drained, seeded and chopped
- 4 15½-ounce cans kidney beans, drained
- 2 6-ounce cans tomato paste
- 5 cups cold water
- 1 teaspoon red wine vinegar
- 3 whole cloves
- 2 bay leaves
- 3 tablespoons chili powder
- 4 drops Tabasco sauce
- 1 teaspoon sugar
- salt and pepper, to taste

In a large skillet, heat 4 tablespoons oil. Brown onions, peppers and garlic until golden. In a separate pan, heat remaining 2 tablespoons oil, brown ground meat in batches; separate meat with fork and cook until all meat is browned. Drain off fat. In a Dutch oven or stew pot, spoon sautéed onion, green peppers, garlic and browned meat. Add tomatoes, kidney beans, tomato paste, water, vinegar, cloves, bay leaves, chili powder and Tabasco sauce. Cover and simmer over low heat 1 hour. Add sugar, salt and pepper to taste. Simmer, uncovered, for 1 hour. Remove cloves and bay leaves before serving.

Marie's Red No~Beans Chili

Serves 4 to 6

- 1 pound ground round
- 1 tablespoon butter
- 2 tablespoons flour
- 1 10-ounce jar red chili sauce
- 1 cup water
- ½ teaspoon garlic powder
- salt, to taste

Brown meat, add flour and mix well. Add chili sauce and a little water at a time, to reach desired thickness, adding more water if necessary. Add garlic powder and salt, and let simmer for 20 minutes, stirring occasionally.

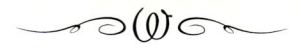

Albuquerque Chili

Serves 8 to 10

- 5 pounds ground beef, round or chuck
- 3 tablespoons butter
- 3 onions, diced
- 4 large green peppers, diced
- 1 garlic clove, minced
- 2 tablespoons olive or vegetable oil
- 6 tablespoons chili powder
- 2 tablespoons salt
- 2 tablespoons oregano
- 1½ tablespoons paprika
- 1½ tablespoons cumin
- 2 28-ounce cans whole tomatoes, drained, seeded and chopped
- 1 28-ounce can tomato purée
- 5 cups water
- 4 15½-ounce cans kidney beans, drained

Brown beef in butter; drain excess fat. In a separate pan, sauté onions, peppers and garlic in vegetable oil and add to beef. Combine all remaining ingredients except kidney beans in large pot. Simmer uncovered for 1½ hours, stirring occasionally. Add kidney beans during last half-hour of cooking; add more water if necessary.

Chili con Carne and Beans

Serves 8
Yield: ½-gallon

**Adapted for your kitchen...
from the original Walgreens recipe!**

*Walgreens Cafeterias
1940's ~ 1960's*

- 2 pounds ground beef, chuck or round
- 2 to 3 tablespoons olive oil or other vegetable oil
- 1 medium onion, coarsely chopped
- ¼ teaspoon oregano
- ¼ teaspoon ground cumin
- 2 tablespoons chili powder
- 1 teaspoon paprika
- 1 teaspoon salt
- ¼ teaspoon black pepper
- ¼ teaspoon cayenne pepper
- 1 6-ounce can tomato paste
- 4 to 6 cups water
- 2 15½-ounce cans red kidney beans

Brown beef in olive oil, stirring frequently. Add onions and continue to sauté until onions are cooked. Add all seasonings, spices, tomato paste, water and kidney beans. Cook slowly, for about 1 to 1½ hours.

Gigi's Goulash

Serves 4 to 6

- 2 medium onions, coarsley chopped
- 2 garlic cloves, minced
- ¼ cup vegetable oil
- 1½ pounds round steak, cut into cubes
- 2 tablespoons paprika
- 2 teaspoons salt
- ¼ teaspoon pepper
- 2 tablespoons flour
- 5 cups hot water
- ⅓ cup red wine vinegar
- 1 bay leaf
- 1 14½-ounce can beef broth
- ¼ cup tomato paste
- 2 teaspoons Worcestershire sauce
- 2 medium potatoes, peeled and cubed
- 2 carrots, peeled and cubed
- 2 zucchini, cubed

sour cream

Sauté onion and garlic in oil until tender. Add beef cubes and brown over high heat, stirring frequently. Stir in paprika, salt and pepper. Slowly add flour and stir until well blended. Add hot water, vinegar and bay leaf. Bring to a boil, cover and simmer for 1½ hours, stirring occasionally. After beef has simmered, stir together beef broth, tomato paste and Worcestershire sauce; add to beef mixture along with potatoes and carrots. Cover and simmer for 15 minutes. Add zucchini and continue to simmer for 30 minutes more. Before serving, remove bay leaf. Top with sour cream.

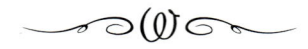

Stuffed Zucchini

Serves 4

- 1 large zucchini

Filling:
- 1 cup ground beef
- 2 tablespoons butter or olive oil
- 1 large onion, chopped
- ½ cup parsley, chopped
- 2 eggs, beaten
- ½ cup bread crumbs

Stuffed Zucchini, *continued on next page.*

Stuffed Zucchini, continued.

Topping:
½ cup Swiss cheese, grated
2 tomatoes, sliced

Preheat oven to 350 degrees. To hollow out zucchini, place on cutting board. Cutting lengthwise, cut oval shape around top and scoop out pulp and seeds. To prepare filling, heat butter in fry pan and brown meat. Set aside. Mix onion and parsley with eggs and bread crumbs; add beef. To bake: Stuff zucchini with filling. Sprinkle with grated cheese; place in 9x13 lightly-greased baking dish. Bake for 30 minutes. Top with sliced tomatoes and bake an additional 10 minutes.

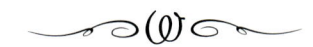

Stuffed, Ripe Plantains ~ Canoas

Serves 8

Adapted for your kitchen... from the original Walgreens recipe!

Walgreen Grills in Puerto Rico, 1960's ~ 1980's

8 ripe plantains (*platanos*)
½ cup olive oil
salt and pepper

Filling:
1 pound ground beef
2 tablespoons olive oil
2 garlic cloves, minced
1 teaspoon salt
¼ teaspoon pepper
fresh cilantro, chopped

Topping:
2 onions, coarsely chopped
3 tablespoons olive oil

To prepare filling, heat oil and cook beef. Season beef with garlic, salt, pepper and cilantro. Cook mixture until beef is thoroughly cooked. Set aside. To prepare plantains, cut plantains lengthwise down one side. Remove plantain, reserving whole plantain skin. Slice plantains and fry in heated oil until soft. Season with salt and pepper and mash. Add the mashed plantain to the stuffing mixture and heat through. Prepare topping: Sauté onions in olive oil until soft. To serve, put stuffing mixture in whole plantain shells. Top with sautéed onions.

Stuffed Cabbage Rolls

Serves 8 to 10

1 large head cabbage

Filling:
- 2 pounds ground sirloin or round
- 1½ cups half-cooked rice
- 1 medium onion, chopped and sautéed in vegetable oil or butter
- ½ cup (or more) canned beef broth
- 2 eggs, small or medium
- salt and pepper, to taste

Tomato sauce:
- 1 28-ounce can stewed tomatoes
- 1 10¾-ounce can tomato soup
- 1 8-ounce can tomato sauce
- 1 small onion, chopped
- ½ cup beef broth (or more)
- ¼ teaspoon garlic powder
- 1 tablespoon sugar (optional)

Combine the filling ingredients, mix thoroughly and set aside. Prepare a large pot of boiling water. Core head of cabbage and parboil 3 to 4 minutes. Remove leaves as they cook and set them aside to cool. Combine the sauce ingredients; cook slowly for 30 minutes to blend flavors. If too sour, add sugar.

Prepare rolls by placing 2 or 3 tablespoons of filling in core pocket, (according to the size of cabbage leaf, large leaves may need more meat), fold and tuck into a pocket roll and place into a Dutch oven, (or heavy pot) that has been lined with cabbage leaves that were broken, too large or small to roll. Place each roll, (as you finish rolling), very close to each other around the pot. Fill in empty spaces with remaining filling. Pour most of the sauce over the rolls, top with remaining cabbage leaves, and pour remainder of sauce over cabbage. Cover, cook on top of stove at medium to low heat for 2 to 3 hours; or bake, uncovered, in 325-degree oven for 2 to 3 hours, basting occasionally. If the cabbage leaves are browning too quickly, cover with foil and vent.

Note: May be prepared ahead and served the next day. Simply heat through in a 325-degree oven before serving.

Kosher Stuffed Cabbage

Serves 8

8 to 10 large cabbage leaves, blanched

Filling:

1½ pounds ground beef
½ cup rice, cooked
1 medium onion, chopped
1 egg
1 teaspoon salt
¼ teaspoon pepper

Tomato sauce:

1 15-ounce can tomato sauce
½ cup brown sugar, packed
¼ cup golden raisins
3 tablespoons vegetable oil
2 tablespoons vinegar or lemon juice
1 bay leaf

Preheat oven to 350 degrees. In a medium bowl, combine beef, rice, onion, egg, salt and pepper; mix well. In the center of each cabbage leaf, place a mound of beef filling. Fold sides of cabbage leaf over filling; then roll up, completely enclosing beef mixture. In a large, deep baking dish, arrange cabbage rolls, seam-side down, in a single layer. In a medium bowl, combine tomato sauce, brown sugar, raisins, oil, vinegar or lemon juice and bay leaf. Pour over cabbage rolls. Cover and bake for 1 hour. Remove bay leaf; serve.

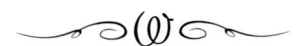

Beef & Cabbage Casserole

Serves 4 to 5

1½ pounds ground beef
1 medium onion, finely chopped
2 tablespoons butter
4 tablespoons mushroom and onion soup mix
1 head cabbage, coarsely shredded
1 10¾-ounce can tomato soup
½ 10¾-ounce can mushroom soup

Preheat oven to 350 degrees. Sauté beef and onions in butter until onions are soft; drain excess fat. Add mushroom and onion soup mix. Line bottom of 9x13-inch pan with half the shredded cabbage. Cover with beef mixture. Add rest of cabbage to cover meat. Mix tomato soup and mushroom soup together and pour over top. Seal with foil; bake for 1¼ hours.

Gladys' Beef & Cheese Casserole

Serves 6

- 2 pounds ground round
- 2 tablespoons butter
- 2 medium onions, finely chopped
- 1 green pepper, finely chopped
- 2 cups celery, finely chopped

salt and pepper, to taste

- 6 ounces medium noodles, cooked per package directions
- ¼ teaspoon Worcestershire sauce
- 1 10¾-ounce can tomato soup
- 1 cup sharp cheddar cheese, grated

Preheat oven to 325 degrees. Brown meat in butter and drain off excess fat. Add onion, green pepper and celery. Cook until tender. Season with salt and pepper to taste. In greased 9x9-inch baking dish, alternate meat and noodles. Mix Worcestershire with tomato soup. Pour over noodles and meat. Sprinkle cheese on top. Bake for 1 hour. Remove from oven. Let stand for 5 minutes before serving.

Penny's Mexican Casserole

Serves 4

- 1 pound ground beef
- 1 tablespoon butter
- 1 package taco seasoning mix
- 1 16-ounce can refried beans
- 8 cups Monterey Jack cheese, grated
- 3 7-ounce cans green chili salsa
- 1 cup sour cream
- 2 4-ounce cans chili peppers, chopped
- 1 onion, chopped
- 2 large tomatoes, chopped

Preheat oven to 350 degrees. Brown ground beef in butter; drain off excess fat. Add taco seasoning and simmer. Spread ground beef in the bottom of a baking dish. Begin by layering refried beans, 6 cups cheese, salsa and sour cream. Then, layer peppers, onions and tomatoes. Finally, add the remaining cheese. Bake, uncovered, for 20 minutes, or until brown.

Liver, Bacon & Onions

Serves 4

Adapted for your kitchen… from the original Walgreens recipe!

Wag's & Humpty Dumpty Restaurants, 1970's ~ 1980's

8 slices bacon
1¼ pounds beef liver, cut in 4 to 6 slices, ¼ to ½-inch thick
1 Bermuda onion, thinly sliced
¼ to ½ cup flour
1 teaspoon salt
¼ teaspoon pepper

Gravy:
1 tablespoon butter and 1 tablespoon flour kneaded together
1 cup canned beef broth
1 tablespoon parsley, minced

To prepare liver, brown bacon slices in skillet and drain on paper towel. Bacon should render 3 tablespoons of drippings. In ½-tablespoon drippings, stir-fry onion slices until soft; lift out with slotted spoon. Combine flour, salt and pepper. Dredge liver slices in seasoned flour. Add remaining drippings to skillet and sauté floured liver slices, only cooking 2 at a time. Remove liver and keep warm with onions. To prepare gravy, add butter-flour mixture to skillet and gradually add broth to make a smooth gravy. To serve, place slice of liver on plate. Top with sautéed onions and 2 slices bacon. Garnish with minced parsley. Pour gravy in bowls and pass to serve over liver.

Uncle Louie's Liver Stew

Serves 4 to 6

1 pound bacon
1 pound calves liver, cubed
2 to 3 onions, sliced
4 to 5 potatoes; peeled, cubed
water, to cover

In a skillet, fry bacon until crispy; drain on paper towels. In same pan, sauté liver in bacon grease; remove from pan and place in stockpot. Then, using the same pan, sauté onions. Add the drained bacon, onions and potatoes to the stockpot and cover with water. Cover pot and simmer 30 minutes to 1 hour, until potatoes are very tender and break apart.

Beef Stew Over Noodles

Serves 6

Adapted for your kitchen... from the original Walgreens recipe!

Corporate Cafeteria, Walgreen Company Headquarters

- 2 pounds beef (chuck, rump, or brisket) cut into 1½-inch cubes
- 2 tablespoons vegetable oil
- 2 medium yellow onions, coarsely chopped
- 5 cups water
- 1 tablespoon tomato paste
- 1 teaspoon Worcestershire sauce
- 1 bay leaf
- 8½ teaspoons rosemary
- 1 pinch black pepper
- 4 carrots, cubed
- 6 small red potatoes, peeled
- 4 celery stalks
- 2 tablespoons Maggi Beef Bouillon granules
- 1 tablespoon each flour and butter kneaded together
- 1 cup frozen green peas
- 1 1-pound package broad noodles, cooked per package directions
- 2 tablespoons butter

Heat oil in stew pot; add meat and sear well until browned on all sides. Add onions and cook until lightly brown. Add water, tomato paste, bay leaf, rosemary and black pepper; cover pot and simmer 2 hours. Add carrots, potatoes and celery. Cover and simmer until vegetables are tender. Add bouillon granules, kneaded flour and butter to thicken, and enough water to replace water that evaporated during stewing. Add frozen peas. Adjust seasonings and heat through. Prepare noodles, mix in butter. Serve hot over hot, buttered noodles.

Easy, Oven~Baked Beef Stew

Serves 4 to 6

- 1½ pounds beef (chuck, rump, or brisket), cut into 1-inch cubes
- 1 15-ounce can whole potatoes
- 1 16-ounce can whole onions
- 1 14½-ounce can carrots
- 1 8½-ounce small can peas
- 1 10¾-ounce can cream of celery soup

Do not brown meat! Combine all ingredients, except soup, in large, greased casserole dish. Add soup. Cover and bake at 325 degrees for 3 hours.

Beef Stew with Fresh Vegetables

Serves 6 to 8

Adapted for your kitchen... from the original Walgreens recipe!

Walgreens Cafeterias 1940's ~ 1960's

- 3 pounds beef (chuck or bottom round), cut into 1 to 1½-inch cubes
- 2 to 3 tablespoons vegetable oil
- ½ cup flour, unsifted
- 1 14½-ounce can tomatoes, drained
- 4 cups canned beef stock, heated
- 12 small white onions
- 2 teaspoons salt
- ¼ teaspoon pepper
- 6 carrots, scraped and cut into 1-inch pieces
- 12 small potatoes, peeled
- 6 celery stalks, cut into 1-inch pieces
- 1 teaspoon Worcestershire sauce

Heat oil in Dutch oven or stewpot. Add beef and brown for 20 to 25 minutes. Remove from heat; add flour and blend. Add tomatoes; mix thoroughly. Stirring constantly, add hot stock. Return to stove, cover and simmer over low heat for 1 to 1½ hours. Add onion, salt and pepper. (Steam carrots and potatoes separately.) Cook approximately 1 more hour or until beef is tender. Add cooked potatoes and carrots, celery and Worcestershire sauce. Cook for another 20 to 30 minutes. Taste for seasoning and serve.

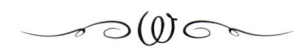

Beef Stew Deluxe

Serves 6 to 8

- 3 pounds round steak, cut into 2-inch cubes
- 1 10¾-ounce can onion soup, undiluted
- 1 10¾-ounce can golden mushroom soup, undiluted
- 1 cup port wine
- 1 7.3-ounce (4¼-ounce drained) jar sliced mushrooms, drained
- 1 teaspoon salt
- ¼ teaspoon pepper
- **rice or noodles, cooked per package directions**

Preheat oven to 300 degrees. Mix steak, onion soup, mushroom soup, wine, mushrooms, salt and pepper; pour into a 3-quart casserole. Cover and bake for 3 hours. Serve over rice or noodles.

Hunter's Stew

Serves 8

- 2 pounds beef, cut into 1½-inch cubes
- 1 8-ounce can tomato sauce
- 2 medium red potatoes, cut into ¼-inch slices
- 2 medium onions, sectioned
- 3 celery stalks, cut into diagonal pieces
- 4 medium carrots
- ⅓ cup quick-cooking tapioca
- 1 tablespoon sugar
- ½ teaspoon basil
- 1 teaspoon salt
- ¼ teaspoon pepper

Preheat oven to 325 degrees. Combine all ingredients in a 2½-quart casserole. Cover and cook for 3½ hours.

Meat & Vegetable Loaf

Serves 6 to 8
Yield: One 1½-pound loaf

Adapted for your kitchen... from the original Walgreens recipe!

Walgreens Cafeterias 1940's ~ 1960's

- 2 pounds lean ground beef
- 1 medium potato, peeled and finely chopped
- 2 carrots, pared and finely chopped
- 2 celery stalks, finely chopped
- 1 medium onion, peeled and finely chopped
- ½ green pepper, finely chopped
- 2 cups bread crumbs
- 1 teaspoon salt
- ¼ teaspoon pepper
- 1 cup milk

Preheat oven to 350 degrees. Chop all vegetables very fine either in food processor or by hand with knife. Mix with all other ingredients. Grease a 9x5-inch loaf pan or a 13x9-inch pyrex glass baking dish, line with waxed paper, and regrease. Pack mixture compactly into pan. Bake for 1 hour, or until done.

Cheese~Stuffed Meat Loaf

Serves 6

- 2 pounds ground beef
- 8 ounces mozzarella cheese, grated
- 2 eggs
- ½ cup Italian-seasoned bread crumbs
- 1 cup tomato juice
- 1 teaspoon salt
- ½ teaspoon oregano
- pepper, to taste
- 2 small onions, minced
- 2 tablespoons vegetable oil
- 8 thin slices boiled ham

Preheat oven to 350 degrees. Combine beef, eggs, bread crumbs, tomato juice, salt, oregano and pepper. Sauté onion in oil until golden brown. Add to meat mixture, mix well. Turn out on a sheet of aluminum foil. Flatten into oblong, about 1-inch thick. Place ham slices in oblong, keeping them about 1-inch from edge. Sprinkle grated cheese on ham. Use foil to fold meat mixture over ham and cheese, close all openings. Turn loaf from foil into a greased, 8x5x3-inch loaf pan. Pat with fingers to fill corners of pan and shape loaf. Bake for 1 to 1½ hours; center will register 150 degrees on meat thermometer.

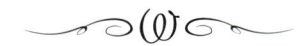

Monday Meat Loaf

Serves 4

- 1½ pounds ground beef
- 1 cup soda crackers, crushed
- 1½ tablespoons onion, chopped
- 2 tablespoons Worcestershire sauce
- 2 teaspoons salt
- ¼ teaspoon pepper
- ¾ cup milk
- 1 egg

Preheat oven to 350 degrees. Combine all ingredients. Shape and place in greased loaf pan. Bake for 1 hour, or until done.

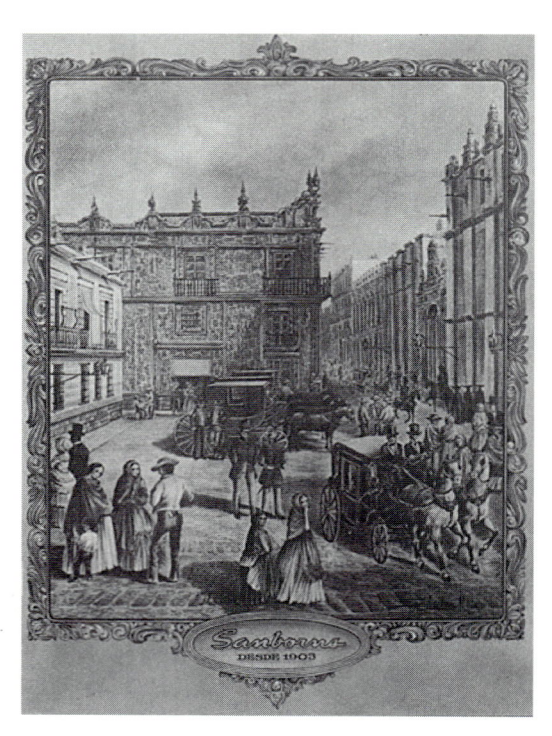

A Sanborns menu featuring an etching of The House of Tiles (circa 1596). The etching was done in 1903, the year the Sanborn brothers opened a drugstore there.

Citrus~Marinated Pork Chops

Serves 8

8 center-cut pork chops
1 tablespoon olive oil
1 tablespoon butter

Citrus marinade:
1 tablespoon Dijon mustard
2 garlic cloves, crushed
1 sprig fresh thyme
2 tablespoons balsamic vinegar
juice of 2 limes
juice of 2 oranges
juice of 1 lemon

Sauté pork chops in olive oil until browned. Meanwhile, mix together all marinade ingredients. Add to pork chops. Simmer, covered, for 10 minutes. Remove chops and keep warm. Reduce marinade to half of its original quantity. Stir in butter. Drizzle marinade over chops, and serve.

Pork Chops with Sage & Onion

Serves 6

6 butterfly pork chops, cut ¾-inch thick, well trimmed
3 tablespoons flour
2 tablespoons vegetable oil or use non-stick cooking spray
3 cups onions, sliced
½ teaspoon salt
¼ teaspoon pepper
1¼ teaspoons sage
½ cup hot water

Sprinkle pork chops with flour. Brown both sides of chops in oil; remove from pan and keep warm. In same pan, sauté onions until lightly browned. Add salt, pepper, sage and hot water. Stir. Arrange chops on top of onions. Cover and simmer for 1 hour and 15 minutes or until tender.

Pork Chops Supreme

Serves 4

- 4 lean center-cut pork chops, cut 1-inch thick
- 1 teaspoon salt
- 4 thin slices onion
- 4 thin slices lemon
- ¼ cup brown sugar, packed
- ¼ cup catsup

Preheat oven to 350 degrees. Season chops well with salt. Place in 9x13-inch pan or baking dish. Top each chop with an onion and lemon slice. Place 1 tablespoon each of brown sugar and catsup on top of each chop. Cover and bake 1 hour; uncover and bake 30 minutes more. Baste occasionally.

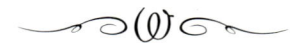

Pork Chops in Spicy Mustard Sauce

Serves 2

- ⅔ pound boneless pork chops, thinly sliced
- 1 pinch seasoned salt
- 1 pinch pepper
- 1 pinch onion powder
- 1 pinch garlic powder
- 2 tablespoons butter
- 4 ounces fresh mushrooms, sliced

Mustard sauce:
- 1 10¾-ounce can Campbell's Golden Mushroom soup
- reserved cooking juices from mushrooms
- 1 tablespoon Gulden's spicy brown mustard
- ½ to 1 teaspoon dried marjoram

Wipe chops with damp paper towel. Season with salt, pepper, onion powder and garlic powder. Set aside. Heat 1 tablespoon butter in skillet and cook mushrooms until brown and tender, about 5 minutes. Set aside in small dish with pan juices. Heat the other tablespoon butter in skillet and brown chops, cooking 3 to 4 minutes on each side. Mix soup, mushroom juices, mustard and marjoram, and pour over chops. Cover and simmer 30 to 40 minutes, or until tender. Uncover and add mushrooms. Heat through.

Pork Chops with Apple Rings

Serves 4

4   5-ounce pork loin chops, ¾-inch thick
salt and pepper, to taste

Ginger-apple sauce:
¼   brown sugar, packed
¼   cup apple juice
¼   cup soy sauce
2   tablespoons catsup
1   tablespoon cornstarch
¼   teaspoon ginger, ground

1   medium apple, Golden Delicious or Cortland
4   sprigs parsley (optional)

Preheat oven to 350 degrees. Arrange chops in a 12x7½x2-inch baking dish; sprinkle with salt and pepper. Bake for 30 minutes. Combine brown sugar, apple juice, soy sauce, catsup, cornstarch and ginger. Core apple and cut into ¾-inch thick slices. Turn chops, place 1 apple ring on each chop, spoon some sauce over each. Return chops to oven and bake for 30 minutes more, until chops are lighty browned; baste with juices once. Garnish pork chops with parsley, and serve with remaining sauce.

Cherry Pork Chops

Serves 4

6   center-cut pork chops
1   tablespoon butter
salt and pepper, to taste

Cherry sauce:
1   cup canned cherry pie filling
2   teaspoons lemon juice
½   teaspoon instant chicken bouillon
⅛   teaspoon mace, ground

parsley (optional)

Brown chops in butter. Season with salt and pepper. In crock pot, stir together cherry pie filling, juice, bouillon and mace. Place browned chops on top of cherry mixture. Cover and cook in crock-pot on low, 4 to 5 hours. Place chops on warm serving platter. To serve, pour a small amount of cherry sauce over chops. Garnish with parsley and serve with remaining sauce.

Pork Chop Casserole

Serves 4 to 6

6 or 7 medium potatoes, sliced
4 center-cut pork chops
1 14¾-ounce can cream-style corn
¾ cup milk
flour
butter
salt and pepper, to taste

Preheat oven to 350 degrees. Place half the sliced potatoes into greased, 3-quart casserole. Sprinkle potatoes with flour, salt and pepper. Dot with butter. Arrange chops over potato layer. Pour 1 can cream-style corn over chops. Add remaining sliced potatoes on top of corn, and sprinkle with flour, salt and pepper. Dot with butter. Pour milk over entire casserole and cover, and bake for 1 hour. Remove cover and bake for 20 to 30 minutes more, or until browned.

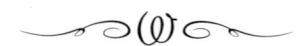

Pork Tenderloin Casserole

Serves 6 to 8

1½ pound pork tenderloin patties
1 cup flour
1 teaspoon salt
1 tablespoon butter
½ pound bacon
1 to 1½ cup chicken bouillon
8 ounces fresh mushrooms, sliced
1 medium onion, sliced
1 tablespoon oregano

Preheat oven to 350 degrees. Combine salt and flour; coat patties. Sauté in butter until brown. Arrange patties in 2-quart casserole. Partially fry bacon, remove from pan, drain and cut into pieces; cover patties with bacon. Combine bouillon with mushrooms and onions. Pour mixture over patties and sprinkle with oregano. Cover and bake for 1 hour.

Kathy's South~of~the~Border Pork Tenderloin

Serves 4 to 6

1 pork tenderloin, trimmed

Spicy brown sugar marinade:
1 cup brown sugar
3 tablespoons chili sauce
3 tablespoons soy sauce
3 tablespoons olive oil
2 tablespoons lime juice
½ tablespoon garlic, minced
salt and pepper, to taste

Spicy Apricot Chutney (see recipe in the *RxCetera ~ Sauces & Garnishes* chapter)

Mix marinade ingredients together in bowl. Place pork in a glass casserole pan and cover with glaze. Refrigerate overnight. Grill or broil pork until cooked as desired. Slice diagonally. Serve with *Spicy Apricot Chutney*.

Pork Loin with Rice & Pigeon Peas

Serves 6 to 8

Adapted for your kitchen... from the original Walgreens recipe!

Walgreen Grills in Puerto Rico, 1960's ~ 1980's

Originally called: Arroz con Gandules y Carne de Cerdo

2 pounds pork loin, cut into 1-inch cubes
3 tablespoons olive oil
2 green peppers, seeded and chopped
2 tomatoes, peeled, seeded and chopped
1 onion, finely chopped
2 garlic cloves, finely chopped
2 sprigs fresh cilantro, finely chopped, or 2 teaspoons dried cilantro
2 cups long-grain rice, uncooked
1 teaspoon salt
2 packages Goya Sazan* (1.41-ounce box) with coriander and achiote
1 pound pigeon peas, cooked (or 1-pound can LaPreferida gandules*)
3 cups water

In Dutch oven or soup pot, sauté pork in olive oil over low heat. Add green peppers, tomatoes, onion, garlic and cilantro. Sauté until tender. Add all remaining ingredients to pot; simmer until water is absorbed and rice is cooked and fluffy. Serve immediately.

Note: *Available in the ethnic or specialty sections of grocery stores.

Garlic~Roasted Pork Loin

Serves 8

3 pound boneless loin of pork, trimmed
2 garlic cloves, thinly sliced
2 tablespoons fresh rosemary (or 2 teaspoons dried)
3 tablespoons olive oil
salt and pepper to taste

Preheat oven to 350 degrees. Make small slits with sharp knife on all sides of pork. Insert garlic and rosemary leaves into slits. Rub meat with olive oil. Sprinkle with salt and pepper. Place meat on a rack in roasting pan. Roast in oven until meat thermometer inserted in roast registers 160 degrees; 1½ to 2 hours. Let stand 15 minutes before carving.

Roasted Pork Loin with Gravy

Serves 6

Adapted for your kitchen... from the original Walgreens recipe!

Robin Hood & Briargate Restaurants, 1970's ~ 1980's

1 4-pound pork loin, boned and rolled
2 teaspoons salt
¼ teaspoon white pepper
2 medium onions, coarsely chopped
2 celery stalks, coarsely chopped
½ teaspoon poultry seasoning
1 teaspoon rosemary

Gravy:
1 cup pan drippings
1 cup flour
2 to 3 cups chicken broth

Preheat oven to 350 degrees. Loin should be at room temperature. Rub loin with salt, pepper, poultry seasoning and rosemary. Place in roasting pan. Cover with chopped vegetables. Roast for approximately 2½ hours or until meat thermometer registers 180 degrees. Remove loin from pan. To make gravy, pour off drippings into a saucepan. For each cup of drippings, blend in 1 cup of flour. Cook until frothy. Slowly add 2 to 3 cups of chicken broth, stirring constantly until smooth. If still lumpy, pour gravy through a strainer. Pour into gravy boat. Carve loin, place slices on platter and serve with gravy.

Pork Steaks a la Criolla

Serves 6

*Adapted for your kitchen...
from the original Walgreens recipe!*

Walgreen Grills in Puerto Rico, 1960's ~ 1980's

Originally called: Chuletas a la Criolla

Criolla:
- 3 tablespoons olive oil or margarine
- 3 tomatoes, peeled, seeded and chopped
- 2 onions, finely chopped
- 2 green peppers, seeded and chopped
- 2 garlic cloves, finely chopped
- 1 teaspoon cumin
- 2 tablespoons flour
- 1 cup chicken soup
- 1 teaspoon salt
- ¼ teaspoon white pepper

Pork steaks:
- 2 pounds Boston Butt cut into 6 blade pork steaks
- 2 tablespoons flour
- 2 teaspoons salt
- pepper, freshly ground
- 4 tablespoons olive oil

Preheat oven to 350 degrees. To make sauce, heat oil in saucepan. Sauté tomatoes, onions, green pepper, garlic and cumin until softened. In another saucepan, dissolve the flour into chicken soup and cook until thickened. Drain vegetables and add to thickened sauce. Salt and pepper to taste. To prepare pork steaks, season flour with salt and pepper. Pat both sides of pork steaks with seasoned flour. Heat oil in fry pan. Sauté pork steaks on both sides until lightly browned. To assemble and bake, place sautéed steaks in a baking dish. Spoon criolla sauce on top of pork steaks; cover with foil and bake for about 1 hour.

Honey Spareribs Zygmun

Serves 6 to 8

6 pounds spareribs, quartered
salt and pepper, to taste

Honey-soy sauce:
1 cup soy sauce
1½ cups catsup
1½ cups honey
5 garlic cloves
1 teaspoon Tabasco sauce

Preheat oven to 400 degrees. Quarter ribs, cutting into sections of 4 each. Arrange ribs on a foil-lined rack that will fit into roasting pan. Bake for 25 minutes; turn and continue baking for 25 more minutes. Meanwhile, place sauce ingredients in food processor. Blend until well-mixed and garlic is minced. Roll ribs in sauce and lower oven to 325 degrees. Bake for 20 minutes, turning after 10 minutes. Serve with warmed, leftover sauce.

Breaded Spareribs in Mustard Gravy

Serves 6 to 8

6 pounds spareribs, cut into sections
2 tablespoons tarragon vinegar
2 tablespoons vegetable oil
dry bread crumbs

Mustard gravy:
3 tablespoons green onion, chopped
3 tablespoons butter
¼ cup lemon juice
2 teaspoons Worcestershire sauce
2 teaspoons prepared mustard
1 dash Tabasco sauce
1 10-ounce can beef gravy

Preheat oven to 350 degrees. Cut ribs into serving pieces; combine vinegar and oil and brush on ribs. Roll in bread crumbs. Arrange ribs on a foil-lined rack that will fit into a roasting pan. Bake for 1½ hours, turning during baking to brown both sides. To make sauce, sauté onions in butter and mix in all other ingredients. Heat thoroughly. Serve spareribs with sauce.

Barbecued Spareribs

Serves 6

Adapted for your kitchen... from the original Walgreens recipe!

Walgreens Cafeterias 1940's ~ 1960's

3 sides spareribs, cut in serving pieces
salt and pepper
1 medium onion

Barbecue sauce:
½ cup honey
½ cup soy sauce
2 garlic cloves, crushed and chopped
3 tablespoons catsup
½ cup water

Wipe spareribs with damp cloth. Sprinkle lightly with salt and pepper. Place in kettle or stew pot, cover with water, drop in whole onion and bring to boil. Reduce heat and simmer for about 1 hour. Drain; place spareribs on rack in roasting pan. Mix ingredients for barbecue sauce. Baste spareribs on both sides and bake in 325-degree oven, basting frequently, for 1 to 1½ hours.

Spareribs & Sauerkraut

Serves 6 to 8

Adapted for your kitchen... from the original Walgreens recipe!

Walgreens Cafeterias 1940's ~ 1960's

5 pounds spareribs, cut in serving size pieces
1 medium onion
salt and pepper

Sauerkraut:
3 14-ounce cans sauerkraut, drained
2 to 4 tablespoons butter or margarine
2 onions, finely minced
¼ cup sugar
1 tablespoon salt
¼ teaspoon pepper
2 medium, raw potatoes, grated

Wipe spareribs with a damp cloth and sprinkle lightly with salt and pepper. Place in large kettle or stew pot and cover with water. Drop in whole onion and bring to boil. Reduce heat and simmer for 1½ hours or until tender. Drain sauerkraut. Place sauerkraut in Dutch oven or stew pot and cover with stock used to cook the spareribs. Heat butter or margarine in a small skillet. Sauté onions until wilted, but not brown. Add to sauerkraut. Add sugar, salt, pepper and grated potatoes; mix well. Cook slowly for 1½ hours. Potatoes will prevent sauerkraut from turning dark. To serve, place serving-size pieces of ribs over portions of sauerkraut.

Scalloped Ham & Potatoes

Serves 6 to 8

- 6 to 8 potatoes, thinly sliced
- 4 cups cooked ham, cubed
- ½ cup flour
- 2 tablespoons butter
- 2 teaspoons salt
- ¼ teaspoon pepper
- 2 cups milk, heated
- ½ teaspoon paprika

Preheat oven to 350 degrees. Generously butter a 9x13-inch baking dish or oval casserole. Layer half the potatoes and sprinkle with salt, pepper and flour; dot with butter and diced ham. Repeat sequence to make three layers. Pour heated milk into pan. Top with paprika and bake for about 1 hour or until potatoes are tender and top is browned. Serve immediately.

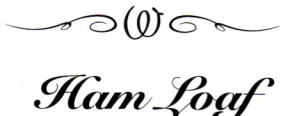

Ham Loaf

Serves 4 to 6

- ¾ pound ground ham
- ½ pound ground beef
- ½ pound ground pork
- 1 cup Pet milk
- ¼ cup catsup
- 2 tablespoons onion, chopped
- ¾ teaspoon dry mustard
- ¾ cup soft bread crumbs
- 1 teaspoon salt
- ¼ teaspoon pepper

Ham basting sauce:
- ½ cup brown sugar
- 2 tablespoons vinegar
- 2 tablespoons water

Preheat oven to 325 degrees. Mix ham, beef, pork, Pet milk, catsup, onion, mustard, bread crumbs, salt and pepper. Shape into loaf and bake for 30 minutes. Combine sugar, vinegar and water in saucepan, and cook for 5 minutes. Bake ham loaf for 1 hour more, basting with sauce every 15 minutes.

Ham Croquettes

Serves 6 to 8

Adapted for your kitchen...
from the original Walgreens recipe!

Walgreens Cafeterias
1940's ~ 1960's

4 cups cooked ham, finely chopped
1 cup bread crumbs
2 eggs
1 cup milk
2 cups cracker crumbs

White sauce:
4 tablespoons butter, margarine or vegetable oil
4 tablespoons flour
2 cups milk, heated to boiling
1 small onion, finely minced

Mix ham and bread crumbs. To prepare sauce, heat butter in saucepan; add flour and cook 5 minutes over low heat until bubbly. Remove from heat and add hot milk, stirring well until mixture is thickened. Return to heat, add minced onion and cook 5 minutes longer over low heat. Remove from heat, combine ham mixture with white sauce, and mix thoroughly. Set aside to cool. Shape ham mixture into small cakes. Combine eggs and milk, and dip cakes into mixture (egg wash); dredge in cracker crumbs. Heat 2 to 3 inches of oil in frying pan or electric skillet to 360 degrees. Fry cakes in hot oil until golden brown. Remove with slotted spoon and drain on wire rack or absorbent paper.

Pineapple~Baked Ham

Serves 12

Adapted for your kitchen...
from the original Walgreens recipe!

Robin Hood & Briargate Restaurants, 1970's ~ 1980's

1 10 to 12-pound ham, bone in
1 pound brown sugar
24 whole cloves
1 quart pineapple juice

Preheat oven to 325 degrees. Be sure ham is thawed, but chilled. Place ham in roasting pan fat side up and bake for about 3 hours. Remove ham, trim skin and score fat. Pat ham with brown sugar, dot with cloves. Increase oven temperature to 425 degrees. Return to oven for about 30 to 45 minutes. Baste frequently, after glaze begins to set, with pineapple juice.

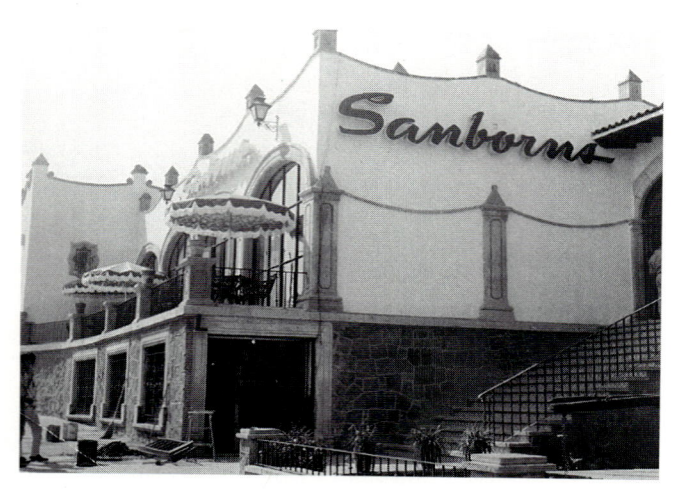

"The Haunted Village" Sanborns in San Angel, Mexico, 1968. "Meet me at Sanborns" was the chain's official slogan.

Veal Piccata de Hudson

Serves 4

1½ pounds veal, round or sirloin, cut ¼ to ½-inch thick
salt and pepper, to taste
flour
3 tablespoons butter
1 tablespoon olive oil
2 garlic cloves, minced
8 ounces fresh mushrooms, sliced
2 tablespoons fresh lemon juice
½ cup dry white wine
2 teaspoons capers, plus 1 teaspoon caper juice (optional)
3 tablespoons parsley, minced
½ lemon, thinly sliced

Sprinkle veal with salt and pepper on both sides, and dust lightly with flour. Heat butter and olive oil in a large skillet. Add veal and brown on both sides. Remove veal from skillet. Add garlic and mushrooms to pan and cook one minute. Return veal to pan. Add lemon juice, white wine, cover and simmer for 20 minutes, or until veal is tender. Add capers. Remove veal and keep warm on serving platter. Add more wine if necessary; scrape around bottom and sides of pan. Heat through and pour sauce over veal. Sprinkle with parsley and garnish with lemon slices.

Santina's Veal Piccata

Serves 3 to 4

¼ cup flour
1 pound leg of veal, sliced into very thin 3x4-inch pieces
¼ cup vegetable oil
2 tablespoons unsalted butter
¼ cup dry white wine
juice of 1 lemon
1 lemon
salt and pepper, to taste

Lightly flour veal on both sides. Shake off excess. In a large, heavy skillet, heat oil and butter. When bubbling, add veal and sauté about 2 minutes on each side. When veal is nearly cooked, sprinkle on lemon juice. Remove veal from pan and keep warm. Add wine to pan and de-glaze over high heat, stirring constantly. Reduce liquid to 3 tablespoons. Pour sauce over veal. Slice lemon paper thin; put slices on each veal scallop. Sprinkle with salt and pepper. Serve immediately.

Fricassee of Veal with Morels

Serves 6 to 8

6 ounces dried morels
1 cup water
5 pounds boneless veal, cut into 1½-inch cubes
salt and black pepper, freshly ground, to taste
all-purpose flour
4 tablespoons butter
2 tablespoons vegetable oil
2 cups dry white wine
16 whole shallots, peeled
3 cups homemade chicken stock or canned broth
1 teaspoon dried thyme
1 bay leaf
2 tablespoons Dijon mustard
3 cups heavy cream
1 1-pound package egg noodles, cooked per package directions

Soak morels in 1 cup of water for 30 minute; drain, reserving liquid; and chop. Strain reserved liquid and set aside. Season the veal pieces with salt and pepper, and dust lightly with flour. Heat butter and oil in large frying pan and brown the pieces of veal in batches.

Transfer the veal cubes to a bowl as they cook. Pour the wine into the pan and cook over high heat for 1 minute, scraping up any browned bits in the pan. Pour mixture into an 8-quart pot. Add the veal, shallots, stock, thyme, bay leaf, chopped morels and morel reserve liquid. Bring to a boil and simmer for 1 hour and 30 minutes, stirring occasionally. Combine the mustard and cream, and stir mixture into a gravy. Cook for 10 minutes; then taste for seasoning. Serve with egg noodles.

Veal Cutlets in Marsala Wine

Serves 6

2 pounds veal cutlets
flour
salt and pepper, to taste
10 tablespoons unsalted butter
1 pound fresh mushrooms, thinly sliced
1½ cups marsala wine
1 cup heavy cream
zest of 1 lemon
parsley, chopped

Pound cutlets with meat mallet to ⅛-inch thickness. Season flour with salt and pepper. Dredge veal in flour mixture and shake off excess. Heat a third of the butter in large skillet. Add veal in single layer. Cook each side 3 minutes, until golden brown on both sides. Remove veal and keep warm on serving platter. Cook remaining cutlets. Add mushrooms to pan, cook and stir until light gold. Add wine to pan. Cook, scraping up brown bits from bottom of pan, and stir until pan juices reduce slightly. Stir in cream, and cook 5 more minutes, or until sauce is thickened. Pour sauce over warm cutlets, sprinkle with lemon zest and parsley. Serve immediately.

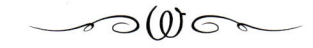

Paprika Veal Cutlets

Serves 6 to 8

Adapted for your kitchen... from the original Walgreens recipe!

Walgreens Cafeterias 1940's ~ 1960's

¼ pound bacon, finely chopped
6 veal cutlets, cut ¾-inch thick
salt and pepper, to taste
2 medium onions, finely chopped
2 tablespoons sweet paprika
1 cup sour cream
1 cup tomato purée

Preheat oven to 375 degrees. Fry bacon in a heavy skillet until done. Add veal cutlets to bacon and rendered fat; brown veal cutlets. Remove cutlets and put in 13x9-inch baking pan. Brown onions in bacon fat, season with salt and pepper. Add paprika, sour cream and tomato purée. Mix, bring to boil, and taste for seasoning. Pour sauce over veal in baking pan. Cover baking pan with foil and bake in a 375-degree oven for 30 to 45 minutes, or until tender.

Veal Chops with Mushrooms in Cream Sauce

Serves 6

- 6 center-cut or loin veal chops
- 1 ounce porcini mushrooms
- 4 cups luke-warm water
- 6 teaspoons butter
- 12 sprigs flat-leaf parsley, leaves only, coarsely chopped
- 2 garlic cloves, chopped
- 1 pound champignon mushrooms (or firm, white mushrooms), chopped
- 3 teaspoons extra-virgin olive oil
- salt and pepper, to taste
- ⅓ cup brandy or white wine
- ¼ cup heavy cream

Soak porcini's in bowl with 4 cups of lukewarm water for half an hour. Drain mushrooms, reserving water. Strain water through paper towels. Melt 4 teaspoons of butter in casserole over medium heat. Add chopped parsley and garlic. Add all mushrooms, and sauté for 5 minutes. Gradually add drained porcini water. Stir and simmer for 10 minutes. Heat oil and remaining butter in skillet over medium heat. Add chops and fry with salt and pepper for 1 minute each side, turning chops a couple of times. Add brandy (or white wine) and let evaporate–about 2 minutes. Transfer chops to the casserole with the mushrooms and over low heat start adding cream, a little at a time, until incorporated. Stir mixture and turn chops. When all of the cream is incorporated, about 10 minutes, transfer chops, in the mushroom sauce, to a platter. Serve immediately.

Veal Scallopini

Serves 6

**Adapted for your kitchen…
from the original Walgreens recipe!**

Robin Hood & Briargate Restaurants, 1970's ~ 1980's

- 2 pounds veal round, sliced into 6 ¼-inch thick pieces
- 1 teaspoon salt
- ¼ teaspoon pepper
- ½ cup flour
- 6 tablespoons butter or margarine
- ½ pound mushrooms, thinly sliced
- 2 medium onions, coarsely chopped
- 1 16-ounce can tomato purée
- 1 tablespoon vinegar
- ¼ to ½ cup Parmesan cheese, grated
- 1 to 1½ cups hot chicken broth

Veal Scallopini, *continued on next page.*

Veal Scallopini, continued.

Preheat oven to 350 degrees. Pound cutlets thin (⅛ to ¼-inch thick); slip cutlets between 2 sheets waxed paper and flatten with a rolling pin or meat mallet. Pound 3 to 4 times per side. Mix salt, pepper and flour, and dredge scallopini in seasoned flour. Heat butter in frying pan and brown 2 pieces at a time, 2 to 3 minutes on a side. Remove to a large baking pan. In another pan, melt remaining butter, and sauté onions and mushrooms until soft. Add unused flour and cook until bubbly. Add hot chicken stock; stir until smooth. Add tomato purée and vinegar; bring to a boil. Pour over browned cutlets. Sprinkle top with Parmesan cheese. Bake for 30 to 40 minutes.

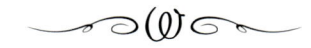

Creamed Veal with Rice

Serves 6 to 8

Adapted for your kitchen... from the original Walgreens recipe!

Walgreens Cafeterias 1940's ~ 1960's

- 3 cups cooked veal, diced
- ½ cup green pepper, diced
- ¼ cup pimentos, diced
- 1 tablespoon margarine or vegetable oil
- 1 cup canned green peas, drained
- 3 hard-boiled eggs, chopped
- 2½ cups rice, cooked per package directions
- 2 cups water
- ½ teaspoon salt

White sauce:
- 4 tablespoons butter, margarine or vegetable oil
- 4 tablespoons flour
- 2 teaspoons salt
- ¼ teaspoon pepper
- 1 pinch cayenne pepper
- 2 cups milk, heated to boiling

Prepare sauce first. Bring milk to boil in a pan. In another saucepan, heat oil and blend in flour and seasonings. Stir constantly; bring to boil. Remove from heat and add boiling milk; stir until smooth. Return to low heat. Add diced veal to sauce. In a separate pan, sauté diced green pepper and pimento in 1 tablespoon margarine. Then combine sautéed peppers and pimento with sauce, along with drained peas and chopped eggs. Bring sauce to boil with all ingredients in it. To serve, place a portion of rice on a plate and ladle creamed veal over rice.

Osso Buco ~ Vincent

Serves 6

Osso buco is a traditional Italian meal of veal shanks and minced vegetables stewed in a white wine sauce with tomatoes, garlic and seasonings.

6	pounds veal shanks
½	cup flour
2	tablespoons olive oil
2	tablespoons butter
1	large green pepper, coarsely chopped
1	carrot, peeled and coarsely chopped
3	sprigs parsley, coarsely chopped
2	medium onions, coarsely chopped
3	celery stalks, coarsely chopped
2	garlic cloves, cut and chopped

Spicy tomato-wine sauce:

1	8-ounce can tomato sauce
½	cup white wine
1	pinch chili sauce
1	pinch dried red peppers

To prepare veal, dredge in flour and fry in olive oil and butter until brown. Remove. Sauté in skillet used to prepare veal. Cook until soft. Place cooked vegetables in a food processor and blend together. To prepare sauce: in the same skillet, simmer tomato sauce, wine, chili sauce and dried red peppers. Add vegetable mixture and veal shanks. Simmer, covered, for 2 hours or bake at 350 degrees for 1 hour. The shanks should be very tender.

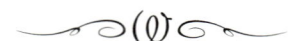

Spring Lamb Stew with Fresh Vegetables

Serves 6 to 8

Adapted for your kitchen... from the original Walgreens recipe!

Walgreens Cafeterias 1940's ~ 1960's

2	pounds lamb shoulder, cut into 1-inch cubes
2	quarts water
3	celery stalks, coarsely chopped
3	medium onions, coarsely chopped
½	cup vegetable oil
½ to ¾-cup flour	
1	cup chicken stock
1 to 2 teaspoons salt	
¼	teaspoon pepper
3	large carrots, coarsely chopped
4	medium potatoes, coarsely chopped
1	10-ounce package frozen peas, thawed and drained

Spring Lamb Stew with Fresh Vegetables, *continued on next page.*

Spring Lamb Stew with Fresh Vegetables, *continued.*

Blanch lamb by pouring 2 quarts of cold water over it in Dutch oven or stew pot; bring to boil and pour into strainer. Rinse lamb thoroughly in cold water. Return meat to Dutch oven or pot, cover with cold water, and bring to boil. Add salt and pepper, reduce heat, and simmer for 1 hour. Add celery and onions and cook until tender. In another saucepan, heat oil and blend in flour, making a roux. Add part of lamb stock from stew pot, stirring constantly, and bring to boil. Add this mixture to stew pot, stirring constantly. Cook carrots and potatoes separately. Add them along with drained peas. Mix, heat thoroughly, and taste for seasoning.

Crown Roast of Lamb with Wild Rice

Serves 8

1   7 to 8-pound crown roast of lamb, all fat removed
juice of 1 lemon
salt and pepper, freshly ground, to taste
½   cup Dijon mustard
2   tablespoons soy sauce
2   garlic cloves, minced
1   teaspoon dried rosemary, crumbled
¼   teaspoon marjoram
wild rice, cooked per package directions
curly lettuce or laurel leaves
May apples

Preheat oven to 325 degrees. Moisten paper towel with lemon juice and rub over lamb. Place on rack in roasting pan and sprinkle with salt and pepper. Cover tips of bones with foil to prevent burning. Crumple additional foil and place in center of roast to retain shape. Using meat thermometer, roast until thermometer registers 120 degrees. Meanwhile, combine next five ingredients (mustard, soy sauce, garlic, rosemary and marjoram) in small bowl and blend well. When 120-degree temperature is reached, discard foil in center of roast and paint inside of meat generously with mustard mixture. Continue roasting until thermometer registers 130 to 135 degrees, or until cooked to desired degree. Baking time should be 1½ to 2 hours. To serve, place crown on a large, round platter and put paper frills on rib bones. Fill center of roast with wild rice; form rice into a mound. Surround roast with curly lettuce or laurel leaves and May apples. Carve like a pie.

Roast Leg of Lamb with Mustard~Ginger Sauce

Serves 8

1   4-pound boned leg of lamb, butterflied and trimmed of visible fat

Red wine marinade:
- 1 cup dry red wine (or ½-cup red-wine vinegar and ¾-cup water)
- ⅓ cup vegetable oil
- 1 bay leaf (about 2 inches long)
- 1 teaspoon dried rosemary
- 1 teaspoon salt
- ½ teaspoon black pepper, freshly ground
- 1 teaspoon garlic, minced

Mustard-ginger basting sauce:
- ½ cup Dijon mustard
- 2 tablespoons soy sauce
- 1 teaspoon dried rosemary
- ½ teaspoon minced garlic
- ¼ teaspoon ground ginger
- 2 tablespoons olive oil

Mix marinade ingredients in a shallow baking dish large enough to hold lamb opened flat. Add lamb. Turn to coat with marinade. Cover and refrigerate at least 4 but not more than 8 hours, turning meat 3 or 4 times.

To make basting sauce, mix all ingredients except olive oil in a small bowl until blended. Gradually whisk in oil until smooth. Place lamb flat on broiler-pan rack (discard marinade). Brush with the sauce. Broil 4 to 5 inches from heat source 10 to 15 minutes per side, brushing with sauce 3 times, until a meat thermometer inserted in thickest part registers 140 degrees for medium-rare. Let stand 15 minutes before slicing.

Lamb Patties with Bacon

Serves 6 to 8

Adapted for your kitchen... from the original Walgreens recipe!

Walgreens Cafeterias 1940's ~ 1960's

2 pounds ground lamb shoulder
2 teaspoons salt
¼ teaspoon pepper
¼ pound sliced bacon
toothpicks

Preheat oven to 350 degrees. Mix ground lamb with seasonings. Shape into patties that are 1-inch thick. Wrap a strip of bacon around outside of each patty and fasten with toothpicks. Place on a greased 15x10-inch baking pan; bake for 45 minutes or until done.

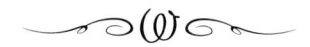

Lamb Croquettes

Serves 6 to 8

Adapted for your kitchen... from the original Walgreens recipe!

Walgreens Cafeterias 1940's ~ 1960's

2 pounds ground lamb shoulder
1½ cups bread crumbs
1 tablespoon Worcestershire sauce
1 tablespoon salt
¼ teaspoon pepper
1 cup milk
2 eggs
2 cups cracker crumbs

White sauce:
4 tablespoons butter, margarine or vegetable oil
4 tablespoons flour
2 cups milk, heated to boiling
1 small onion, finely minced

Mix ground lamb with bread crumbs, Worcestershire sauce, salt and pepper. Set aside. To prepare sauce, heat butter, blend in flour and cook 5 minutes. Remove from heat and add hot milk, stirring well. Mixture will be thick. Return to heat for 5 minutes, add minced onion; stir constantly. Combine lamb mixture with sauce and mix thoroughly. Set aside to cool. Form lamb mixture into cakes. Combine eggs and milk, and dip cakes into mixture (egg wash); dredge in cracker crumbs. Heat 2 or more inches of oil to 360 degrees in deep fryer. Deep fry until golden brown. Remove from oil and drain on wire rack or absorbent paper.

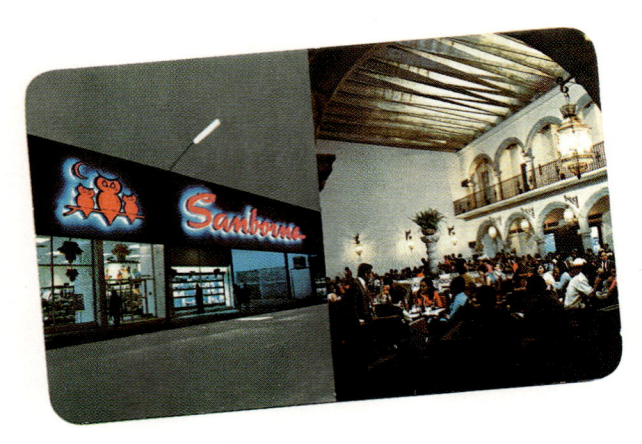

A 1970's postcard of Sanborns in Puebla, Mexico. The dining room was in an authentic, reconstructed 17th century colonial patio.

Calzone ~ Italian Easter Pie

Yield: 2 pies

Dough:
- 1½ cups flour
- 1 teaspoon baking powder
- ½ teaspoon salt
- ½ cup butter
- 2 eggs
- ¼ cup milk

Filling:
- 1 pound Italian sausage
- 2 pounds Italian ricotta cheese
- 1 8-ounce package shredded mozzarella cheese
- 3 eggs, slightly beaten
- 1 stick pepperoni, thinly sliced
- parsley, to taste

Glaze:
- 1 egg yolk, beaten
- 1 teaspoon milk

Preheat oven to 375 degrees. Cook and cool sausage; remove casings and crumble. Combine sausage with remaining filling ingredients; mix well and set aside. For dough, sift dry ingredients, work in butter until mealy like pie crust. Add milk to eggs and mix into dry ingredients, until it forms a ball. Add more flour if too sticky. Makes two balls of dough. Roll out dough to large circle. Fill one half of circle with half of filling. Fold other half of circle over filling to cover. Flute edges, repeat with other ball of dough and remaining filling. Place on greased cookie sheet. Bake for 35 to 40 minutes. Mix glaze ingredients. Brush pies with glaze while still hot.

Meal ~ in ~ One

Serves 4

- 1 1-pound Eckrich sausage, cut into 1-inch pieces
- ¼ cup olive oil
- 5 potatoes, peeled and cubed
- 1 small head cabbage, cored and chopped
- 1 small onion, chopped (optional)
- salt and pepper, to taste

Brown sausage in olive oil in Dutch oven. Add potatoes, cabbage, onion, salt and pepper. Cover and simmer for 40 minutes, stirring occasionally.

Spanish Sausage with Rice

Serves 6 to 8

Adapted for your kitchen... from the original Walgreens recipe!

Walgreen Grills in Puerto Rico, 1960's ~ 1980's

Originally called: Arroz con Longaniza

2 pounds Longaniza sausage (may substitute a good Italian sausage), sliced into 1-inch pieces
3 tablespoons olive oil
2 green peppers, seeded and chopped
2 tomatoes, peeled, seeded and chopped
1 onion, finely chopped
2 garlic cloves, finely chopped
2 sprigs fresh cilantro, finely chopped, or 2 teaspoons ground cilantro
1 teaspoon salt
2 packages Goya Sazan* (1.41-ounce box) with coriander and achiote
2 cups long-grain rice, uncooked
3 cups water

Sauté sausage in olive oil. Add green peppers, tomatoes, onion, garlic and cilantro. Sauté until tender. Add salt, Sazan, rice and water. Cook over low heat, covered, until water is absorbed and rice is cooked and fluffy. Serve immediately.

Note: *Available in the ethnic or specialty sections of grocery stores.

Smoked Sausage & Sauerkraut

Serves 6

1 1-pound smoked sausage, sliced diagonally
6 teaspoons cornstarch
3 cups water
¾ cup onion, chopped
2 tablespoons butter
2 14-ounce cans sauerkraut, drained
5 tablespoons brown or white sugar
1 teaspoon salt
1 teaspoon caraway seeds

Mix cornstarch with ¼-cup water. Set aside. Sauté chopped onions in butter until tender. Add sauerkraut, sugar, salt, caraway seeds and remaining water. Cook until soft. Stir in cornstarch and water mixture. When thickened, add cooked sausage and heat thoroughly; for approximately 15 minutes.

Country Sausage, Biscuits & Gravy

Serves 6

An original Hazelwood recipe!

1 1-pound package pork sausage (breakfast sausage)
1 stick butter
¼ cup flour
2 cups whole milk
salt and pepper, to taste
Bisquick biscuits, prepared per package directions

Heat 1 tablespoon butter in medium skillet. Crumble sausage into skillet and cook over medium heat until lightly browned, stirring occasionally. Drain well. Melt remaining butter in frying pan. Add flour and stir to blend. Gradually add milk (may add more to thin gravy, if necessary). Stir in sausage, salt and pepper. Serve with biscuits.

Note: A classic "rib sticker" country breakfast.

Sunday Brunch Casserole

Serves 8 to 10

1 1-pound package pork sausage
6 slices sourdough or day-old white bread
3 to 4 tablespoons butter or margarine, softened
1 8-ounce package shredded cheddar cheese
½ medium sweet red pepper, cut into thin strips
¼ cup green onion tops, sliced
3 eggs, beaten
1 10¾-ounce can cream of asparagus soup, undiluted
2 cups milk
½ teaspoon Dijon mustard
¼ teaspoon pepper

Preheat oven to 300 degrees. Heat 1 tablespoon butter in medium skillet. Crumble sausage into skillet and cook over medium heat until lightly browned, stirring occasionally. Drain well. Remove and discard crusts from bread, if desired. Spread remaining butter on bread, cube and place in lightly greased 13x9x2-inch baking dish. Sprinkle cheese, sausage, red pepper and onions (in order) over the bread cubes. In a bowl, beat eggs. Mix in soup, milk, mustard and pepper. Pour over bread mixture. Cover and refrigerate overnight. Bake, uncovered, 1 hour, or until knife comes out clean. Let stand for 5 minutes before cutting.

Christmas Breakfast Strata

Serves 8

- 1   1-pound package pork sausage
- 1   tablespoon butter or margarine
- 1   dozen eggs
- 2   cups milk
- 1   6-ounce box seasoned croutons
- 1   onion, chopped
- 1   cup mushrooms, sliced
- 2   cups cheddar or Swiss cheese, shredded

Heat butter in medium skillet. Crumble sausage into skillet and cook over medium heat until lightly browned, stirring occasionally. Drain well. Grease a 9x13-inch pan. Beat eggs and milk together. Place croutons on bottom of pan. Pour egg and milk mixture over croutons. Top with other ingredients. Refrigerate overnight or up to 24 hours. To prepare for a meal, cover and bake at 350 degrees for 30 minutes. Uncover and bake for 15 minutes more. Let set 5 minutes before cutting.

Egg~Sausage Soufflé

Serves 6

- 1   1-pound package pork sausage
- 1   tablespoon butter or margarine
- 6   eggs, beaten
- 2   cups milk
- 1   cup sharp cheddar cheese, shredded
- 2   slices bread, cubed
- 1   teaspoon dry mustard
- ½   teaspoon salt

Preheat oven to 350 degrees. Heat butter in medium skillet. Crumble sausage into skillet and cook over medium heat until lightly browned, stirring occasionally. Drain well. Mix remaining ingredients together. Add the sausage. Pour in a greased 8x8-inch pan, cover and refrigerate overnight. Bake, uncovered, for about 45 minutes, or until done.

Pennebaker's "Little Pig" Soufflé

Serves 4

- 1   1-pound package pork sausage
- 1   tablespoon butter or margarine
- 4   eggs, beaten
- 2   cups milk
- 1   teaspoon dry mustard
- 6   slices bread, cubed
- 2   cups cheddar cheese, shredded

Heat butter in medium skillet. Crumble sausage into skillet and cook over medium heat until lightly browned, stirring occasionally. Drain well. Beat eggs, adding milk and mustard. Grease medium-size glass baking dish. Mix bread crumbs and cheese together and place in dish. Layer sausage over bread crumbs and cheese. Pour milk and eggs over sausage. Refrigerate overnight. To prepare for a meal, bake at 325 degrees for 1 hour, or until done.

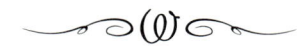

Egg~Sausage Casserole

Serves 6 to 8

- 1   1-pound package pork sausage
- 1   tablespoon butter or margarine
- 6   eggs, beaten by hand
- 2   cups milk
- 5   slices day-old white bread, cubed
- 2   dashes cayenne pepper
- ½   teaspoon dry mustard
- **butter or non-stick vegetable oil spray**
- ¾   cup sharp cheddar cheese, grated

Preheat oven to 325 degrees. Heat butter in medium skillet. Crumble sausage into skillet and cook over medium heat until lightly browned, stirring occasionally. Drain well. Combine all ingredients except cheese in large bowl. Butter or spray, with non-stick vegetable oil, a 13x9-inch baking dish. Sprinkle cheese on top before baking. Bake for 45 minutes.

Note: May be prepared one day before serving.

Wag's Breakfast Croissant

Serves 1

*Adapted for your kitchen...
from the original Walgreens recipe!*

*Wag's &
Humpty Dumpty Restaurants,
1970's ~ 1980's*

1 croissant
1 egg, scrambled
1 tablespoon butter or margarine
2½ ounces shaved ham, heated
¼ cup Velveeta or Cheese Whiz cheese, melted
parsley (optional)

Cut croissant open and place in toaster oven to warm; but do *not* toast. Scramble 1 egg in tablespoon butter or margarine. Place egg on bottom half of croissant; add heated, shaved ham. Top with melted cheese. Cover sandwich with top of croissant. Garnish with parsley, and serve.

Sweet Onion Quiche

Serves 6

1 tablespoon olive oil
3 cups sweet onions, thinly sliced
2 tablespoons butter
2 tablespoons shallots or scallions (green onions), minced
salt and pepper, freshly ground, to taste
nutmeg, to taste
¼ cup Swiss cheese, grated and lightly packed
3 large eggs, blended with whole milk (or half-and-half) to make 1½ cups of liquid
1 9-inch pre-baked pie shell

Preheat oven to 375 degrees. Heat olive oil in large sauce pan. Sauté sliced onions until soft, but not brown. In a separate pan, heat butter and sauté shallots (or scallions) briefly. Add to onions and continue cooking until mixture is tender. Season with salt, pepper and nutmeg. Let cool. Strew all but 2 tablespoons grated cheese in pie shell. Add onions to egg-milk mixture and pour into pie shell, up to ¼-inch of rim. Sprinkle with reserved cheese. Bake for 35 minutes, until puffed and brown. Cool slightly before cutting.

Kathy's Quiche

Serves 6

- 1 8-inch unbaked pie shell
- 4 slices of bacon
- 1 medium onion, sliced
- ¾ cup of milk
- 2 eggs, beaten
- ½ cup cheddar cheese, grated
- ½ teaspoon salt
- ½ teaspoon pepper
- 2 tablespoons parsley, chopped
- 1 pinch sugar
- 1 pinch nutmeg
- 1 dash red pepper

paprika

Preheat oven to 350 degrees. Chill pie shell, or place in freezer 4 to 5 minutes. Fry bacon until crisp; drain and reserve drippings. Crumble bacon. Cook onion in bacon drippings until transparent, stirring frequently. Combine eggs, milk, ¼-cup cheese, salt, pepper, parsley, sugar, nutmeg and red pepper in a large mixing bowl. Stir in bacon and onion and pour mixture into pie shell. Sprinkle with cheese and paprika. Bake in 350-degree oven for 30 minutes or until knife inserted in middle comes out clean. Cool slightly before cutting.

Texas Eggs

Serves 18

- 3 dozen eggs
- ½ cup milk
- ¼ cup butter, melted
- 2 cans cream of mushroom soup, undiluted
- ½ cup sherry
- ½ pound sharp cheddar cheese, shredded

paprika

Whisk eggs with milk. Scramble lightly in butter, just to soft stage. Layer scrambled eggs in flat, buttered baking dish. Mix soup and sherry. Spread over eggs. Sprinkle with cheese and paprika. Cover and refrigerate for 8 hours or longer. Bake, uncovered, at 250 degrees for 40 minutes to 1 hour or until bubbly and hot.

Fresh Spinacheese Omelette

Serves 1 to 2

Adapted for your kitchen... from the original Walgreens recipe!

Wag's & Humpty Dumpty Restaurants, 1970's ~ 1980's

3 eggs, at room temperature
3 shakes Lawry's seasoned salt
1½ to 2 tablespoons vegetable oil
½ cup fresh spinach, sautéed
¼ cup Velveeta or Cheese Whiz cheese, melted
parsley

Whisk together eggs and Lawry's seasoned salt. Heat oil; pour egg mixture into pan, while continually shaking pan in a circular motion. Sprinkle in half the sautéed spinach. Flip omelette over and continue to shake until set on both sides. Place omelette on warm plate, and sprinkle rest of sautéed spinach on one half of it. Pour half the cheese over the spinach. Fold omelette closed, and pour rest of cheese across the top. Garnish with parsley, and serve.

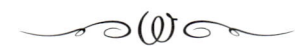

Ham & Cheese Omelette

Serves 1 to 2

Adapted for your kitchen... from the original Walgreens recipe!

Wag's & Humpty Dumpty Restaurants, 1970's ~ 1980's

3 eggs, at room temperature
3 shakes Lawry's seasoned salt
1½ to 2 ounces vegetable oil
¼ cup shaved ham, chopped and heated
¼ cup Velveeta or Cheese Whiz cheese, melted
parsley

Whisk together the eggs and Lawry's seasoned salt. Heat oil; pour egg mixture into pan. Add half of the ham, while continually shaking pan in a circular motion. Let side set; flip omelette over and continue shaking until set on both sides. Place omelette on warm plate, and add the remaining ham to one half of it. Pour half the cheese over ham. Fold the omelette closed, and pour rest of cheese across the top. Garnish with parsley, and serve.

Western Omelette

Serves 1 to 2

Adapted for your kitchen... from the original Walgreens recipe!

Wag's & Humpty Dumpty Restaurants, 1970's ~ 1980's

2   tablespoons butter
¾   cup green peppers, diced ¼-inch
1¾ cup onions, diced ¼-inch
1   cup shaved ham, chopped
1½ to 2 ounces vegetable oil
3   eggs, at room temperature
3   shakes Lawry's seasoned salt
parsley

In 2 tablespoons butter, sauté diced green peppers, onions and chopped shaved ham until soft; set aside. Heat oil. Whisk together eggs and salt; pour into hot oil. Add pepper, onion, ham mixture to eggs, while continually shaking pan in a circular motion. When one side is set, flip the omelette over to set other side. Remove omelette from pan; fold closed. Garnish with parsley, and serve.

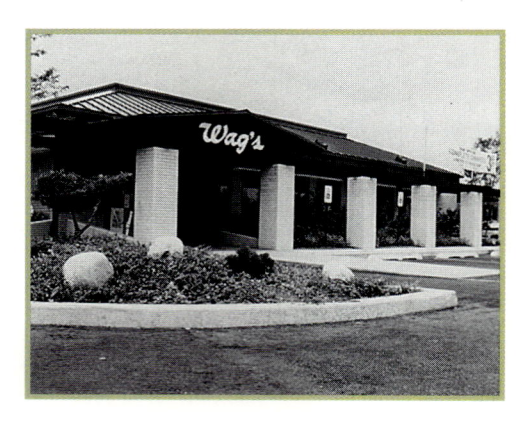

Wag's, Walgreens most successful restaurant chain, prospered with careful planning and tireless effort. In 1976, to ensure success, the company started its own restaurant manager training school.

Facing Page: *Italian Chicken with Polenta*
Photo: Scott Lanza, 1995
Stylist: F. Lynn Nelson

POULTRY

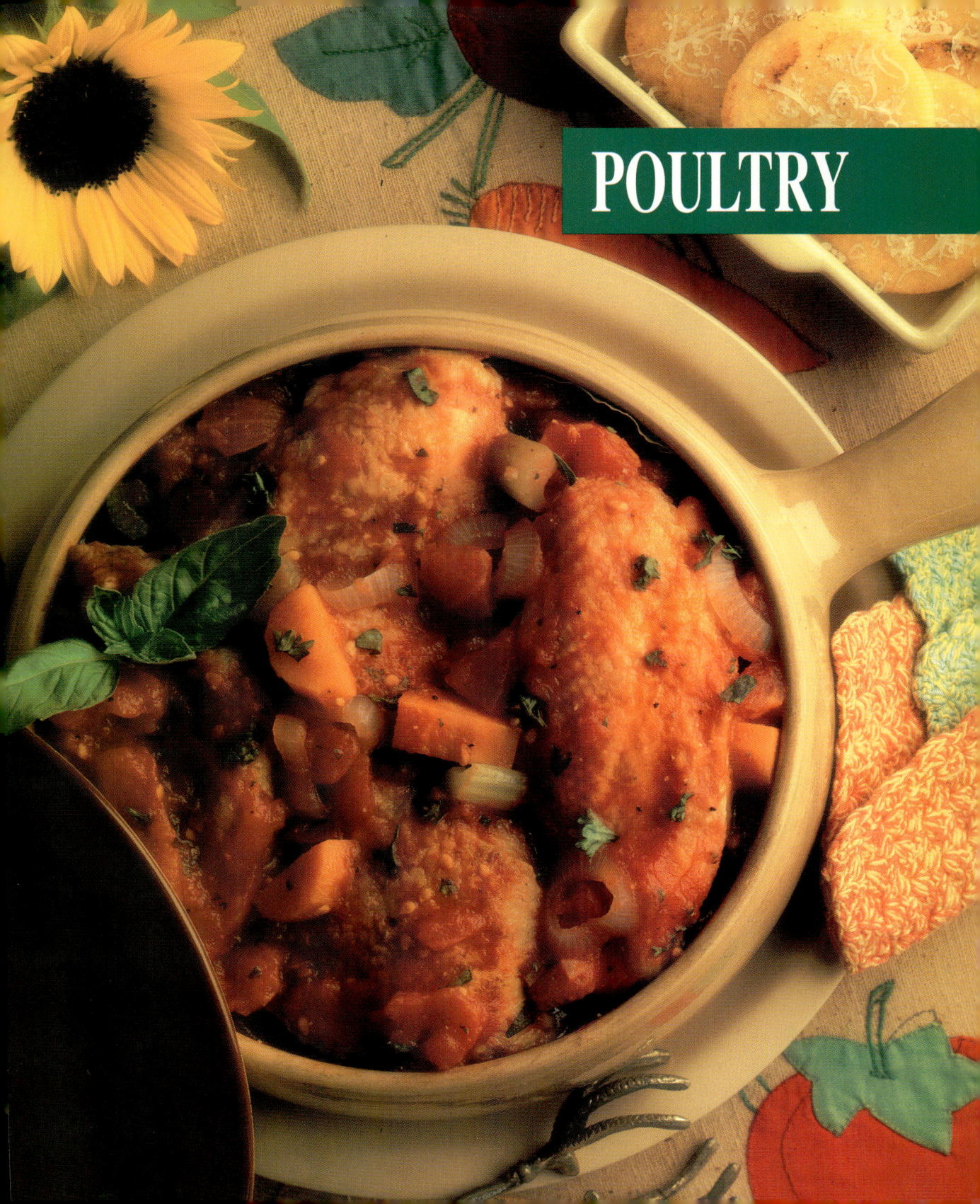

Wag's & Humpty Dumpty
Freestanding Favorites...
The Family Restaurants

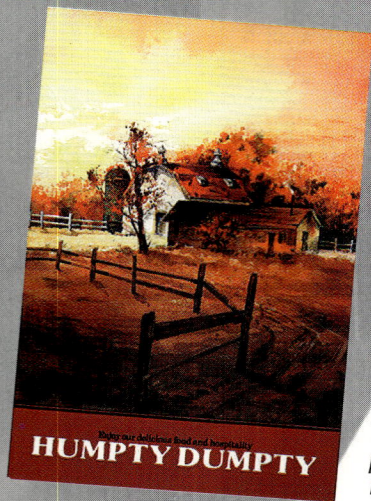

The Humpty Dumpty coffee shops, purchased in 1976, provided the recipe for Wag's tasty omelet.

During 1976, as America celebrated its Bicentennial, Walgreens was ushering in a new era of independence with the opening of *Wag's*, a chain of freestanding restaurants. Named after the company's stock exchange letters, *WAG*, and free from the bonds of the drugstore, this newest investment was pleasant, affordable and accessible ~ and open 24 hours a day! Walgreens also acquired four *Humpty Dumpty* restaurants the same year, bringing the Wag's idea to Arizona.

Ahead of its time, with quality and health in mind, the Wag's menu included freshly-brewed coffee and the "best breakfast in town," ice-cream specialties, all-you-can-eat specials and bread baked right in the kitchen! In 1981, *Appeteasers* and low-cal entrées (on the *Feelin' Fit...Feelin' Good* menu) were added; and Wag's won the *National Restaurant Association's Great Menu Award* for its children's menu. More than a coffee shop, Wag's was a much-loved family affair, and went on to become Walgreens most successful food service venture.

Cinnamon Chicken with Couscous

Serves 6 to 8

- 1 tablespoon butter
- 1 tablespoon olive oil
- 4 pounds chicken parts
- 2 cups onion, chopped
- 8 small yellow onions
- 2 garlic cloves, crushed
- 1 6-ounce can tomato paste
- 3 cinnamon sticks
- 2 navel oranges, peeled and coarsely chopped
- 2 14½-ounce cans chicken broth
- 2 chicken bouillon cubes
- 1 teaspoon salt
- ¼ teaspoon pepper
- 2 10-ounce boxes couscous
- ½ cup golden raisins
- ½ cup pine nuts
- 2 large tomatoes, quartered
- 1 large yellow pepper, julienne

Melt butter in olive oil in a Dutch oven over medium-high heat. Add half the chicken pieces; brown on both sides, about 5 minutes. Remove to plate. Brown remaining chicken in pan drippings and remove to plate. Discard drippings. In pan, mix chopped onion, yellow onions, garlic, tomato paste, cinnamon sticks, oranges, broth, bouillon, salt and pepper; mix well. Return chicken to pan. Cover and bring to boil. Reduce heat and simmer for 1 hour.

Prepare the couscous per package directions, adding the golden raisins and pine nuts, along with couscous, to the boiling water. Cover and let set according to package directions. Spoon couscous onto heated serving platter and top with chicken pieces. In saucepan, add tomatoes and yellow pepper and simmer until pepper is tender and crispy, about 5 to 10 minutes. To serve, put couscous and chicken on pasta plates and spoon sauce over top.

Chicken Saltimbocca

Serves 4 to 5

- 6 chicken breasts, boned, skinned and halved
- ½ cup dry bread crumbs
- 2 tablespoons Parmesan cheese, grated
- 2 tablespoons parsley, chopped
- ¼ cup butter or margarine, melted
- 2 tablespoons oil
- 6 thin slices of prosciutto (Italian ham)
- 6 slices mozzarella cheese

Preheat oven to 350 degrees. Put chicken breasts between two pieces of wax paper and pound thin. Combine bread crumbs with Parmesan cheese and parsley. Dip chicken lightly in melted butter or margarine and then in seasoned bread crumbs. Brown chicken in oil and put in baking dish. Put 1 slice of prosciutto and 1 slice of mozzarella cheese on each piece of chicken and bake about 20 minutes, or until cheese has melted.

Chicken Cacciatore ~ A Garlic Lover's Recipe

Serves 2 to 4

- 1 pound chicken breasts, boned, skinned and cut into pieces
- 3 tablespoons vegetable oil
- 1 medium yellow onion, chopped
- 1 large whole bulb garlic, peeled and chopped
- 1 10¾-ounce can Campbell's tomato soup
- 1 cup Chianti wine
- 1 teaspoon oregano
- ½ teaspoon salt
- 1 green pepper, cut into strips
- 8 ounces thin spaghetti, cooked per package directions

Heat vegetable oil in large frying pan; add chicken, stirring often until no longer pink. Add chopped onion and garlic. Stir in undiluted tomato soup, Chianti, oregano and salt. Bring to a boil and reduce heat. Simmer partly covered 15 to 20 minutes, stirring occasionally. Then add green pepper; simmer for an additional 15 minutes. To serve, divide spaghetti among plates and top with cacciatore mixture. Serve immediately.

Note: This quantity is a large serving for two. However, if you want a smaller meal, make more spaghetti and stretch to serve four. Also, stove fan may be needed during cooking as garlic smell may be strong.

Chicken Milanese

Serves 8

10 chicken breasts, boned and skinned
½ cup flour
4 eggs, beaten
3 tablespoons parsley, chopped
2 to 3 cups bread crumbs
Wesson oil
3 tablespoons olive oil
paprika, to taste
garlic salt, to taste
salt and pepper, to taste
butter (optional)
parsley, chopped (optional)

Preheat oven to 350 degrees. Wash chicken breasts; dry with paper towels. Put flour in a paper bag. Add 2 pieces of chicken at a time; shake, thoroughly coating chicken. Combine beaten eggs and parsley. Dip chicken in egg mixture, roll in bread crumbs, flatten with hand and roll again until thoroughly coated. Let sit for 15 minutes. Put ½-inch Wesson oil in bottom of skillet. Add 3 tablespoons of olive oil. Sprinkle chicken with paprika, garlic salt, salt and pepper. Fry chicken 5 minutes on each side until golden. Remove from skillet and put on cookie rack on top of cookie sheet. Bake for 20 minutes. May drizzle butter and parsley on top before baking.

Papa's Only Chicken Meal

Serves 6 to 8

6 chicken breasts, boned, skinned and cut into strips
olive oil
1 small onion, thinly sliced
1 garlic clove, thinly sliced
1 14½-ounce can Italian plum tomatoes
1 15-ounce can baby peas
salt and pepper, to taste
mashed potatoes or rice, prepared

Heat enough olive oil to cover bottom of electric frying pan and sauté onions. Add garlic until golden. Remove onion and garlic. Fry chicken breasts until golden. Add tomatoes and onion-garlic mixture. Add peas. Simmer until peas are cooked. Add salt and pepper. Serve with mashed potatoes or rice.

Italian Chicken with Polenta

Serves 8

- 2 small broilers or fryers, cut up
- 2 tablespoons olive or salad oil
- ½ cup onions, sliced
- 2 garlic cloves, minced
- 1 cup carrots, diced
- 1 cup celery, diced
- 2 tablespoons parsley
- 1 teaspoon salt
- ½ teaspoon pepper
- ½ teaspoon dried basil
- 1 bay leaf
- 1 14½-ounce can whole tomatoes, drained
- 1 15-ounce can tomato sauce

Polenta:
- 4 cups water
- 1 pinch of salt
- 2 cups cornmeal

Heat oil in Dutch oven and add chicken. Brown chicken on all sides and remove from pot. Add onions, garlic, carrots, celery, parsley, salt, pepper, basil and bay leaf. Sauté until golden brown. Add tomatoes and tomato sauce, mashing tomatoes with fork. Bring to a boil and simmer for about 20 minutes. Add browned chicken and cook for 45 minutes to 1 hour. While chicken is cooking, bring water and salt to a boil. Reduce to a simmer and gradually stir in cornmeal. Cook for 15 to 20 minutes, stirring constantly. Pour polenta into a moistened 1½-quart dish. Let stand for 5 minutes. Invert dish onto serving platter. Slice polenta; serve with chicken.

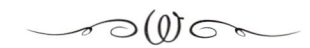

Chicken Fajita Potatoes

Serves 4

- 4 large (2 pounds) baking potatoes
- 1 medium red or green sweet pepper, cut into bite-size strips
- 1 small (¼-cup) onion, chopped
- 2 tablespoons margarine or butter
- 1 tablespoon taco seasoning mix
- 6 ounces chicken breast, boned, skinned, cooked and cut into strips
- ½ cup cheddar cheese, shredded
- ½ cup Monterey Jack cheese, shredded

Chicken Fajita Potatoes, *continued on next page.*

Chicken Fajita Potatoes, continued.

1   2¼-ounce can sliced, pitted, ripe olives, drained
2   tablespoons green chilies, diced
1   cup salsa
dairy sour cream (optional)
guacamole (optional)
salsa (optional)

Scrub potatoes with a brush; pat dry. Prick skins with a fork. Arrange potatoes on a 9-inch microwave-safe pie plate. Cover loosely with wax paper. Cook on 100 percent power (high) for 15 to 18 minutes, or until tender; turn the dish twice during cooking. Meanwhile, prepare the filling. Heat margarine in a medium saucepan, cook sweet pepper and onion over medium heat until tender. Add taco seasoning mix. Cook and stir for 1 minute. Remove from heat. Stir in chicken, cheeses, olives and chili peppers. Cut a lengthwise slit in top of each potato. Press potatoes open. Divide chicken mixture among potatoes. Spoon ¼-cup salsa over each potato. Cover loosely with wax paper. Microwave on high for 5 to 7 minutes, or until heated through. If desired, serve with sour cream, guacamole and salsa.

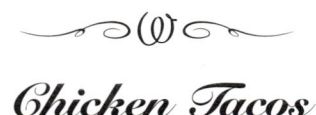

Chicken Tacos

Serves 2

Adapted for your kitchen... from the original Walgreens recipe!

Sanborns, Mexico, 1946 ~ 1984

Originally called: Tacos de Pollo

4   corn tortillas
2   tablespoons vegetable oil
1   cup chicken, cooked and shredded
4 to 8 wooden toothpicks
½   cup refried beans (frijoles)
1   tablespoon cotija cheese* or Parmesan cheese, grated
2   totopos* (deep-fried tortillas) or tostados
½   cup prepared guacamole
6 to 8 lettuce leaves
6 to 8 sprigs Chinese parsley (fresh cilantro)

Heat 1 tablespoon oil in fry pan; briefly sauté tortillas. Remove; fill with chicken, securing top with a wooden toothpick. Add remaining oil to fry pan; sauté filled tortillas to desired degree of crispiness. Drain on paper towel. To serve, prepare platter, placing fried tortillas in the center. On one side, mound refried beans with cheese grated on top. On the other side, make a bed of lettuce leaves. Put guacamole on lettuce and stick two totopos or tostados in mound of guacamole. Lay sprigs of Chinese parsley over top.

Note: *Available in the ethnic or specialty sections of grocery stores.

Totopo Jalisciense ~ Crisp Chicken Tortilla

Serves 6

Adapted for your kitchen... from the original Walgreens recipe!

Sanborns, Mexico, 1946 ~ 1984

- 6 flour tortillas, uncooked
- 4 tablespoons vegetable oil
- 4 tablespoons refried black or red beans
- 1½ cups lettuce, shredded
- 1 pound chicken breast, boned, skinned, boiled and shredded
- 2 ripe avocados, peeled, seeded and sliced
- 1 7-ounce jar green (poblano) chilies, sliced
- 1 Mexican jijomate* (a small, green tomato with a leaf around it) or substitute 1 small tomato, sliced
- 4 ounces cotija* cheese or ½-cup Parmesan cheese, grated
- 1¼ cups vinegar

Heat oil and pan-fry tortilla, not too crisp. Remove. Portion each of the following ingredients among the cooked tortillas (totopos). Start with refried beans; then add shredded lettuce. Top with chicken pieces. Then arrange avocado slice on tortillas (totopos) and top avocado with green chili. As garnish, arrange jijomate or tomato slice on uncovered piece of tortilla. Grate cotija or Parmesan cheese on tomato. The entire tortilla should be completely covered. Pass the vinegar separately at the table after plates are served.

Note: *Available in the ethnic or specialty sections of grocery stores.

Chicken Enchiladas Suiza

Serves 10 to 12

- 3 chicken breasts, boned, skinned, chopped and sautéed
- 1 12-ounce jar salsa sauce
- 1 4-ounce can green chilies, chopped
- 1 half pint carton half-and-half
- 3 tablespoons olive oil
- 1 12-pack tortillas
- 1 large onion, chopped
- 1 16-ounce package Monterey Jack cheese, shredded

Preheat oven to 350 degrees. Combine first 3 ingredients. Pour half-and-half in bowl. Heat oil in fry pan; lightly brown tortilla in oil. Dip tortilla in half-and-half and fill with chicken mixture. Roll with seam side down. Place in 9x13-inch pan. Pour remaining half-and-half over tortillas. Top with onions and cheese. Bake for 25 to 30 minutes.

Swiss Chicken Enchiladas

Serves 4

Adapted for your kitchen... from the original Walgreens recipe!

Sanborns, Mexico, 1946 ~ 1984

Originally called: Salsa Suiza (Swiss Sauce)

- 3 10-ounce bottles Old El Paso green chili enchilada sauce
- 1 pint heavy whipping cream
- ½ pound Chihuahua cheese*, grated
    or 1-pound package shredded cheese with taco seasoning
- 4 tortillas, uncooked
- 1 tablespoon vegetable oil
- 1 cup chicken breast, boned, skinned, cooked and hand shredded

Preheat broiler. Whip the cream, then blend in the bottles of green sauce until smooth. Heat oil in skillet and sauté tortillas, one at a time. Drain on paper towel. Put tortillas on foil-lined broiler pan. Fill tortillas, layering with shredded chicken, then the green sauce and cream mixture, topped with Chihuahua cheese or shredded cheese with taco seasoning. Set tortillas under the hot broiler, only until cheese melts. Serve immediately.

Note: *Available in the ethnic or specialty sections of grocery stores.

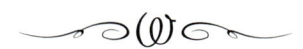

Szechwan Chicken Over Steamed Rice

Serves 4 to 6

Adapted for your kitchen... from the original Walgreens recipe!

Corporate Cafeteria, Walgreen Company Headquarters

- 1 pound chicken breasts, boned and skinned, julienne
- 2 cups and 2 tablespoons vegetable oil
- 2 carrots, peeled and cut on bias
- 2 celery stalks, cut on bias
- 2 medium onions, peeled, julienne
- 1 green pepper, seeded, cut in cubes
- ½ red pepper, seeded, cut in cubes
- 1 cup homemade Szechwan sauce or 10-ounce bottle San-J sauce
- ¼ pound fresh pea pods
- 1 8¾-ounce (4⅜-ounce drained) can baby corn, drained
- 2 cups water
- 2 tablespoons cornstarch
- 2 cups rice, cooked per package directions

Heat 2 cups of oil in an electric skillet or deep fat fryer to 350 degrees. Put the chicken strips in a wire cooking basket; lower chicken into oil and cook until no longer pink. Remove and set aside. In a wok or a deep-fry pan, heat the other 2 tablespoons oil, sauté carrots, then celery and peppers, then onions, followed by pea pods and baby corn. When the vegetables are almost done, add meat, water and Szechwan sauce; bring to boil. Dissolve corn starch in a small amount of water. Add to chicken; stir to thicken. Serve over steamed rice.

Chicken or Pork Chow Mein ~ Shanghai Style

Serves 4 to 6

Adapted for your kitchen... from the original Walgreens recipe!

Corporate Cafeteria, Walgreen Company Headquarters

- 1 pound chicken breasts (or lean pork), boned, skinned and thinly sliced
- ¾ cup bottled Cantonese sauce
- 2 tablespoons vegetable oil
- 1½ tablespoons fresh garlic, chopped
- 1 tablespoon fresh ginger, peeled and chopped
- 1 medium yellow onion, julienne
- 1 cup carrots, julienne
- 1 cup celery, julienne
- 1 cup Chinese cabbage (bok choy), chopped
- 1 cup water
- ¼ cup bottled Chow Chow sauce
- ¼ cup green onion, cut in 2-inch pieces on a diagonal
- 1 12-ounce package chow mein noodles

Marinate chicken (or pork) in ¼-cup Cantonese sauce for 1 hour or longer. Heat wok or frying pan over high heat. Add oil, garlic, ginger and chicken (pork); stir-fry until lightly browned. Add onion, carrot, celery, bok choy; stir-fry for one minute. Add water, Chow Chow sauce, remaining Cantonese sauce and mix thoroughly until hot. Add green onion and remove from heat. Serve over chow mein noodles.

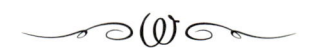

Chicken Hot Dish

Serves 8

- 3 cups chicken breasts, boned, skinned and cooked
- 2 10¾-ounce cans cream of chicken soup
- ½ cup milk
- 1 8-ounce can water chestnuts, drained and sliced
- 1 5-ounce can chow mein noodles
- 1 cup celery, diced
- 2 tablespoons onion, chopped
- 1 teaspoon lemon juice
- ½ cup Miracle Whip salad dressing
- ½ cup cashews, for topping

Preheat oven to 350 degrees. Combine all ingredients except cashews in large bowl. Spread in 2-quart casserole. Top with cashews. Bake until bubbly, approximately 1 hour.

Soul Chicken Stir-Fry with Black-Eyed Peas

Serves 4 to 6

- ¾ cup salad dressing (Miracle Whip) or mayonnaise
- 1 tablespoon and 1 teaspoon jerk (spicy Caribbean) seasoning
- 1 garlic clove, minced
- 4 large chicken breasts, boned, skinned, halved and cut into strips
- 1 15½-ounce can black-eyed peas, drained and rinsed
- 1 15¼-ounce can whole kernel corn, drained
- 4 green onions, cut into 1-inch strips
- 1 small red pepper, cut into strips

rice, cooked per package directions and heated

Mix salad dressing, jerk seasoning and garlic. In a large skillet, heat mixture on medium heat until just simmering. Add chicken; sauté, cooking and stirring, about 3 minutes, until chicken is no longer pink. Add remaining ingredients. Stir-fry about 5 minutes more. Serve over hot rice

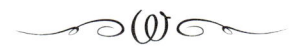

Oven-Barbecued Chicken

Serves 8

- 2 frying chickens, skinned and cut up
- ¾ cup onions, chopped
- ½ cup margarine
- ¾ cup catsup
- ¼ cup water
- 2 tablespoons lemon juice
- 2 tablespoons sugar
- 3 tablespoons Worcestershire sauce
- 1 tablespoon prepared mustard

salt and pepper, to taste

Preheat oven to 350 degrees. Sauté onions in margarine. Add remaining ingredients, except chicken, and simmer 15 minutes. Place chicken pieces in roasting pan; pour sauce over. Cover and bake for 30 minutes. Uncover and bake another 30 to 45 minutes, basting several times.

Dixie Fried Chicken

Serves 6 to 8

Adapted for your kitchen... from the original Walgreens recipe!

Corky's late 1960's, early 1970's

Robin Hood & Briargate Restaurants, 1970's ~ 1980's

2 2½-pound chickens, cut up
ice water, salted
1 cup flour
1 teaspoon salt
¼ teaspoon white pepper
⅛ teaspoon cayenne pepper
lard, oil or vegetable shortening, for deep-frying

Gravy:
3 tablespoons flour
1 to 1½ cups milk
salt and pepper, freshly ground

mashed potatoes and hot biscuits, prepared

Soak chicken pieces in salted ice water for one hour or more. Remove from salted water, rinse and shake dry. Fill an electric skillet or deep fat fryer 1 to 1½-inches; heat to 360 degrees. Season flour with salt, pepper and cayenne. Dredge chicken pieces, both sides, in seasoned flour (may also coat chicken by shaking in a brown paper bag), shaking off excess flour. Prop in hot fat and deep fry 6 to 8 minutes. Turn and cook other side. Turn one more time and cook until chicken is browned and also tender when forked. Drain on paper towel and then transfer to warm serving platter. To prepare gravy, pour off all but 2 tablespoons fat from skillet; add 3 tablespoons flour and cook until bubbly. Gradually stir in milk, stirring until gravy is thickened. Season with salt and freshly ground pepper. Serve with chicken, mashed potatoes, peas and hot biscuits.

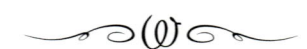

Deep~Fried Chicken

Serves 6 to 8

Adapted for your kitchen... from the original Walgreens recipe!

Walgreens Cafeterias 1940's ~ 1960's

3 frying chickens, cut up

Batter:
1 egg
1 cup milk
½ cup water
1 teaspoon sugar
1 teaspoon salt
1½ cups flour

1 cup cracker crumbs

Deep-Fried Chicken, continued on next page.

Deep-Fried Chicken, *continued.*

Beat egg; add milk and water. Sift together sugar, salt and flour. Mix seasoned flour with liquids; blend until creamy. Batter should be consistency of heavy cream. Heat 1 to 2 inches of oil in heavy skillet, electric skillet or deep fat fryer; to 350 to 375 degrees. Pat chicken pieces dry, dip in batter and sprinkle lightly with cracker crumbs. Fry in deep fat until golden brown. Remove from fat with tongs or a slotted spoon and place on a wire rack.

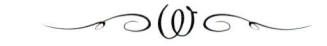

Chicken Robin Hood

Serves 6

Adapted for your kitchen… from the original Walgreens recipe!

Robin Hood & Briargate Restaurants, 1970's ~ 1980's

2	2½-pound fryers, cut up
1	cup flour
1	dash cayenne pepper
1	teaspoon salt
¼	teaspoon white pepper
4	tablespoons oil
4	tablespoons butter
2	medium onions, coarsely chopped
1	pound fresh mushrooms, stems removed, coarsely chopped
1	green pepper, seeded and coarsely chopped
2	tablespoons chicken base or bouillon
2	14½-ounce cans chicken broth, heated to boiling
1	28-ounce can tomatoes, squeezed dry, seeded and chopped
½	cup sherry
	rice pilaf, prepared

Preheat oven to 350 degrees. Mix flour with cayenne, salt and white pepper. Dredge chicken pieces in ½-cup of the flour, reserving other ½-cup. Heat 2 tablespoons oil and 2 tablespoons butter and sauté chicken pieces until lightly browned. Remove chicken to a baking dish. In another saucepan heat remaining 2 tablespoons oil and 2 tablespoons butter. Sauté onions, mushrooms, green peppers and chicken base until soft. Add remaining ½-cup flour; blend and cook until bubbly. Add hot chicken broth gradually and bring to a boil. Reduce heat. Add squeezed, chopped tomatoes. Add sherry and stir. Pour sauce over chicken in baking dish. Bake for 30 minutes. Serve with rice pilaf.

Puerto Rican Chicken with Rice

Serves 8

Adapted for your kitchen… from the original Walgreens recipe!

Walgreen Grills in Puerto Rico, 1960's ~ 1980's

Originally called: Arroz con Pollo

1   2½-pound chicken, skinned and cut into serving-size pieces
½   teaspoon white pepper
¼   teaspoon garlic powder
1   teaspoon salt
1½ cups sofrito (*see recipe below*) or 12-ounce bottle Goya sofrito*
2   packages Goya Sazan* (1.41-ounce box) with coriander and achiote
1   quart water
1½ pounds white rice, uncooked
1½ tablespoons stuffed olives, chopped

Sofrito:
1   cup onion, coarsely chopped
1   cup green pepper, coarsely chopped
1   garlic clove, finely minced
½   cup olive oil

Season chicken with salt, pepper and garlic powder. Next, prepare sofrito. Combine sofrito ingredients in a skillet and cook until vegetables are tender. Heat olive oil in a soup or stew pot. Fry chicken until lightly browned. Add the sofrito, chopped olives and water. Reduce heat and simmer until chicken is tender. Add rice and Sazan; mix and cook over medium-low heat until rice is fluffy, and all the water is absorbed.

Note: *Available in the ethnic or specialty sections of grocery stores.

Chicken with Artichokes & Wild Rice

Serves 4

1   whole chicken or 8 pieces of chicken
    salt, pepper and paprika, to taste
5 to 6 tablespoons of butter or margarine
1   14½-ounce can artichoke hearts, drained
1   small onion, minced
½   pint fresh or 7-ounce jar sliced mushrooms
½   cup sherry
1   teaspoon dried rosemary
1   tablespoon corn starch
1½ cups chicken broth
1   package Uncle Ben's long grain & wild rice,
        cooked per package directions (optional)

Chicken with Artichokes & Wild Rice, continued on next page.

Chicken with Artichokes & Wild Rice, *continued.*

Preheat oven to 350 degrees. Sprinkle chicken with salt, pepper and paprika to taste. In a skillet, brown chicken in 3 tablespoons butter or margarine. When brown, transfer to 2-quart casserole dish. Arrange drained artichoke hearts between chicken pieces, add remaining butter to drippings in skillet. Add onions, sauté until tender. Add mushrooms. Cook for about 2 minutes. Stir in sherry and rosemary. Cook a few minutes. Dissolve corn starch with little chicken broth; add dissolved corn starch and remaining chicken broth. Stir until thickened. Cook 5 minutes and pour over chicken. Cover and bake for 45 minutes to 1 hour. Serve with long grain & wild rice.

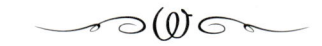

Chicken a la King

Serves 6

Adapted for your kitchen... from the original Walgreens recipe!

Walgreens Cafeterias 1940's ~ 1960's

3 cups chicken, cooked and cubed
3 tablespoons pimentos, diced
2 tablespoons green pepper, chopped
¼ pound mushrooms, sliced
2 tablespoons oil

Velouté sauce:
6 tablespoons butter, margarine, or oil
6 tablespoons flour
1 teaspoon salt
¼ teaspoon pepper
2 cups milk
2 cups canned chicken broth
1 tablespoon sherry

6 patty shells

Bring milk and chicken stock to boil. In another saucepan heat margarine or oil; blend flour and seasoning, stirring constantly. Bring to boil. Remove from heat. Add boiling milk, stirring until smooth. Return to heat, bring to boil, stirring constantly. Combine cubed chicken with sauce. Sauté diced green peppers, pimentos and mushrooms in 2 tablespoons oil. Combine with cream sauce. Mix thoroughly and bring to a boil. Season to taste. Spoon chicken into patty shells and serve.

Smith's Crab~Stuffed Chicken

Serves 8

- 4 large chicken breasts, boned, skinned and halved
- ¼ cup butter or margarine
- ¼ cup all-purpose flour
- ¾ cup milk
- ¾ cup chicken broth
- ⅓ cup dry, white wine
- ¼ cup onion, chopped
- 1 6-ounce can crab meat, drained, cleaned and flaked
- 1 7-ounce (4-ounce drained) can chopped mushrooms, drained
- ½ cup saltine crackers, coarsely crumbled
- 2 tablespoons parsley, snipped
- ½ teaspoon salt
- 1 dash pepper
- 1 cup process Swiss cheese, shredded

paprika

Preheat oven to 350 degrees. Place each chicken piece, boned side up, between 2 pieces of wax paper. Pound lightly with meat mallet to ⅛-inch thick. In saucepan, melt 3 tablespoons of butter; blend in flour. Add milk, broth and wine all at once; cook and stir until bubbly. Set aside. In skillet, cook onion in remaining 1 tablespoon butter until tender. Stir in crab, mushrooms, cracker crumbs, parsley, ½-teaspoon salt and dash of pepper. Stir in 2 tablespoons of the sauce. To stuff chicken, top each chicken piece with ¼-cup crab mixture. Fold sides in and roll up. Place seam side down in 12x7½x2-inch baking dish. Pour remaining sauce over. Bake, covered, for 1 hour. Uncover; top with cheese and a little paprika. Bake 2 more minutes.

Bacon~Wrapped Chicken Breasts

Serves 6 to 8

- 4 whole chicken breasts, boned, skinned and halved
- 8 bacon slices
- 4 ounces chipped beef
- 1 10¾-ounce can golden or cream of mushroom soup
- ½ pint sour cream

paprika

Preheat oven to 275 degrees. Wrap each chicken breast half in bacon. Cover the bottom of a greased 8x12-inch baking dish with chipped beef. Arrange chicken on top of this. Blend soup and sour cream and pour over chicken breasts. Sprinkle with paprika. Refrigerate at this point, if desired. Bake, uncovered, for 3 hours.

Texas Chicken Breast Cutlets

Serves 4

4 chicken breasts, boned and skinned
1½ cups dry bread crumbs or cracker crumbs, finely crushed
½ cup grated Parmesan or Romano cheese
2 tablespoons parsley flakes
½ teaspoon garlic salt
2 eggs, beaten
1 tablespoon water
4 tablespoons corn oil
1 cup sliced mushrooms
½ cup butter, melted
½ to ¼-cup lemon juice
thin lemon slices
parsley sprigs

Preheat oven to 350 degrees. Divide each chicken breast into 2 cutlets. Combine bread or cracker crumbs, cheese, parsley flakes and garlic salt. Mix beaten eggs and water together. Dip each cutlet into egg mixture, then into crumbs. Heat oil in large skillet and brown cutlets on each side until golden brown. Remove cutlets to flat baking dish. Sauté mushrooms briefly in oil used to brown cutlets. Spoon mushrooms over cutlets. In small saucepan, melt butter and add lemon juice. Pour over chicken and mushrooms. Bake for 20 to 25 minutes (allow 30 to 35 minutes if prepared ahead and cooled). Garnish with lemon slices and sprigs of parsley.

Lil's No~Peek Chicken Breasts

Serves 6

1¾ cups quick-cooking rice (uncooked)
½ cup water
6 chicken breasts or 1 whole chicken, cut up
1 10¾-ounce can cream of chicken soup
1 10¾-ounce can cream of mushroom soup
1 10¾-ounce can cream of celery soup
1 7-ounce (4-ounce drained) can chopped mushrooms
1 package onion soup mix

Preheat oven to 325 degrees. Place rice in 9x13x2-inch baking pan. Pour water over rice. Place chicken on top. Combine undiluted soups and add mushrooms. Pour on top of chicken and rice. Sprinkle onion soup on top. Cover with foil and bake for 1½ hours.

Julie's Chicken Breasts Divan

Serves 8

1 bunch fresh broccoli
3 to 4 tablespoons butter or margarine
8 single chicken breasts
1 cup mayonnaise
2 14½-ounce cans chicken broth
1 teaspoon curry powder
¼ cup lemon juice
4 ounces cheddar cheese, shredded
bread crumbs

Preheat oven to 350 degrees. Blanch broccoli. Heat butter in skillet. Sauté chicken breasts on both sides, only until lightly browned. Arrange broccoli in dish; then arrange chicken. Mix mayonnaise, chicken soup, curry powder and lemon juice; pour over chicken and broccoli. Top with cheese. Sprinkle with crumbs for color. Bake for 20 to 30 minutes or until hot.

Marinated, Grilled Chicken Breasts with Citrus Salsa

Serves 4 to 6

4 chicken breasts, boned, trimmed and lightly pounded

Tequila marinade:
¼ cup lime juice
¼ cup olive oil
2 jalapeno peppers, seeded and sliced very thinly
1 tablespoon Tequila

Citrus salsa:
1 orange, chopped
1 grapefruit, chopped
4 scallions (green onions), chopped
1 cup yellow and red cherry tomatoes, chopped
¼ cup fresh cilantro, chopped
zest of 1 orange
zest of 1 lime

lettuce leaves

Combine all the marinade ingredients. Marinate chicken for 1 hour. Remove from marinade and charcoal-grill until done. Meanwhile, combine all the salsa ingredients and refrigerate. To serve, place chicken on a bed of lettuce and spoon salsa on top.

Chicken Breasts in White Wine

Serves 4

4 chicken breasts (1⅓ to 1½ pounds total, bone in)
2 teaspoons chef's salt
1 teaspoon dry tarragon
2 to 3 garlic cloves
2 to 3 tablespoons shortening
    (preferably 1 tablespoon butter and 1 to 2 tablespoons "high-smoking-point" shortening, like peanut oil, lard or chicken fat)
1 cup white white
1 tablespoon parsley, finely chopped
¼ teaspoon black pepper, freshly ground
½ teaspoon sugar; or, to taste
Juice of ½ lemon (optional)

Chef's salt:
1 cup salt
1 tablespoon paprika
1 teaspoon black pepper, freshly ground
¼ teaspoon white pepper
¼ teaspoon celery salt
¼ teaspoon garlic salt (*not* garlic powder)

Mix chef's salt ingredients well and keep in covered jar.

Bone breasts: with a sharp knife, cut bones away from breast meat.
The easiest way to do this is as follows: Place breast skin-side down and press with your palm–be careful not to cut yourself on the small bones! Hold knife flat, parallel with the thin bone of breast, and cut immediately under bones. After bones are loosened from meat, pull them to the side and cut off tendon at shoulder, where wing joins breast.

Prepare chicken: sprinkle both sides of chicken breasts with chef's salt and tarragon. 30 minutes before serving time, crush garlic cloves with flat side of knife. Heat 1 tablespoon butter and 1 tablespoon other shortening in skillet over high heat. Add crushed garlic. When fat is hot, add breasts, skin-side down; add remaining shortening. Cook 2 or 3 minutes. Reduce heat to medium, cover skillet, and cook 5 minutes. Add ¼-cup wine in small amounts, pouring it around chicken, but not on it! Loosen breasts in case they stick to the pan. Cover and cook another 10 minutes. Add remaining wine, parsley, pepper, sugar and (optional) lemon juice. Cover, increase heat to high and cook 2 or 3 more minutes.

Move to serving platter, and spoon pan juices over chicken. (There will be very little juice, but it will be very tasty.) Serve at once.

Sautéed Lemon Chicken Breasts

Serves 6

*Adapted for your kitchen...
from the original Walgreens recipe!*

Corporate Cafeteria, Walgreen Company Headquarters

- 6 chicken breasts, boned and skinned
- 1 egg
- ¾ cup water
- 1 cup bread crumbs
- ½ teaspoon garlic powder
- 2 sprigs parsley, finely chopped
- 4 tablespoons margarine
- 1 cup chicken stock
- ¼ cup lemon juice or juice of 1 lemon squeezed
- 6 lemon slices

rice pilaf or a vegetable, prepared

Combine egg and water in a shallow bowl; set aside. Combine bread crumbs, garlic powder and chopped parsley. Flatten chicken breasts between two sheets of wax paper with a meat mallet or plate. Place in egg-water mixture. Shake off excess and place each breast in the bread crumb mixture, coating both sides. Put coated breasts on wax paper sheets. Melt margarine in frying pan; sauté until lightly browned on both sides. Add stock and lemon juice; cook covered 5 minutes more. Remove breasts to serving plates. Top each with lemon slice. Serve with rice pilaf or a vegetable.

Chicken Breasts in Sour Cream & Sherry

Serves 4

- 4 chicken breasts
- 1 7.3-ounce can (4½-ounce drained) sliced mushrooms, drained
- 1 10¾-ounce can cream of mushroom soup
- ½ soup can sherry
- 1 cup sour cream

paprika, to taste

Preheat oven to 350 degrees. Arrange chicken in a shallow baking pan; do not overlap pieces. Cover with mushrooms (do not use juice). Combine mushroom soup, sherry and sour cream. Stir until well blended. Pour over chicken, completely covering it. Dust with paprika. Bake for 1½ hours.

Alpine~Dressed Chicken Breasts

Serves 6 to 8

6 chicken breasts, boned, skinned and halved (to make 12 pieces)
salt and pepper, to taste
1 6-ounce package Swiss cheese slices
1 10¾-ounce can cream of chicken soup
1 10¾-ounce can cream of celery soup
1 soup can water
1 8-ounce package Pepperidge Farm seasoned stuffing mix
¾ cup melted margarine

Preheat oven to 350 degrees. Arrange chicken in a greased, shallow baking dish. Season with salt and pepper. Layer slices of Swiss cheese over chicken. Combine soups and water, pour over cheese and chicken evenly. Toss stuffing and butter or margarine (melted) and spoon over all. Bake, covered with foil or a lid, for 1 hour. Uncover and bake 30 minutes more.

California Crunch Chicken Breasts

Serves 4

4 chicken breasts, boned
salt and pepper, to taste
1 8-ounce container sour cream
1 10-ounce box cheese crackers, rolled into crumbs
¼ pound butter or margarine

Preheat oven to 350 degrees. Season chicken breasts with salt and pepper. Dip each into sour cream and roll in cheese cracker crumbs. Place in casserole dish and pour melted butter over all. Bake, covered, for 1 hour; uncover, bake for an additional 15 minutes.

Jarlsberg Chicken Breasts with Dressing

Serves 6

- 4 whole chicken breasts, boned, skinned and halved
- 8 slices Jarlsberg cheese
- pepper, to taste
- garlic powder, to taste
- 1 10¾-ounce can cream of chicken soup
- ¼ cup white wine
- ½ to ¾-cup fresh mushrooms, sliced and sautéed
- 2 cups Pepperidge Farm stuffing mix
- ⅓ cup butter, melted

Preheat oven to 350 degrees. Place chicken in 9x13-inch Pyrex dish. Place one slice of cheese on each piece of chicken. Season with pepper and garlic powder. Spread soup, wine and mushrooms over top. Cover with stuffing mix; drizzle melted butter over all. Bake, uncovered, for 40 minutes to 1 hour.

Chicken & Chive Crescent Squares

Serves 4

- 1 8-ounce container crescent rolls
- 3 ounces cream cheese, softened
- 2 cups chicken, cooked and cubed
- ¼ teaspoon salt
- ⅛ teaspoon pepper
- 2 tablespoons milk
- 1 tablespoon chives or onions, chopped
- 1 tablespoon pimento, chopped
- 2 tablespoons margarine, melted

Preheat oven to 350 degrees. On greased cookie sheet, separate 8 crescent rolls into 4 rectangles. Seal perforations. Mix remaining ingredients, except margarine, together. Spoon equal portions of chicken mixture onto center of each rectangle. Pull four corners of dough to center and seal chicken mixture in dough. Brush tops with melted butter. Bake for 20 minutes, or until golden brown.

Crisp, Baked Chicken Breasts

Serves 6

6 chicken breasts, boned and halved
2 tablespoons butter
½ teaspoon garlic powder
salt and pepper, to taste
3 cups corn flakes or Rice Krispies, coarsely crumbled

Preheat oven to 350 degrees. Melt butter in heated oven, in shallow baking pan. Sprinkle chicken with garlic powder, salt and pepper. Dip in butter to cover. Dip in crumbs, pressing firmly. Bake, uncovered, about 30 minutes.

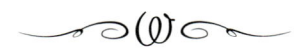

Cheddar~Baked Chicken Soufflé

Serves 8

4 cups chicken, cooked and diced
8 slices white bread
½ pound fresh mushrooms, sliced
¼ cup butter
1 8-ounce can sliced water chestnuts
½ cup mayonnaise
8 slices sharp cheddar cheese
4 eggs, well beaten
2 cups milk
1 teaspoon salt
1 10¾-ounce can golden or cream of mushroom soup
1 10¾-ounce can cream of celery soup
1 2-ounce jar pimentos, finely cut
2 cups coarse bread crumbs, buttered

Line a large 10x15-inch buttered baking pan with bread. Top with chicken. Heat butter in a small skillet and cook mushrooms in butter for 5 minutes. Pour mushrooms over chicken. Add water chestnuts and dot with mayonnaise. Cover with cheese. Combine eggs, milk and salt. Pour mixture over all. Mix soups and pimentos, and spoon over mixture. Cover with foil and refrigerate overnight. Bake in a preheated, 350 degree oven for 1½ hours. Uncover and sprinkle with crumbs. Bake 15 minutes or more.

Chopped Chicken with Noodles

Serves 6

Adapted for your kitchen... from the original Walgreens recipe!

Walgreens Cafeterias 1940's ~ 1960's

3 cups chicken, cooked and diced
½ pound wide noodles, cooked per package directions

Velouté sauce:
4 tablespoons butter, margarine or oil
4 tablespoons flour
1 teaspoon salt
¼ teaspoon pepper
3 cups canned chicken broth

Cook noodles in boiling, salted water until tender. Drain and rinse thoroughly in cold water. Bring chicken stock to boil. In another saucepan heat butter, margarine or oil; blend in flour and seasoning, stirring constantly. Bring to a boil. Remove from heat, add chicken broth, and stir until smooth. Return to heat and bring to a boil, stirring constantly. If mixture is too thick, add more chicken broth. Add chicken and cooked noodles. Mix and heat thoroughly. Season to taste.

Creamed Chicken on a Biscuit

Serves 6 to 8

Adapted for your kitchen... from the original Walgreens recipe!

Walgreens Cafeterias 1940's ~ 1960's

4 cups chicken, cooked and cubed

Velouté sauce:
1½ cups milk
1½ cups chicken broth
4 tablespoons butter, margarine, or oil
4 tablespoons flour
1 teaspoon salt
¼ teaspoon pepper

6 to 8 biscuits or patty shells

Bring milk and chicken broth to boil. In another pan heat margarine or oil; blend in flour and seasonings, stirring constantly. Bring to boil and remove from heat. Add hot liquid, stirring until smooth. Return to heat and bring to boil. Add cubed chicken, bring to boil, and season to taste. Serve over biscuits or pour creamed chicken mixture into patty shells.

Chicken~Green Bean Casserole

Serves 6 to 8

- 1 10¾-ounce can cream of mushroom soup
- ½ cup milk
- 1 teaspoon salt
- 3 cups chicken, cooked and chopped
- 1 10-ounce package frozen French-style green beans, thawed
- 1 14-ounce can chop suey vegetables, drained
- ⅓ cup onions, chopped (optional)
- 1 3½-ounce can crispy, fried onion rings
- **Parmesan cheese (optional)**

Preheat oven to 350 degrees. Mix soup, milk and salt; combine with chicken, beans, vegetables and onions. Pour into greased casserole dish. Bake for 45 minutes. Top with onion rings and bake 10 minutes longer. Parmesan cheese may be sprinkled on top before serving.

Chicken & Rice Casserole

Serves 6

- 1 10¾-ounce can cream of celery soup
- 1 10¾-ounce can cream of asparagus soup
- 2 10¾-ounce cans cream of chicken soup
- 1 cup rice, uncooked
- 8 to 10 chicken pieces (breasts, legs or thighs)
- ¼ pound butter (optional)

Preheat oven to 350 degrees. Mix all soups and rice together and pour into buttered 9x13-inch pan. Place chicken on top of mixture. Pat of butter on each piece optional. Bake for 1½ hours or until done.

Chicken Miracle Casserole

Serves 8

- 4 cups chicken breasts, boned, skinned, cooked and cut up
- 1 teaspoon salt
- 2 cups celery, chopped
- 2 tablespoons lemon juice
- 4 hard-boiled eggs, chopped
- ½ small jar pimentos
- 1½ cups Miracle Whip
- 1 cup cheese, grated
- 1 small package potato chips

Preheat oven to 400 degrees. Mix first seven ingredients well and place in greased 9x13-inch baking dish. Cover with plastic wrap and refrigerate overnight. To cook, sprinkle with cheese and crushed potato chips. Bake for 40 minutes.

Chicken Crescent Roll Casserole

Serves 4 to 6

- 2 cups chicken, cooked and diced
- 1 10¾-ounce can cream of potato soup
- 1 cup milk
- ¼ teaspoon Lawry's seasoned salt
- ½ teaspoon salt
- ¼ teaspoon pepper
- ½ 3½-ounce can crispy, fried onion rings
- 8 ounces cheddar cheese, shredded
- 4 Pillsbury crescent rolls

Preheat oven to 375 degrees. Mix together chicken, soup, milk, seasoned salt, salt, pepper, onion rings and half the cheddar cheese (4 ounces). Pour into 9x13-inch casserole dish. Bake for 20 minutes. Remove from oven, and cover with crescent rolls and the other half of the cheddar cheese. Bake, uncovered, for 15 minutes and serve.

Margaret's Terrific Turkey Casserole

Serves 6

3 cups turkey (or chicken), cooked and diced
2 10½-ounce cans chicken soup or
    10¾-ounce cans cream of chicken soup
1 cup milk
1 10-ounce package frozen, mixed peas and carrots, thawed
⅓ to ½-cup pimento, chopped (optional)
1 7-ounce package elbow macaroni, cooked per package directions
Parmesan cheese, grated, to taste

Preheat oven to 325 degrees. Mix chicken soup and milk in large saucepan; heat until smooth. Add turkey, frozen peas and carrots and pimentos. Drain macaroni and add. Mix together and place in large, greased casserole dish. Sprinkle with Parmesan cheese. Bake for 30 to 40 minutes.

Turkey~Broccoli Pie

Serves 8

An original Hazelwood recipe!

2 cups turkey, cooked and chopped
2 tablespoons butter
¼ cup onion, chopped
2 tablespoons flour
¼ teaspoon salt
½ teaspoon garlic powder
1¼ cups milk
1 3-ounce package cream cheese, softened
1 egg, beaten
1 10-ounce package frozen, chopped broccoli (or fresh, chopped)
1 frozen 2-piece pie crust
8 ounces smoked cheddar cheese

Preheat oven to 350 degrees. Heat butter in skillet and brown onion; add turkey. Stir until warmed, a few minutes. Stir in flour, salt and garlic powder. Add 1¼ cups milk and cream cheese, cook until smooth. Stir 1 cup of mixture into beaten egg. Return mixture to skillet. Cook over medium heat until thickened, 1 to 2 minutes. Add broccoli. Prepare pie crust. Pour mixture into pie crust. Arrange cheese slices on top. Put on top crust and crimp edges; cut vent slits on top of crust. Bake for 45 minutes.

Turkey Chili

Serves 3 to 4

1½ pounds ground turkey
1 or 2 tablespoons oil
1 medium onion
2 14½-ounce cans tomatoes, diced
1 11½-ounce can V-8 juice
1 can dark kidney beans
2 tablespoons Lawry's chili seasonings

Heat oil in skillet and sauté onion. Add turkey and brown. Add remaining ingredients. Simmer 30 to 40 minutes.

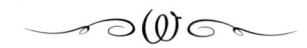

Roast Duckling with Orange Sauce

Serves 4 to 6

An original Hazelwood recipe!

1 duck, cleaned

Orange sauce:
⅓ cup brown sugar
⅓ cup sugar
1 tablespoon cornstarch
1 tablespoon orange rind, grated
1 cup orange juice
¼ teaspoon salt
rice pilaf or wild rice, prepared

Preheat oven to 325 degrees. Combine all orange sauce ingredients in a saucepan, stir over low heat until sugars dissolve. Simmer until transparent, about 3 minutes. Roast duck for 2½ to 3 hours. During last 30 minutes baste duck with orange sauce. Serve with rice pilaf or wild rice.

Note: An excellent Sunday dinner! And a favorite at Hazelwood!

Apricot~Glazed Cornish Hens

Serves 2

2 Rock Cornish game hens, cleaned
¾ cup apricot preserves
2 tablespoons orange juice
rind from ½ orange, cut into strips
salt and paprika, to taste
wild rice, prepared

Preheat oven to 350 degrees. Mix apricot preserves, orange juice and orange rind in small bowl. Remove giblets from hen. Place hens on rack in roasting pan, sprinkle lightly with salt and paprika. Roast hens for 1 to 1½ hours. Baste frequently with apricot mixture during last 30 minutes. Serve with wild rice.

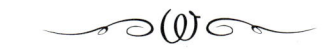

Donna Erickson's Pheasant

Serves 4 to 6

3 cups pheasant, boned, cleaned and cooked
2 eggs, beaten
2 cups corn flake crumbs
1 teaspoon ground pepper
1 teaspoon garlic salt
3 tablespoons butter
1 cup onions, sliced
1 cup mushrooms, sliced
2 cups chicken broth
½ cup white wine
2 tablespoons flour
2 tablespoons butter

Dip pheasant in beaten eggs, then in corn flake crumbs seasoned with pepper and garlic salt. Heat butter in skillet. Fry pheasant until brown; then remove from pan. Sauté onions and mushrooms in same pan until tender. Add cooked pheasant and chicken broth. Cook covered for 2 hours. Add wine and simmer 30 more minutes. Knead flour and butter together. Drop into pan and stir until sauce thickens. Serve immediately.

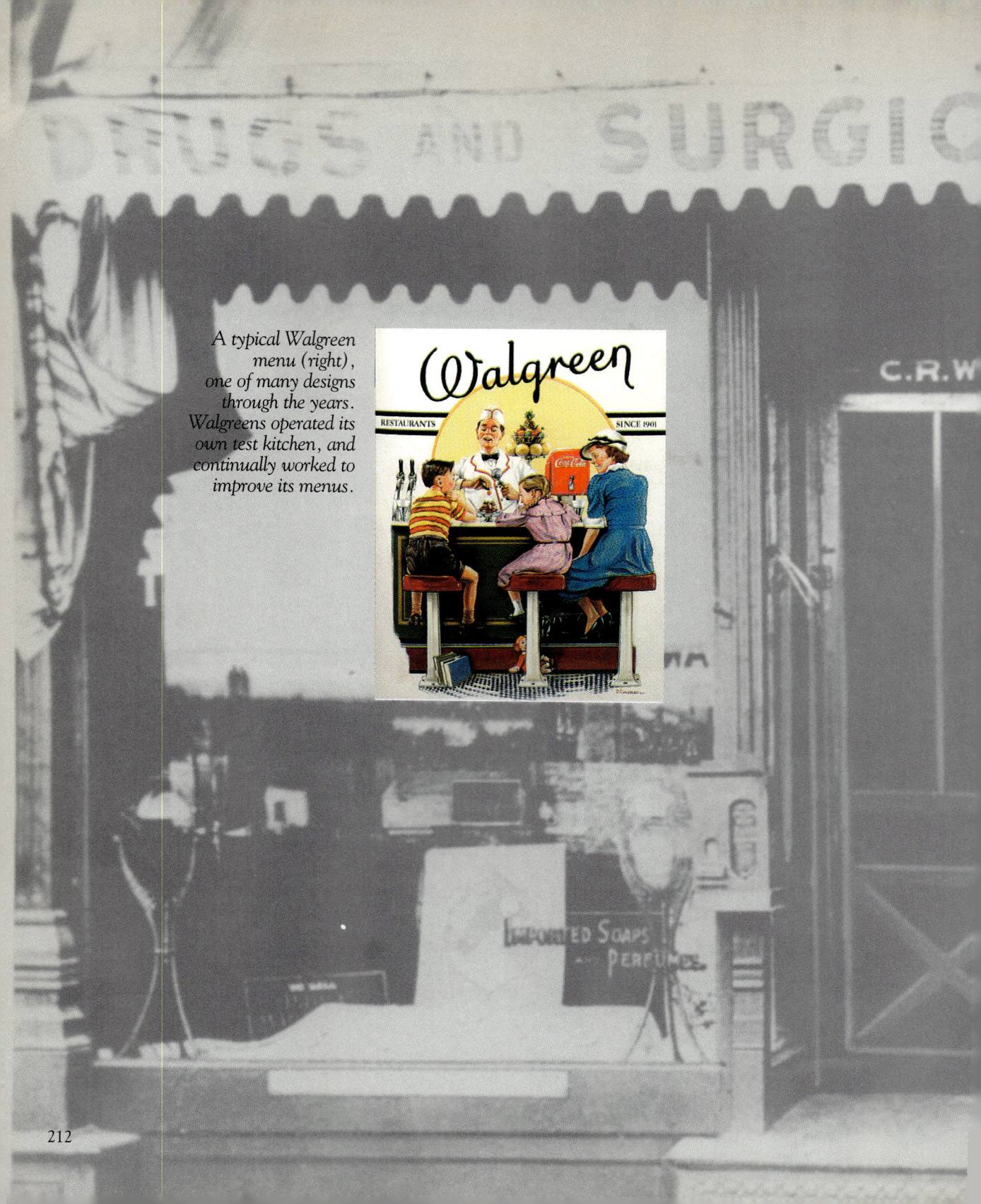

A typical Walgreen menu (right), one of many designs through the years. Walgreens operated its own test kitchen, and continually worked to improve its menus.

Welcome to Walgreens!
HISTORICAL HIGHLIGHTS

Walgreens long, successful food service history began in about 1915, in the kitchen of Myrtle R. Walgreen, wife of founder Charles R. Walgreen, Sr. Walgreen, Sr. was so disappointed that he had to shut down the fountain during the winter because of a lack of sales, that he began to think of ways to keep it open and profitable. He and Myrtle came up with the idea of serving hot, homemade meals. To keep the work manageable, they offered one hot sandwich and soup selection for each day of the week.

The year-round soda fountain became so popular, that Walgreens expanded it to other stores, opening up the first Commissary in 1916, to keep up with the demand.

During the 1920's, as Walgreens experienced remarkable growth, its fountains became famous throughout the nation. After the invention of Walgreens Double-Rich Chocolate Malted in 1922, patrons crowded the counters and "meet me at Walgreens for a shake and sandwich" became the popular bywords.

Walgreens opened its first full-fledged, in-store cafeterias in the late 1930's. In the 1960's, fountains were phased out and the cafeterias became beautifully-decorated, full-service grills. In the late 1960's a fast-food chain, Corky's, was opened, as well as the company's first freestanding restaurant, Robin Hood. And in 1976, Walgreens opened its most successful food service venture ever ~ Wag's, freestanding, family-style restaurants.

Walgreens sold the flourishing division in 1988, to concentrate on its pharmacy business.

"There is no drugstore in the world so modern or as complete."
Charles R. Walgreen, Sr., 1937, commenting to reporters about the 200 East Flagler, Miami store.

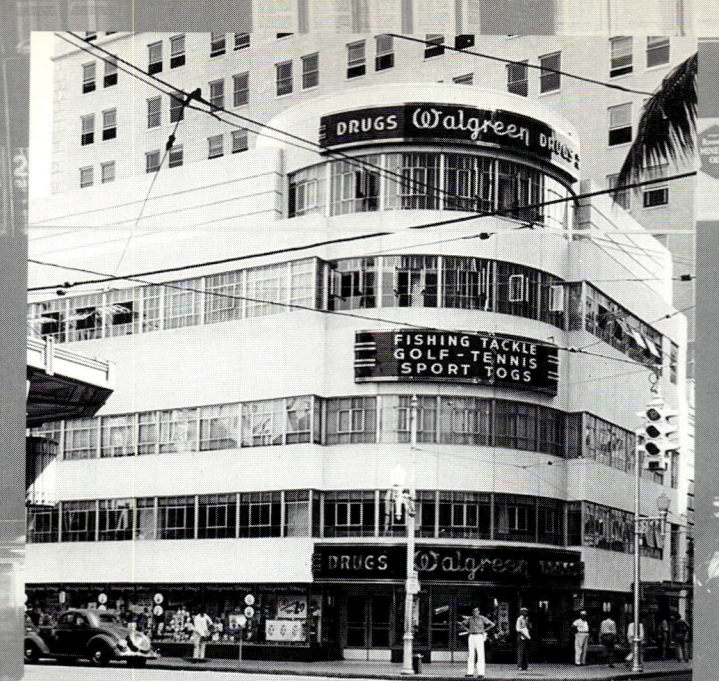

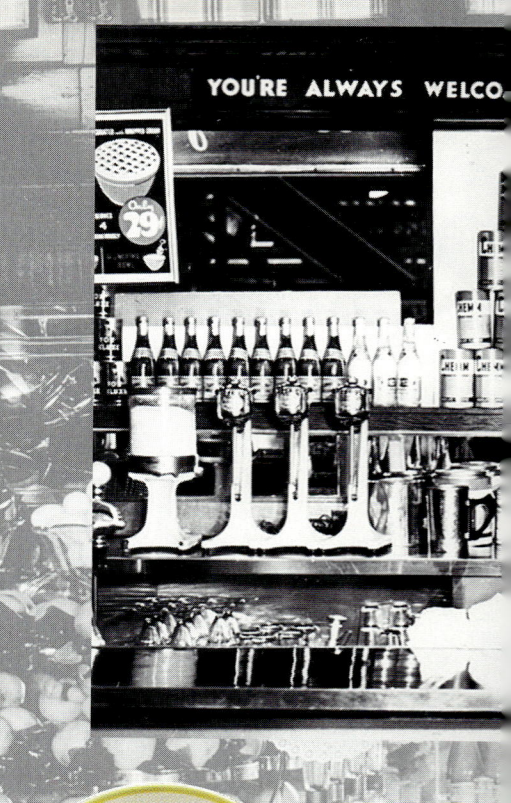

When it opened in 1937, the five-story, air-conditioned Walgreens at 200 East Flagler Avenue in Miami, Florida (*above*), was the largest in the company, and an engineering feat. Its sporting goods basement was created below the water table by sinking a huge, preformed concrete "boat."

A drug store took up the entire first floor, and included an 80-foot long, white oak soda fountain and separate dining area. On the top floor was an ice cream plant capable of producing 600 gallons a day. Two balconies encircled the store's interior. The glass-enclosed, sound-proof radio studio, used for in-store entertainment, was on the first balcony. On the second balcony, was a 700-capacity restaurant with a state-of-the-art kitchen, for preparing full-course meals.

The Flagler Avenue store was also the scene of many exciting events through the years. Its huge restaurant doubled as the area's largest banquet hall and actually catered to several weddings. During World War II, during the coastal blackouts, Walgreens attracted nightly crowds because it was one of the few buildings in the area to remain open. The store used blackout shades and turned off the window display lights.

The store closed recently, in the spring of 1995.

A plate from Humpty Dumpty (above).

Walgreens acquired four of the Arizona-based Humpty Dumpty restaurants in 1976. They used Wag's menu.

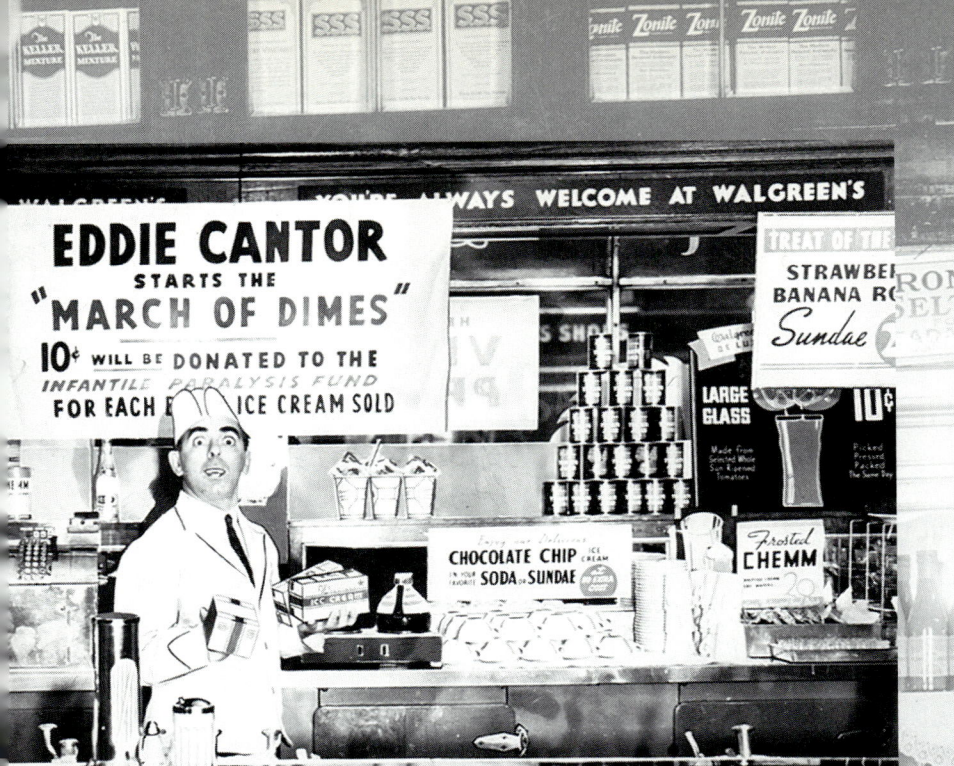

A Wag's coffee mug (above).

Walgreens opened Wag's in 1976. With special menus geared toward kids and healthy eating, Wag's went on to become the company's most successful restaurant chain.

Walgreens joined Eddie Cantor, star of Camel Caravan radio program and founder of the March of Dimes, in sponsoring the Infantile Paralysis Fund in 1939 (above).

Through the years, Walgreens has reached out to many local communities, coming to the aid of many worthy causes.

An early 1930's "Inner Toast" promotion (right).

A Walgreens invention, Inner Toast sandwich rolls were created with a special device that was slipped inside the roll, toasting it internally.

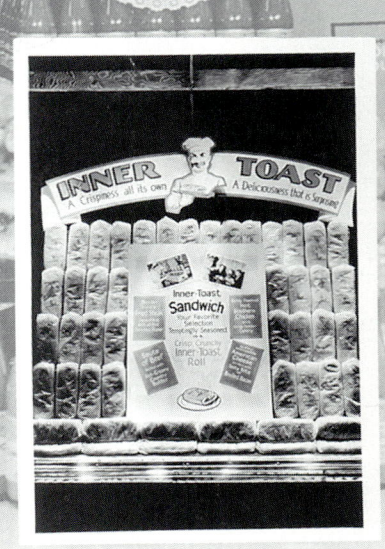

215

WALGREENS at the 1933~34 CHICAGO WORLD'S FAIR

The mid 1930's was an era of hard times for the entire nation. But in defiance of it all, the 1933-34 Chicago World's Fair gave everyone a reason to smile. Dubbed "A Century of Progress," the celebration marked the 100th anniversary of Chicago's incorporation as a village. On opening night, in keeping with the theme of scientific progress, the lights were turned on with energy captured from Arcturus, a star forty light years away!

Walgreens had the only drugstores at the fair, and they worked to capacity every day. The soda fountains were very popular refreshment stops, and unlike other concessionaires, Walgreens never raised its prices. Each of Walgreens four drugstores at the fair won acclaim and each was judged architecturally distinctive. The interiors utilized contemporary show-cases, lighting techniques and bright colors, and the soda fountains were constructed (for the first time anywhere) with metal frames and porcelain enamel surfaces.

The 23rd Street Plaza entrance store was the largest and had a revolving sign. Extremely popular, its glass and chrome interior was airy and bright. And its circular fountain room

The 23rd Street Walgreens fountain, a technological wonder with its backbar aquarium, seated 100 patrons (right).

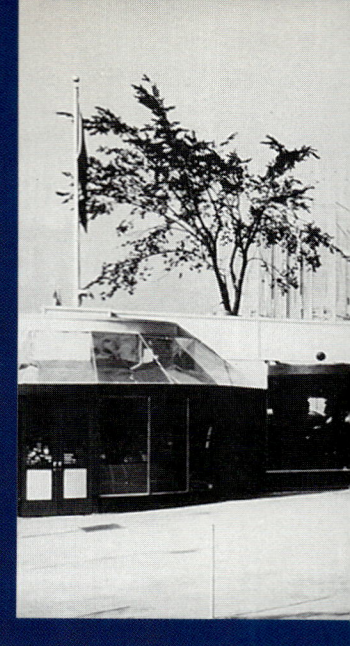

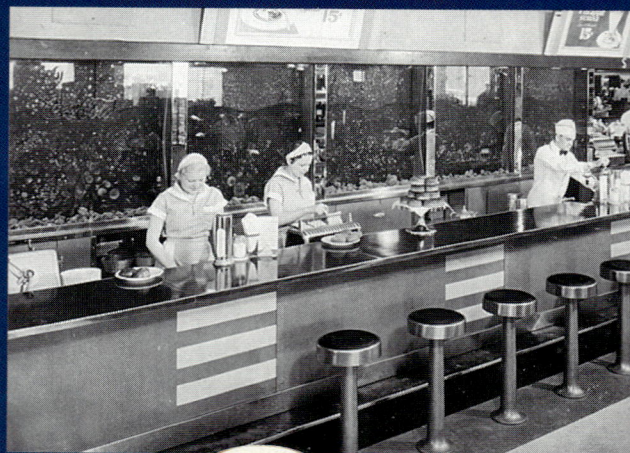

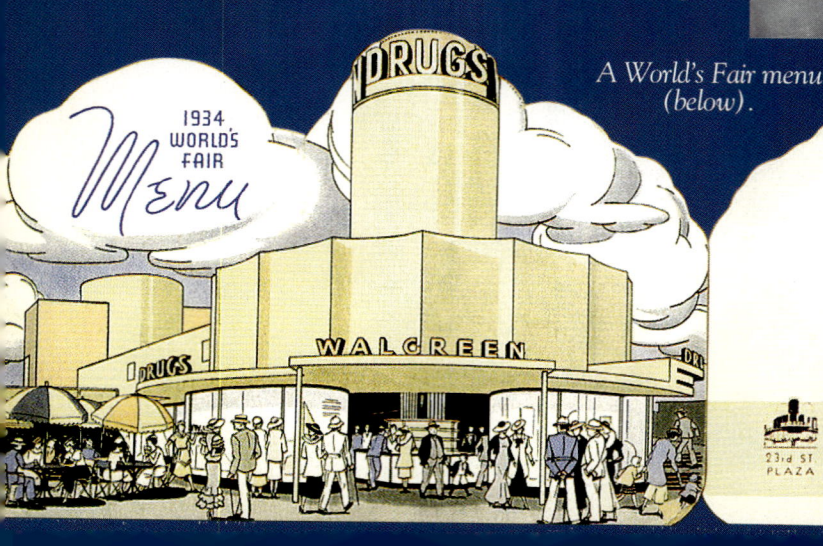

A World's Fair menu (below).

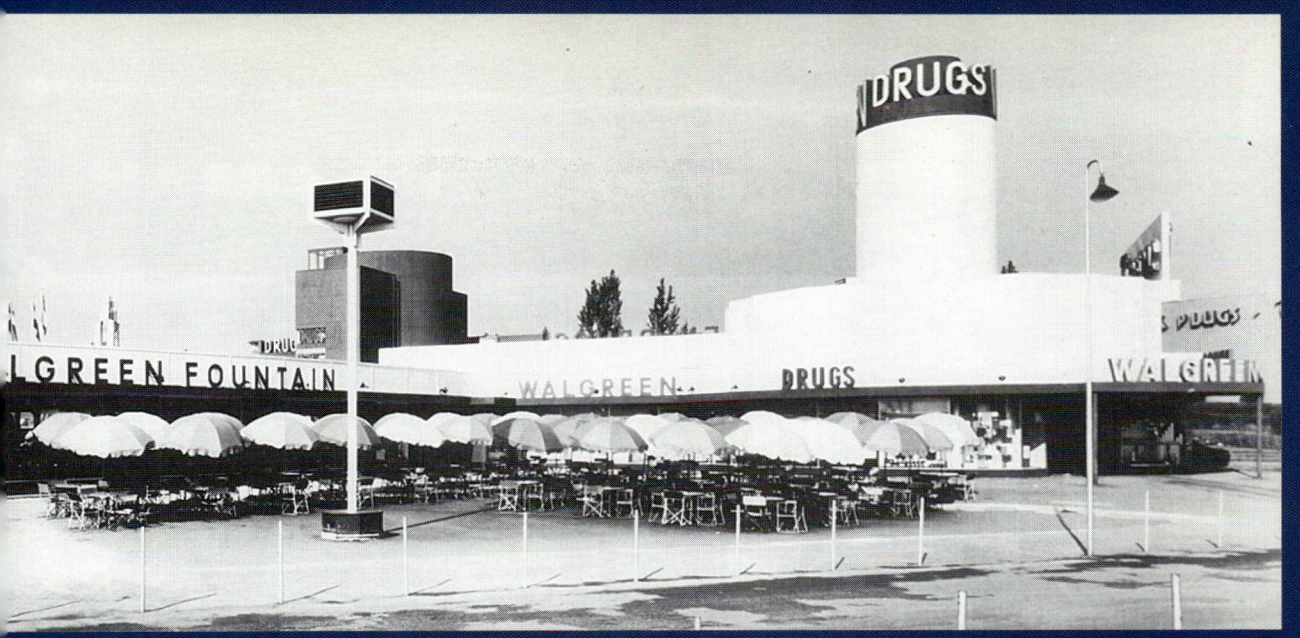

The Walgreens at the 23rd Street Plaza entrance, with its revolving "Walgreen Drugs" sign (above).

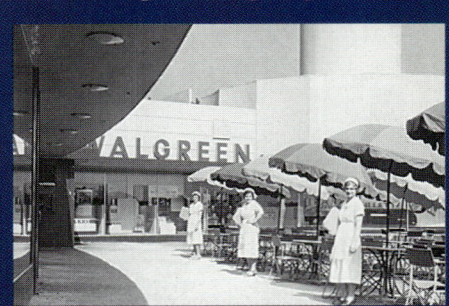

featured a giant glass aquarium which was built into the wall behind the 100-stool soda bar.

The store inside the Hall of Science at the 18th Street entrance had a small lounge where visitors could rest and watch a ten-minute movie ~ a tour of Walgreens laboratories, which demonstrated how the company made its products. Two more stores opened in the summer of 1933.

Despite the depression and many doubts, the exposition was a success. Total fair gate receipts and concession sales topped $36 million. But Walgreens success at the fair measured far beyond income. The positive exposure ensured the company of millions of regular customers.

Waitresses ready to serve (above).

WALGREEN GARDEN MENU

Fox's De Luxe Turkey Sandwich, Tomato and Lettuce Garnish . . . 30c

REFRESHING BEVERAGES
Fresh Fruit Orange Freeze......20c
De Luxe Orangeade or Lemonade..................15c
Schlitz Beer............stein 15c

DELICIOUS SANDWICHES
Sugar-Cured Baked Ham........15c
Harding's Corned Beef Sandwich......................15c
Kraft's American Cheese......15c

All sandwiches on white or rye bread

Dish of Walgreen's Vanilla Ice Cream...10c

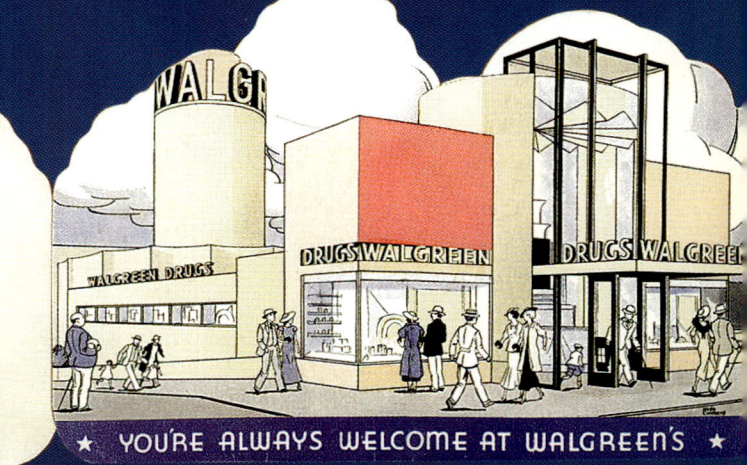

THERE ARE 480 WALGREEN DRUG STORES

★ YOU'RE ALWAYS WELCOME AT WALGREEN'S

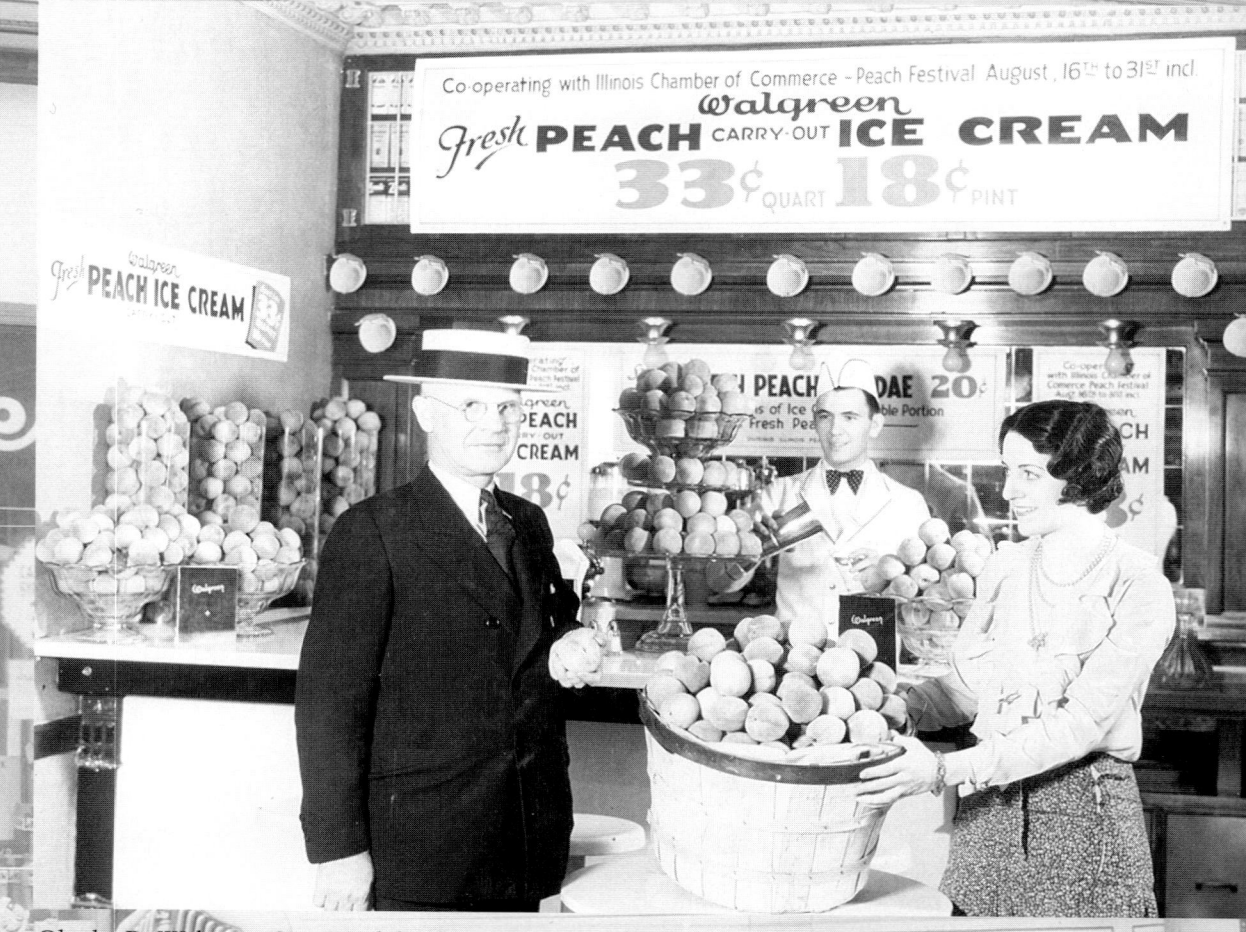

Charles R. Walgreen, Sr., joined the Illinois Chamber of Commerce Peach Festival promotion in the 1920's. The fountains featured fresh peach ice cream to eat in or carry out, at yes, only 18¢ a pint and 33¢ a quart (above).

Beginning in 1913, the ice cream was made in the basement of Walgreens second store. To keep up with the demand, Walgreens opened its first Commissary in 1916, which included an ice cream plant. In 1950, Walgreens completed the new Commissary, which processed more than a thousand gallons of ice cream per hour!

In the true spirit of the company, it is interesting to note that Walgreen, Sr. spared no expense in obtaining quality ingredients. For example, he once bought a registered bull for the farm that supplied the Walgreen-owned creamery. The result was a herd of top-quality dairy cattle which produced the finest milk available for his extra-rich ice cream.

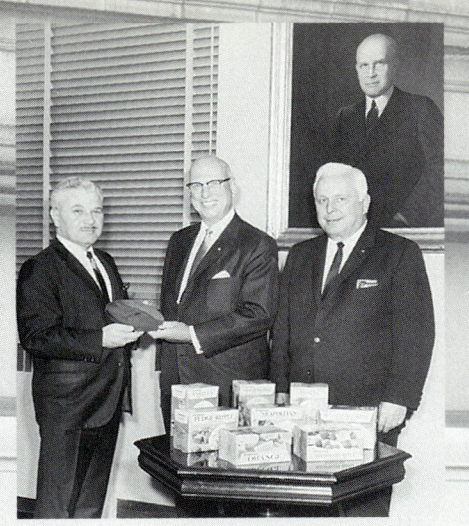

Chairman Charles R. Walgreen, Jr., with president Alvin Borg, receiving Ice Cream World's Gold Scoop Award for advertising excellence (left).

Walgreens rectangular ice cream boxes won first place, nationwide, for design in 1966.

A coffee mug from Robin Hood (right).

Walgreens first line of freestanding restaurants, Robin Hood and counterpart Briargate, featured medieval decor.

The Walgreens ice cream plant at 500 East 40th Street, Chicago, in the 1950's (right).

The large tank first mixed and pasteurized the cream. Then a "viscolizer" used pressure to break it down into fine particles. Finally, cooler coils lowered the ice cream's temperature to 40 degrees for a 48-hour period before freezing.

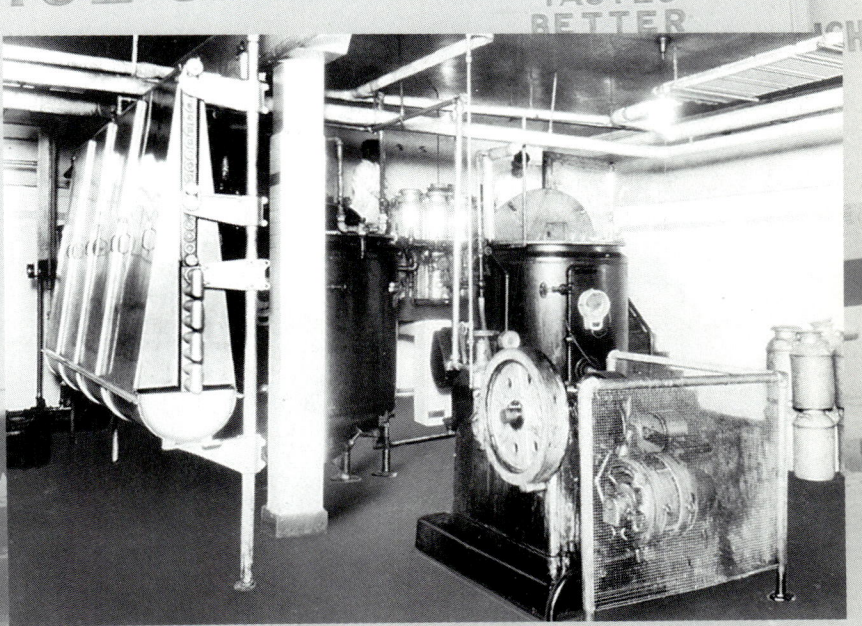

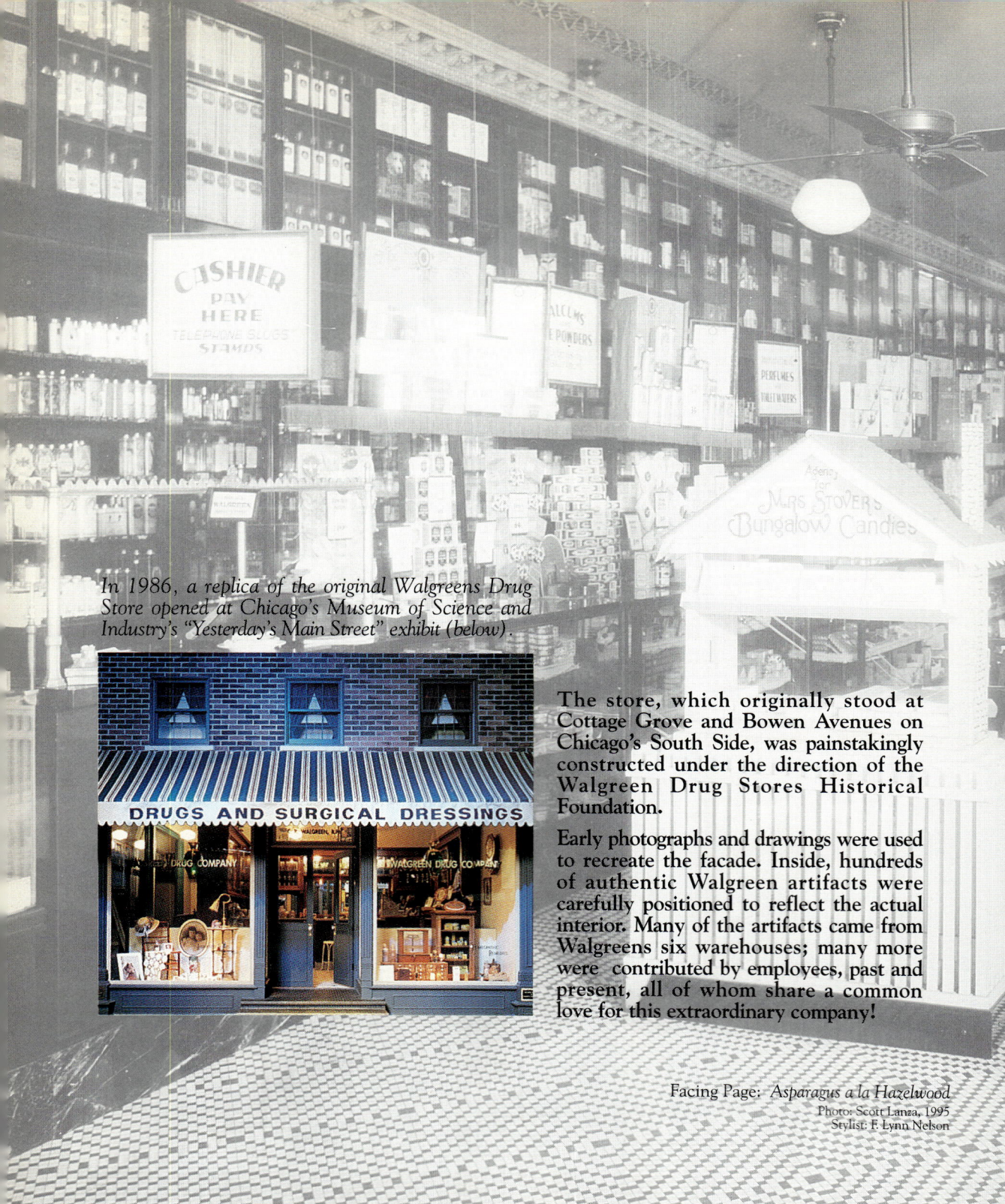

In 1986, a replica of the original Walgreens Drug Store opened at Chicago's Museum of Science and Industry's "Yesterday's Main Street" exhibit (below).

The store, which originally stood at Cottage Grove and Bowen Avenues on Chicago's South Side, was painstakingly constructed under the direction of the Walgreen Drug Stores Historical Foundation.

Early photographs and drawings were used to recreate the facade. Inside, hundreds of authentic Walgreen artifacts were carefully positioned to reflect the actual interior. Many of the artifacts came from Walgreens six warehouses; many more were contributed by employees, past and present, all of whom share a common love for this extraordinary company!

Facing Page: *Asparagus a la Hazelwood*
Photo: Scott Lanza, 1995
Stylist: F. Lynn Nelson

VEGETABLES

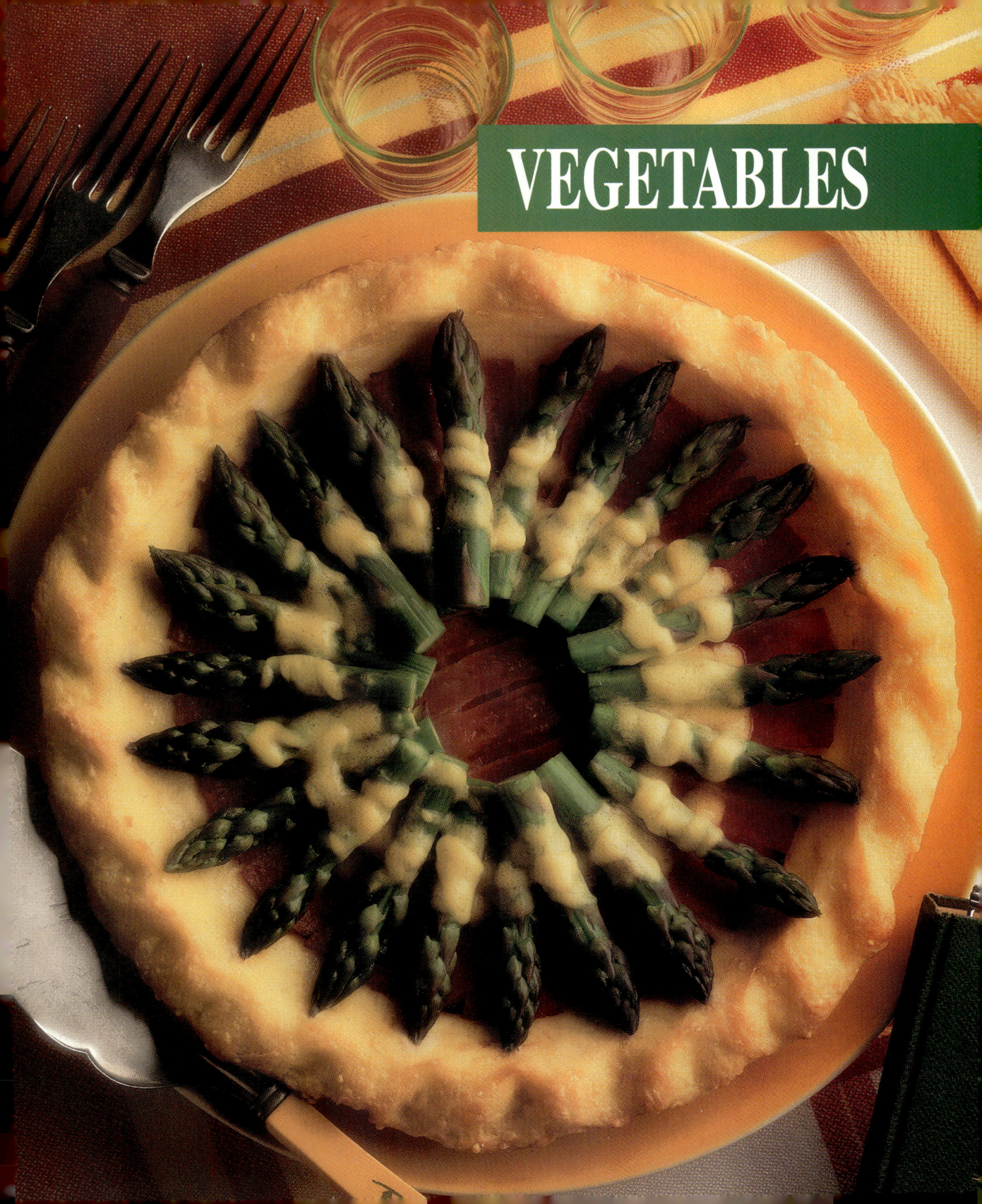

The Cafeterias
In the Store, They Stood on Their Own

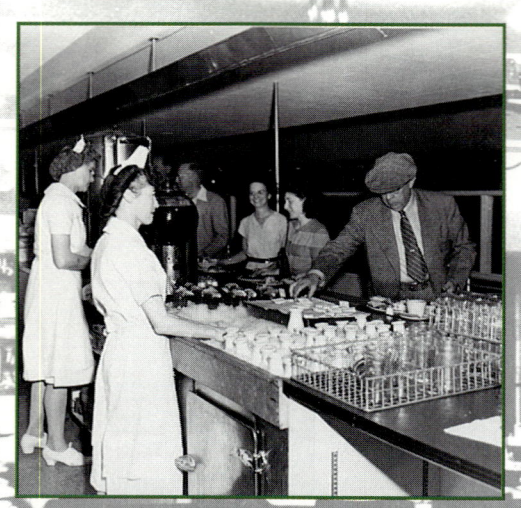

Generations of fond memories recall...the food was good, the coffee always hot, and the waitresses all knew your name.

Walgreens cafeterias evolved out of a need to provide much more than the soda fountain fare and cater to ever-increasing crowds. The first opened in the late 1940's and early 1950's in Walgreens stores at 200 East Flagler Avenue in Miami, Canal Street in downtown New Orleans and in the basements of three Chicago Walgreens ~ Randolph & State Streets, Madison & State Streets (where the present stores still attract noonday crowds), and the Merchandise Mart. Soon, they spread throughout the country. The largest cafeteria Walgreens built was in (of course) a Texas store.

The cafeterias were adjoined but separate from the drugstore and soda fountain. They quickly became very popular and eventually absorbed the old fountains. Although the cafeterias were converted to more-elaborate grills in the 1960's, for many Americans, these beloved eateries remained a favorite meeting place.

Mexican Black Bean Pizza

Serves 2 to 4

- 1   10-ounce refrigerated pizza crust
- 1   15-ounce can black beans, rinsed and drained
- 3   tablespoons olive oil
- 5   tablespoons cilantro or parsley, chopped and divided
- 1   teaspoon ground cumin
- 1   teaspoon Mexican chili powder
- 1   teaspoon red hot pepper (Tabasco) sauce
- 1   garlic clove
- ½   small onion, chopped
- ½   cup Monterey Jack cheese, grated
- ½   cup cheddar cheese, grated
- ½   cup olives, sliced
- ½   cup green onion, chopped
- 2   medium tomatoes, seeded and chopped
- 1   tablespoon jalapeño pepper, seeded and chopped
- 1½   tablespoons red pepper, diced (optional)
- 1½   tablespoons green pepper, diced (optional)
- ½   cup sour cream, half-and-half or plain yogurt
- ¼   cup green (*verde*) taco sauce

chunky salsa

Preheat oven to 425 degrees. Press rolled-out pizza dough into a greased, 9x12-inch or 9x13-inch baking pan. Bake crust for 5 minutes, or until light, golden brown. In a food processor, combine and pureé black beans, olive oil, 2 tablespoons cilantro, cumin, chili powder, pepper sauce, garlic and onion.

Spread puréed bean mixture over partially-baked crust. Sprinkle cheddar and Monterey Jack cheese, olives, green onion, tomatoes, jalapeño pepper, 3 tablespoons cilantro, and red and green peppers on pizza. Bake for about 12 to 15 minutes, or until done.

To serve pizza, garnish with chunky salsa and cut like a pie with pizza cutter. In a bowl, combine sour cream and taco sauce; serve mixture with pizza.

Vegetarian Chili in a Tortilla Bowl

Serves 6

*Adapted for your kitchen...
from the original Walgreens recipe!*

Corporate Cafeteria, Walgreen Company Headquarters

1 tablespoon vegetable oil
2 medium onions, chopped
1 green pepper, seeded and chopped
1 teaspoon jalapeño peppers, seeded and minced
2 medium zucchini, cubed
1 14½-ounce can whole tomatoes, drained and crushed
1 15½-ounce can kidney beans
1 8-ounce can garbanzo beans (chickpeas)
1 jicama, peeled and diced
3½ ounces Burgundy wine
1 tablespoon Worcestershire sauce
1 teaspoon dry mustard
1 teaspoon celery seed
1 tablespoon chili powder
1 teaspoon black pepper
2 teaspoon fennel seed
2 cups water
salt, to taste
2 tablespoons butter or margarine
2 tablespoons flour
3 medium red potatoes, boiled, peeled and cubed
6 10-inch Azteca tortilla bowls, prepared per package directions
sour cream or plain yogurt

Heat oil in a large pot; sauté onions, green peppers and jalapeño peppers, until onions turn clear. Add all the remaining ingredients except the potatoes, tortilla bowls and sour cream. Bring to a boil and cook until zucchini is tender and the flavors are blended. Make a roux by combining butter and flour; cook over low heat. Add roux to thicken mixture, and then add the boiled, cubed potatoes. Adjust the seasonings, to taste, and remove from pot. Serve in tortilla bowls; garnish with sour cream.

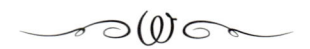

Yams with Grand Marnier

Serves 6 to 8

An original Hazelwood recipe!

6 to 7 medium size yams
1 cup Karo corn syrup
1 cup Grand Marnier "Triple Orange" liqueur
1 stick sweet butter

Yams with Grand Marnier, *continued on next page.*

Yams with Grand Marnier, continued.

Preheat oven to 325 degrees. Peel and slice yams into 1-inch discs. Parboil in water for ½-hour. Drain. Pour yams into a 2 to 3-quart glass casserole dish. Pour corn syrup and Grand Marnier over yams. Slice butter into enough sections to cover the yams evenly. Cover and bake for at least 1½ to 2 hours, or until tender.

Candied Sweet Potatoes

Serves 4

Adapted for your kitchen... from the original Walgreens recipe!

Robin Hood & Briargate Restaurants, 1970's ~ 1980's

4 medium sweet potatoes, unpeeled

Brown sugar syrup:
- 2 cups water, heated to boiling
- 1 cup brown sugar
- 1 dash salt
- 1 dash nutmeg
- 2 tablespoons butter
- 2 tablespoons cornstarch
- ¼ cup cold water

Preheat oven to 375 degrees. Cover sweet potatoes with water and boil in skins until soft, about 30 minutes; then plunge sweet potatoes into cold water and remove skins. Cut sweet potatoes in half lengthwise; put into buttered baking dish. Prepare syrup. Boil water; add brown sugar, salt and nutmeg. Dissolve corn starch in cold water. Add to boiling mixture and simmer for 15 minutes. Add butter. Pour syrup over sweet potatoes. Bake for 20 minutes. Baste sweet potatoes while they are baking to glaze them.

Galesburg Rutabaga Bake

Serves 6 to 8

- 1 large (3-pound) rutabaga (Swedish turnip), peeled and diced
- 3 tablespoons butter
- 1½ cups apples, peeled and sliced
- ⅔ cup brown sugar
- ¼ teaspoon cinnamon
- ⅓ cup all-purpose flour

Preheat oven to 350 degrees. Cook, drain and mash rutabaga with 1 tablespoon butter. Combine ⅓-cup brown sugar and cinnamon, and mix with apple slices. Arrange alternate layers of rutabaga and apples in greased 2-quart casserole. Mix the flour, ⅓-cup brown sugar and 2 tablespoons butter together until crumbly. Sprinkle over casserole. Bake for 1 hour.

Yummy Yellow Squash Casserole

Serves 6 to 8

- 1 large or 2 small butternut or buttercup squash
- 1 small onion, chopped
- ½ green or red pepper, chopped
- ¼ teaspoon salt
- ¼ teaspoon pepper
- ¼ teaspoon celery salt
- ¼ teaspoon marjoram (optional)
- 1 tablespoon butter or margarine
- 1 large tomato, sliced
- ⅓ to ¼-cup bread crumbs, buttered

Preheat oven to 350 degrees. Peel squash, cut in half and scoop out seeds. Cut squash in small pieces and simmer in a minimum amount of water until soft. Drain well. Mash squash with chopped onions, pepper, salt and spices. Add 1 tablespoon butter. Pat down in a greased casserole. Arrange sliced tomato on top and sprinkle with buttered bread crumbs. Bake for 20 to 30 minutes, or until crumbs are browned.

Note: Casserole may be prepared the night before, without the bread crumbs, and refrigerated. To prepare for serving, add the bread crumbs and follow baking instructions.

Patty Pan Squash Supreme

Serves 8

- 6 slices bacon
- 8 patty pan squash
- 1 small onion
- ½ cup cheddar cheese, grated
- ½ teaspoon salt
- ½ teaspoon dry marjoram
- ½ pint light sour cream
- 1 cup Chablis wine

Preheat oven to 325 degrees. Hollow out squash, removing seeds and pulp. Discard seeds, dice pulp and set aside. Cook bacon until crisp; drain, crumble. Add bacon to squash pulp, add all remaining ingredients, except wine. Divide the filling into 8 portions and fill each hollowed-out squash. Pour the Chablis wine into a 9x9-inch glass baking dish; place squash in dish. Bake for 45 minutes.

Glazed Squash Rings

Serves 4 to 6

- 2 acorn squash
- ½ cup packed brown sugar
- ¼ cup butter or margarine
- 2 tablespoons water
- 1 dash of nutmeg

salt and pepper, to taste

Preheat oven to 350 degrees. Cut squash crosswise into 1-inch slices. Remove seeds. Arrange in single layer in shallow, greased baking dish. Season with salt and pepper. Cover and bake until almost tender, about 30 minutes. In saucepan, combine brown sugar, margarine, water and nutmeg; stir and cook until bubbly. Spoon over squash. Bake uncovered until tender, about 25 to 30 minutes. Place squash in serving dish. Spoon sauce over top.

Zucchini with Green Pepper & Dill

Serves 4

- 4 small (1-pound) zucchini, cut into ¼-inch slices
- 2 tablespoons vegetable oil
- 2 green onions, sliced
- 1 small green pepper, chopped
- ¼ teaspoon dried dill weed
- ⅛ teaspoon garlic powder

salt and pepper, to taste

Heat oil in a large pan or skillet. Add zucchini, onions, green pepper and seasonings. Cover and simmer until zucchini is tender, about 10 minutes, stirring occasionally. Adjust seasoning, if necessary, before serving.

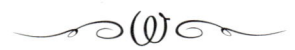

Fried Zucchini

Serves 6 to 8

- 1 large or 2 medium zucchini, cut into ¼-inch slices
- butter or margarine
- seasoned breadcrumbs, finely crushed

Heat 2 tablespoons butter in a large, hot skillet. Place zucchini slices in skillet; do not overlap. Sauté briefly; flip slices over. Sauté other side briefly; sprinkle with breadcrumbs. Flip slices again; sprinkle with breadcrumbs. Sauté until zucchini is tender and crumbs are light brown, about 1 minute. Move cooked slices to a warm platter. Repeat process until all slices have been cooked.

Heavenly Onion Casserole

Serves 6 to 8

2 tablespoons butter or margarine
3 medium sweet Spanish onions, sliced
8 ounces fresh mushrooms, sliced
1 cup Swiss cheese, shredded
1 10¾-ounce can cream of mushroom soup
1 5-ounce can evaporated milk
2 teaspoons soy sauce
6 to 8 slices French bread, ½-inch thick
6 to 8 thin slices Swiss cheese

In a large skillet, melt butter over medium-high heat. Sauté onions and mushrooms until tender. Place in a 12x7½x2-inch baking dish or 2-quart casserole. Sprinkle shredded cheese on top. Combine soup, milk and soy sauce; pour over cheese. Top with bread and cheese slices. Cover and refrigerate 4 hours or overnight. Bake, loosely covered, at 375-degrees for 30 minutes. Uncover and bake 15 to 20 minutes longer, or until heated through. Let stand 5 minutes before serving.

Note: Try this dish as an accompaniment to a hearty roast, with plain, fresh vegetables and a simple salad.

Balsamic Roasted Onions

Serves 4

1 large red onion
¼ cup balsamic vinegar
¼ cup olive oil
salt and pepper, to taste

Preheat oven to 375 degrees. Cut onion from top to bottom (against the rings), into 4 to 6 sections. Arrange sections on baking dish. Combine vinegar, olive oil, salt and pepper. Sprinkle onion sections with combined ingredients. Bake, uncovered, for 45 minutes.

Roasted Sweet Onions

Serves 4

2 8-ounce sweet onions, cut into 8 wedges each (or an equivalent amount of smaller sweet onions)
3 garlic cloves, peeled and thinly sliced
3 bay leaves
8 sprigs fresh parsley
3 sprigs fresh sage, 4 inches long
2 sprigs fresh oregano
8 sprigs fresh basil
½ teaspoon kosher salt
½ teaspoon black pepper, freshly ground
¼ cup balsamic vinegar
¼ cup extra-virgin olive oil

Preheat oven to 500 degrees. Place onion wedges in single layer in shallow baking dish. Sprinkle with garlic and herbs. Season with salt and pepper, and drizzle evenly with vinegar and olive oil. Roast for 8 to 10 minutes, until onions are lightly caramelized, and barely tender. Remove from oven and let cool. Serve at room temperature.

Auntie's Onion Pie

Serves 6 to 8

1 cup saltine crackers, crumbled
¼ cup butter, melted
2 cups yellow onions, thinly sliced
2 tablespoons butter
2 tablespoons vegetable oil
2 large eggs
¾ cup milk
salt and pepper, to taste
½ cup cheddar cheese, grated

Preheat oven to 350 degrees. Mix together cracker crumbs and melted butter. Press into a 9-inch glass pie plate. Sauté onions in butter and oil until rings separate and are glossy. Pour into pie plate. Mix eggs, milk, salt and pepper until blended. Pour over onions. Sprinkle cheese on top. Bake for 30 minutes, in middle of oven. Test with knife. Let stand 10 minutes. To serve, slice like a pie.

Florentine Crepe Cups

Serves 6

Crepes:
- 3 eggs, slightly beaten
- ⅔ cup flour
- ½ teaspoon salt
- 1 cup milk
- 2 tablespoons margarine or butter, melted

Filling:
- 1½ cups sharp cheddar cheese, shredded
- 3 tablespoons flour
- 3 eggs, slightly beaten
- ⅔ cup real mayonnaise
- 1 10-ounce package frozen, chopped spinach, thawed and drained
- 1 7-ounce (4-ounce drained) can chopped mushrooms, drained
- salt and pepper, to taste
- 6 bacon slices, cooked and crumbled ~ reserve some for garnish

Preheat oven to 350 degrees. Prepare the crepes. To make the batter, combine eggs, flour, salt and milk. Beat until smooth. Let stand 30 minutes. For 12 crepes, pour 2 tablespoons of batter into a hot, lightly greased 8-inch skillet. Cook on one side only, until underside is lightly browned. Prepare the filling. Toss cheese with flour, add remaining ingredients; mix well. To fill the crepes, fit crepes into greased muffin tins and fill with cheese mixture. Bake for 40 minutes, or until set. Garnish with bacon to serve.

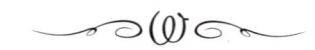

Spinach~Cheddar Pie

Serves 8

- 1 10-ounce package frozen, chopped spinach, thawed and drained
- 3 eggs, beaten
- 16 ounces small-curd cottage cheese
- ¼ cup melted butter
- 1 cup sharp cheddar cheese, grated
- 1 small onion, finely chopped
- 3 tablespoons flour
- 1 teaspoon salt

Preheat oven to 325 degrees. In medium-size bowl, beat eggs, add remaining ingredients. Pour into greased 9-inch pie pan. Bake 1 hour and 15 minutes. Remove from oven. Let stand for 5 minutes before slicing, to serve.

Sea Breeze Spinach Mold

Serves 8

- ¼ cup cold water
- 1 10½-ounce can beef consommé or broth
- 2 envelopes unflavored gelatin
- ¼ teaspoon salt
- 2 tablespoons lemon juice
- 1 cup mayonnaise
- 1 medium onion, quartered
- 4 eggs, hard-cooked and quartered
- 1 10-ounce package frozen, chopped spinach, thawed and drained
- ½ pound bacon, cooked and crumbled ~ reserve some for garnish

Pour the cold water and ¼-cup beef consommé into blender and sprinkle with gelatin. Let stand until the gelatin is softened. Heat the remaining beef broth in a saucepan until boiling. Add to the blender and cover. Process at low speed until gelatin is dissolved, using a rubber spatula to push gelatin granules into the broth mixture. Add the salt, lemon juice and mayonnaise; process until well blended. Add the onion and cover. Process at high speed until the onion is chopped. Add the spinach and eggs and cover. Process at high speed just until the eggs are chopped. Stir in bacon and turn into a greased 6-cup mold. Chill until firm. To serve, unmold and garnish with bacon.

Spinach & Egg Casserole

Serves 8

Adapted for your kitchen... from the original Walgreens recipe!

Walgreens Cafeterias 1940's ~ 1960's

- 2 cups fresh spinach, cooked, drained and chopped (or frozen, chopped spinach, thawed and drained)
- 4 eggs, hard-boiled and sliced
- ½ to ⅔-cup cheese, grated
- ½ cup bread crumbs

White sauce:
- 2 tablespoons margarine or butter
- 2 tablespoons flour
- ⅛ teaspoon white pepper
- 1 cup milk

Preheat oven to 450 degrees. Prepare sauce. Melt margarine in pan. Add flour and seasonings, and blend. Gradually add milk, stirring to avoid lumps. Cook until smooth and thick. Meanwhile, cover bottom of greased baking dish with half the crumbs. Add a layer of spinach, then sliced eggs, then white sauce mixture and finally, cheese. Repeat, covering top with remaining crumbs. Bake until heated-through and browned, about 15 minutes.

Spinach~Stuffed Tomatoes

Serves 8

8 medium unpeeled tomatoes
1 to 2 teaspoons salt
8 slices bacon
2 10-ounce packages frozen chopped spinach
1 pinch garlic powder
1 pinch nutmeg
1 pinch salt
1 pinch pepper
¾ cup breadcrumbs
4 tablespoons butter, melted
8 tablespoons sour cream

Preheat oven to 350 degrees. Cut a thin slice from top of tomato. Scoop out pulp and discard. Sprinkle inside with salt and drain upside down 1 hour. Cook bacon and crumble. Cook spinach until just thawed; drain well. Add bacon, spices and crumbs. Fill tomatoes with spinach mixture. Drizzle with melted butter and refrigerate until needed. Bake in a buttered dish for 20 minutes. Top each with 1 tablespoon sour cream.

Fire & Ice Tomatoes

Serves 6 to 8

6 large tomatoes, thickly sliced
¼ onion, finely chopped
2 teaspoons basil

Red wine vinaigrette:
¼ cup red wine vinegar
¾ cup olive oil
1 garlic clove, finely minced
1 teaspoon Worcestershire sauce
2 teaspoons salt
½ teaspoon pepper
½ teaspoon sugar

Arrange tomato slices in layers in serving bowl. Mix together onion, basil and part of salt. Sprinkle over tomatoes and continue layering. In jar, combine the rest of the ingredients and pour over tomatoes. Chill, covered.

Fried Green Tomatoes

Serves 6

1 tablespoon brown sugar
1 cup all-purpose flour
1 egg, beaten
¼ cup milk
1 cup seasoned, dry bread crumbs
4 to 6 medium green tomatoes, sliced about ½-inch thick
3 tablespoons butter or margarine
1 tablespoon vegetable oil

Combine sugar and flour, and place on shallow plate. Combine the egg and milk in small bowl. Place dry bread crumbs on a plate. Dip both sides of each tomato slice into the sugar-flour mixture. Then dip both sides of each tomato into egg-milk mixture. Finally, dip both sides of each tomato into the bread crumbs. In a skillet, heat butter or margarine and oil over medium-high heat. Fry tomatoes until brown on both sides, but firm enough to hold their shape. Serve tomato slices hot.

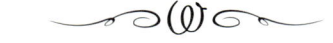

Scalloped Tomatoes

Serves 4

Adapted for your kitchen… from the original Walgreens recipe!

Robin Hood & Briargate Restaurants, 1970's ~ 1980's

4 large firm, ripe beef steak tomatoes, peeled and sliced ¼-inch thick
¾ teaspoon salt
⅛ teaspoon pepper
¼ teaspoon sugar
1 cup bread crumbs
2 tablespoons butter

Preheat oven to 350 degrees. In a buttered baking dish, put successive layers of tomatoes, sprinkled with salt, pepper, bread crumbs and sugar. On last layer of tomatoes put several bits of butter, then dust with pepper and a little sugar. Strew with bread crumbs, cover and bake for 30 minutse. Remove lid and bake until brown.

Spinach~Artichoke Dish

Serves 4 to 6

- 1   8½-ounce can artichoke bottoms, drained
- ½   stick of butter
- 2   packages frozen chopped spinach, cooked and drained
- 8   ounces mozzarella cheese, freshly grated
- 1   teaspoon lemon juice

bread crumbs, buttered

Preheat oven to 350 degrees. Place artichoke bottoms with their cut sides up in bottom of a 7x11-inch baking dish. Melt butter and add spinach, cheese and lemon juice. Top with bread crumbs. Bake for 20 minutes.

Stuffed Artichokes

Serves 8
One half per person

- 4   large artichokes
- 1   cup Italian bread crumbs, seasoned
- 1   cup Romano cheese, grated
- 3   teaspoons salt

pepper, to taste

- 1   teaspoon oregano
- ⅛   teaspoon red pepper, if desired
- 3   tablespoons olive oil
- 1   garlic clove

vinaigrette dressing, prepared

Using scissors, cut artichoke tips straight across to remove thorns. Cut remaining thorns off the artichoke. Remove stem. Soak in cold water. While artichokes are soaking, prepare stuffing by combining bread crumbs, cheese, 1 teaspoon of salt, pepper, oregano and red pepper. Mix thoroughly. While holding them by the base, open the artichokes by pounding against the sink or cutting board. Rinse under cold water, but do not dry. Take each artichoke by the base and scoop it into the mixture. Drizzle 1 tablespoon of the oil over tops of the 4 artichokes and dip into mixture again. Fill a 5-quart pan with water, enough to reach halfway up artichokes. Add garlic, 2 teaspoons salt and 2 tablespoons olive oil to the water. Bring to boil, reduce heat and cover. Do not let boil dry; continue adding water as needed. Cook 45 minutes. Pull leaf to check; artichokes are done when leaves pull off easily. Drain when done. Serve with vinaigrette dressing.

Hot, Spiced Beets

Serves 4 to 6

Adapted for your kitchen… from the original Walgreens recipe!

Walgreens Cafeterias 1940's ~ 1960's

2 pounds boiled fresh beets, peeled and sliced or two 16-ounce cans beets, drained (reserve juice)
½ cup sugar
1 teaspoon whole cloves
3 tablespoons vinegar
reserved beet juice

Slice beets and add sugar, cloves, vinegar and beet juice. Bring to a boil and simmer for 15 minutes. Serve immediately or cover with wax paper to keep beets from turning dark.

Creole Corn

Serves 4

Adapted for your kitchen… from the original Walgreens recipe!

Walgreens Cafeterias 1940's ~ 1960's

2 cups fresh whole kernel corn cut from the cob or canned whole kernel corn, drained
1 medium yellow onion, finely chopped
1 large sweet green pepper, cored, seeded and finely chopped
¼ cup butter or margarine
1 14½-ounce can tomatoes, with pulp and juice
salt and pepper, to taste

Heat butter in saucepan; cook onions, pepper and corn for about 10 minutes. Add remaining ingredients and cook until tender. Season with salt and pepper.

Fort Myers Corn Casserole

Serves 4 to 6

8 tablespoons butter
1 14¾-ounce can cream-style corn
1 15¼-ounce can kernel corn
1 8-ounce container sour cream or plain yogurt
1 8½-ounce box Jiffy corn muffin mix

Preheat oven to 350 degrees. Mix all ingredients together. Pour into greased 2-quart casserole. Bake at 350 degrees for 45 minutes to 1 hour, uncovered. Test with knife; casserole is done when knife comes out clean.

Broccoli Soufflé de Norman

Serves 8 to 10

- ¼ cup onion, chopped
- 6 tablespoons butter
- 6 tablespoons flour
- ½ cup water
- 1 8-ounce jar Cheese Whiz
- 2 10-ounce packages frozen chopped broccoli, thawed and drained
- 3 eggs, well beaten
- ½ cup Ritz cracker crumbs

Preheat oven to 325 degrees. Sauté onions in 4 tablespoons butter, stir in flour. Add water and cook over low heat, 2 to 3 minutes. Remove from heat. Stir in cheese, broccoli and eggs, and mix gently until blended. Pour into greased casserole dish. Cover with cracker crumbs and dot with remaining butter. Bake for 40 to 45 minutes.

Sandy's Broccoli Soufflé

Serves 8 to 10

- 2 packages frozen chopped broccoli, thawed
- 6 tablespoons butter
- ¼ cup onion, finely chopped
- ¼ cup water
- 2 tablespoons flour
- 1 8-ounce jar Cheese Whiz
- 3 eggs, well beaten
- ¼ cup Saltine crackers, crushed

Preheat oven to 325 degrees. Heat 4 tablespoons butter in skillet and sauté onions. Add water and flour and cook until thickened. Add broccoli and Cheese Whiz. Add eggs; mix well and pour into buttered casserole. Brown crackers in remaining 2 tablespoons butter and sprinkle on top of casserole. Bake for 30 minutes.

Party Broccoli

Serves 6 to 8

Also works well as an appetizer!

- 2 tablespoons butter
- 2 tablespoons onion, minced
- 1½ cups sour cream
- 2 teaspoons sugar
- 1 teaspoon vinegar
- ½ teaspoon poppy seeds
- ½ teaspoon paprika
- ½ teaspoon salt
- 1 dash cayenne pepper
- 1 bunch broccoli, cooked and drained
- ½ cup cashew nuts, crushed

Melt butter in saucepan. Add onion, and sauté. Remove from heat and stir in sour cream, sugar, vinegar, poppy seeds and spices. Arrange broccoli on a platter. Top with sauce and sprinkle with cashews.

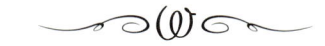

Broccoli Ring with Carrots

Serves 10 to 12

Also works well as an appetizer!

- 2½ pounds fresh broccoli, trimmed and steamed
- 2 ounces Parmesan cheese (½-cup grated)
- 1 onion, chopped
- 1 tablespoon butter
- 4 eggs
- ¼ cup heavy cream
- 1½ teaspoons salt
- ¼ teaspoon pepper
- ¼ teaspoon nutmeg
- 2½ cups baby carrots, cooked

Preheat oven to 350 degrees. Steam broccoli 10 to 15 minutes until tender, rinse immediately with cold water, drain and set aside. Cook chopped onion in butter until tender. In a food processor or blender pureé broccoli; add all ingredients to bowl, except cooked carrots, and process until thoroughly blended. Turn mixture into heavily buttered 2 to 2½-quart ring mold. Place in baking pan filled with 1-inch hot water. Bake on middle oven rack for 30 to 40 minutes or until a knife inserted in the center comes out clean. Unmold and fill center with cooked carrots.

Asparagus a la Hazelwood

Serves 4 to 6

An original Hazelwood recipe!

1	cup water
½	cup butter
½	teaspoon salt
⅛	teaspoon white pepper
1	cup all-purpose, unbleached flour
1	cup Gruyére or Swiss cheese, grated
4	eggs
¼	pound ham, sliced
½	pound asparagus, sliced into 4 to 5-inch spears
1	cup *Hollandaise Sauce*

(see recipe in the *RxCetera ~ Sauces & Garnishes* chapter)

Preheat oven to 375 degrees. In a medium-size saucepan combine the water, butter, salt and pepper. Bring to a boil. Add the flour and cheese. Stir well to make dough. Remove pan from heat and beat in the eggs, one at a time until paste is smooth. This dough makes what is called a gougére. To prepare, grease a large au gratin or 10-inch pie pan. Smooth the dough over the bottom of the pan. Make a well in the center of the dough, building the dough up around the edges. Slice the ham into ½x2-inch pieces. Lay the ham in the center of the dough, overlapping each piece. Bake for 30 minutes. In the meantime, prepare the asparagus and Hollandaise sauce. 5 minutes before the gougére comes out of the oven, blanch or steam the asparagus until tender, about 3 to 5 minutes. Take the gougére out of the oven and place the asparagus on top of the ham. Spoon the Hollandaise sauce over the asparagus and serve immediately.

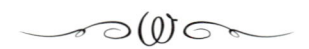

Cold Asparagus with Walnuts

Serves 6 to 8

1½	pounds fresh asparagus
1	cup walnuts, finely chopped
1½ to 2	tablespoons walnut or sesame oil
¼	cup cider vinegar
¼	cup soy sauce
⅓	cup sugar

pepper, to taste

Cook asparagus covered, in boiling water, for 6 to 7 minutes, or until just tender. Drain well, and arrange on serving platter. Whisk remaining ingredients until well-blended. Pour over asparagus, lifting asparagus, so dressing penetrates. Sprinkle with pepper. Chill.

Sesame Asparagus

Serves 4

1 pound asparagus
1½ teaspoons peanut oil
2½ tablespoons sesame oil
½ medium bulb fennel, diced
½ large red pepper, diced
½ large yellow pepper, diced
2½ tablespoons rice vinegar
4 scallions (green onions), thinly sliced
crushed red pepper flakes, to taste
salt, to taste
2 tablespoons cilantro, minced

Cook asparagus in boiling, salted water for about 6 minutes. Drain and run under cold water to keep color green. Heat oils in skillet until very hot. Add fennel and peppers. Heat through, about 2 minutes. Add vinegar and asparagus. Heat about 2 more minutes. Remove from heat and add scallions, salt, crushed red pepper and cilantro. Serve hot.

Vegetable Casserole

Serves 6 to 8

Adapted for your kitchen... from the original Walgreens recipe!

Walgreens Cafeterias 1940's ~ 1960's

2 cups potatoes, diced
2 cups carrots, diced
1 cup string beans, cut small
1 cup celery, chopped
1 cup fresh peas
1 onion, coarsely chopped
salt, to taste
1 cup bread crumbs

White sauce:
2 cups reserved vegetable liquid, hot
4 tablespoons butter
4 tablespoons flour
1 teaspoon salt
¼ teaspoon white pepper
1 dash cayenne

Vegetable Casserole, *continued on next page.*

Vegetable Casserole, continued.

Preheat oven to 350 degrees. Put vegetables in Dutch oven; cover completely with water. Bring to a boil and simmer for 10 to 15 minutes or until vegetables are tender. Drain, reserving 2 cups of liquid. Put vegetables in greased casserole. Prepare white sauce. Melt butter and add flour until bubbly, but not brown. Slowly add hot vegetable liquid, stirring until smooth and thick. Add salt, white pepper and cayenne pepper. Pour sauce over vegetable. Sprinkle with bread crumbs and bake for about 20 minutes, or until lightly browned.

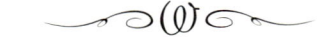

Roman Casserole

Serves 6 to 8

- 3 small Italian eggplants, sliced ½-inch thick
- 2 teaspoons salt
- 3 cups small, red potatoes, quartered
- olive oil, enough to drizzle from spout and also for ½-inch coverage of pan to sauté eggplant
- 2 medium onions, sliced
- 2 medium green peppers, roasted and sliced
- 3 medium tomatoes, sliced
- 1 teaspoon oregano
- 1 teaspoon basil
- salt and pepper, to taste
- ½ cup Parmesan cheese (optional)

Sprinkle salt on both sides of sliced eggplant and let sit for 30 minutes, then rinse well and pat dry. Meanwhile, place potatoes on a baking sheet and sprinkle with olive oil. Bake at 400 degrees for 20 to 25 minutes, or until brown. Sauté egg plant in ½-inch olive oil, and brown; drain on paper towels. Preheat oven to broil. Roast peppers whole under broiler for approximately 25 minutes or until surface is blistered and charred. Scrape charred skin; then slice. To assemble, line baking dish with sliced onions, then drizzle with olive oil. Place roasted peppers on top of onions, then alternate slices of eggplant with tomatoes. Season with oregano, basil, salt and pepper. Sprinkle with Parmesan cheese, if desired. Bake at 400 degrees for 30 minutes, or until bubbly.

Dutch Red Cabbage

Serves 4 to 6

Adapted for your kitchen… from the original Walgreens recipe!

Robin Hood & Briargate Restaurants, 1970's ~ 1980's

- 1 medium red cabbage, outer leaves and hearts removed, shredded
- 1 large onion, cut in half and thinly sliced
- 3 tablespoons butter
- 2 tablespoons sugar
- ½ teaspoon salt
- 1 cup water
- ¼ cup vinegar
- 1 cup applesauce
- 2 tablespoons cornstarch
- ¼ cup water

Melt butter in Dutch oven; add sliced onions. Cover pan and allow to steam for about 5 minutes. Add shredded cabbage in three layers. Sprinkle each layer with sugar and a little salt. Add cup of water and spread applesauce on top of cabbage. Cover pan and allow cabbage to steam for about 30 minutes. Add vinegar and mix thoroughly. Dissolve cornstarch in ¼-cup water and add to cabbage. Mix until cornstarch cooks and thickens, about 5 minutes. Season to taste.

The Best Creamed Cabbage

Serves 6

- 1 head cabbage (approximately 4 pounds), coarsely chopped
- 1 cup water
- 1 8-ounce package cream cheese
- 2 tablespoons butter or margarine
- 1 large onion, chopped
- 1 pound fresh mushrooms, sliced

salt and pepper, to taste

Cook cabbage over medium heat in a pot with the water until the cabbage is tender. Drain any extra water. Add the cream cheese to the cabbage while the cabbage is still hot. Stir until cheese melts. Set aside. In frying pan, with butter, cook chopped onion over low heat, until tender. Add the sliced mushrooms. Cook for about 10 minutes. Combine the onion and mushrooms with the cabbage and cream cheese in the pot. Season to taste.

Sherwood Forest Sauerkraut

Serves 6 to 8

Adapted for your kitchen... from the original Walgreens recipe!

Robin Hood & Briargate Restaurants, 1970's ~ 1980's

2	16-ounce jars sauerkraut, drained
2	tablespoons butter
1	large onion, very finely chopped
2	tablespoons sugar
1	teaspoon salt
¼	teaspoon white pepper
1	potato, peeled and grated
1	quart water

Heat butter in Dutch oven; sauté onions until soft but not brown. Remove from heat; add sugar, salt, white pepper, raw potatoes and cold water. Mix well. Alternately add one layer of onion mixture and one layer of sauerkraut. If necessary, add more cold water so sauerkraut is completely covered. Bring to boil; reduce heat and cook slowly for 10 minutes. Season to taste.

Carrot Bourbonade

Serves 4 to 6

8	medium carrots, peeled and cut in diagonal slices
2	teaspoons butter
2	teaspoons light brown sugar
⅛	teaspoon salt
2	tablespoons bourbon
1	teaspoon fresh dill or ¼-teaspoon dried dill

Combine butter, brown sugar and salt. Heat slowly until butter melts. Add carrots; cover, and cook slowly for 10 to 15 minutes, until just tender. Add bourbon and cook over low heat, uncovered, for 1 minute. Sprinkle with dill and serve.

Mary's Marmalade~Glazed Carrots

Serves 4 to 6

8	carrots, peeled and sliced
¼	cup orange marmalade
1	tablespoon butter

Cook carrots in water for 10 to 15 minutes, or until tender. Add marmalade and butter. Toss gently; serve hot. Great when prepared ahead and reheated.

Mint~Glazed Carrots

Serves 4

Adapted for your kitchen...
from the original Walgreens recipe!

Robin Hood
& Briargate
Restaurants,
1970's ~ 1980's

6 to 8 large carrots, peeled and sliced
1½ cups boiling water
½ teaspoon salt
2 tablespoons brown sugar
2 tablespoons butter
2 tablespoons fresh mint leaves, chopped

Preheat oven to 350 degrees. Cut large carrots in quarters lengthwise and in half crosswise. Add carrots and salt to boiling water. Cook until tender, about 10 to 15 minutes. Drain; put in baking dish. Sprinkle with brown sugar, dot with butter and bake for 45 minutes. Remove from oven and sprinkle with fresh mint.

Knox County Carrot Casserole

Serves 6

10 or 12 carrots, peeled and sliced
1 cup celery, finely cut
1 medium onion, diced
salt

White sauce:
½ cup butter or margarine
½ cup flour
4 cups milk
½ teaspoon mustard
salt and pepper, to taste
½ pound Velveeta cheese, cubed

4 slices bread
2 tablespoons butter

Preheat oven to 350 degrees. Cook carrots, celery and onion separately in salted water and drain. Mix together. Prepare white sauce: melt butter in pan, blend in flour slowly. Add milk and cook until thickened, stirring constantly. Remove from stove; add mustard, salt and pepper. Stir in cheese cubes, mixing well, until melted. In a buttered, square casserole, arrange half the vegetables and half the white sauce. Then add remaining vegetables and white sauce. Butter and score bread (be careful not to cut all the way through); cut off the crusts. Place slices on top of casserole. Bake for 30 minutes, or until brown.

Mushrooms in Wine Sauce

Serves 8 to 10

- 6 tablespoons butter
- ½ pound mushrooms, sliced
- 2 medium onions, finely chopped
- 1 garlic clove, minced
- 2 tablespoons chili sauce
- 1 tablespoon Escoffier Diable Sauce
- ½ teaspoon flour
- 1 pinch dried marjoram
- 1 pinch dried thyme
- 4 drops Tabasco sauce
- 2 dashes Worcestershire sauce
- 5 ounces dry red wine
- 1 bouillon cube, dissolved in ¼-cup water

salt and pepper, freshly ground, to taste
parsley, minced

Tenderloin Deluxe (see recipe in the *Meats ~ Beef* chapter)
Béarnaise Sauce (see recipe in the *RxCetera ~ Sauces & Garnishes* chapter)

Melt butter in a large skillet. Add mushrooms, onions and garlic. Sauté until onions are soft. Add remaining ingredients except for parsley and mix well. Barely simmer for about 10 minutes. Serve in separate, individual crocks or serving bowls with *Tenderloin Deluxe* and *Béarnaise Sauce*.

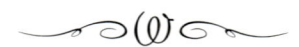

Swiss Baked Mushrooms

Serves 6

Also works well as an appetizer!

- 6 tablespoons butter
- 2 medium onions, chopped
- 1½ pounds mushrooms, sliced
- ¼ cup sherry
- ¼ teaspoon white pepper
- 2 cups (8 ounces) Swiss cheese, shredded

paprika, to taste

Preheat oven to 425 degrees. Melt butter in 12-inch frying pan over medium heat. Add onions and mushrooms. Cook, stirring frequently, until mushrooms are soft and liquid evaporates. Stir in sherry and white pepper. Continue cooking and stirring for 1 minute. Put mushrooms in a shallow baking dish, and cool slightly. Sprinkle Swiss cheese over mushroom; sprinkle paprika on top. Bake, uncovered, for 8 to 10 minutes, until hot and bubbly.

Crumb~Topped Mushrooms

Serves 6

Also works well as an appetizer!

- 3 slices firm-textured white bread, crust removed
- 5 tablespoons butter
- 1½ pounds small, whole mushrooms
- 2 garlic cloves, minced
- ½ cup parsley, chopped

Preheat oven to 425 degrees. Place slices of firm-textured white bread (no crust) in blender and whirl to make 1 cup crumbs; set aside. Melt 2 tablespoons butter in frying pan over medium heat. Add whole mushrooms. Cover and cook 4 minutes. Uncover, turn heat to high, and cook, stirring constantly, until liquid evaporates. Arrange mushrooms in a lightly greased, shallow baking dish. Melt 3 tablespoons butter in frying pan over medium heat. Add bread crumbs, minced garlic and chopped parsley. Mix well and heat through. Distribute evenly over mushrooms. Bake for 8 to 10 minutes, or until crumbs are lightly browned.

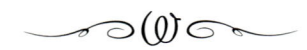

Mushroom Supreme

Serves 6

Also works well as an appetizer!

- 1 pound mushrooms, cleaned
- Pam cooking spray
- 2 beef bouillon cubes
- ½ cup hot water
- 4 tablespoons butter
- 2 tablespoons flour
- ½ cup half-and-half
- 2 teaspoons salt
- 1 dash ground pepper
- ½ cup bread crumbs
- ¾ cup Parmesan cheese

Preheat oven to 350 degrees. Sauté mushrooms in pan with Pam cooking spray. Dissolve bouillon cubes in hot water. In another pan, melt butter; blend in flour and cook over medium heat until bubbly. Add the bouillon-water mixture slowly until thickened and smooth. Add mushrooms. Melt butter. Blend with flour. In medium size bowl, add half-and-half, salt, pepper and beef broth. Add mushroom mixture. Mix. Place mushroom mixture in lightly greased 9x9-inch baking dish. Mix bread crumbs with Parmesan cheese. Sprinkle on top. Bake for 30 minutes.

Boston Baked Beans

Serves 4 to 6

**Adapted for your kitchen...
from the original Walgreens recipe!**

*Robin Hood
& Briargate
Restaurants,
1970's ~ 1980's*

- 1 pound dry navy beans
- 2 quarts cold water
- ½ pound salt pork or bacon, cut into cubes
- 2 garlic cloves, crushed
- 1 medium onion, coarsely chopped
- 3 tablespoons dark brown sugar
- 2 teaspoons salt
- ¼ teaspoon pepper
- ½ cup molasses
- ½ teaspoon dry mustard
- ¼ cup catsup
- 2 tablespoons beef base or bouillon cubes

Preheat oven to 275 degrees. Check beans for stones. Wash beans; soak overnight in 2 quarts of cold water. Bring to a boil in the same water; simmer for 1½ hours, or until tender. Drain, reserving 2 cups of the liquid. Place half the salt pork or bacon in a roasting pan. Mix all the spices. Mix 2 cups liquid from bean pot with spices. Stir this mixture back into bean pot. Pour beans over salt pork. Cover top of beans with other half of pork or bacon. Bake for 4 to 5 hours, adding more water if needed.

China Bean Bake

Serves 4 to 6

- 1 10-ounce package frozen cut green beans, blanched
- 1 10¾-ounce can cream of mushroom soup
- ½ cup celery, cut diagonally
- 1 8-ounce can water chestnuts
- 1 4-ounce can pimentos
- 1 tablespoon soy sauce
- ¾ cup chow mein noodles

Preheat oven to 375 degrees. Mix all ingredients together except chow mein noodles. Top with chow mein noodles. Bake for 45 minutes.

Calico Baked Beans

Serves 8 to 10

An original Hazelwood recipe!

½	pound bacon, cut up
4	large onions, cut in rings
2	garlic cloves, cut fine
⅓	cup catsup
¼	cup vinegar
¾	cup brown sugar
¼	teaspoon dry mustard
1	15¼-ounce can baby green lima beans, drained
1	15½-ounce can kidney beans, drained
1	15½-ounce can butter beans, drained
1	15½-ounce can great northern beans, drained
1	16-ounce can pork and beans

Preheat oven to 350 degrees. Fry together bacon, onions and garlic. Mix together catsup, vinegar, brown sugar and dry mustard. Add liquid mixture to fried bacon and simmer for 20 minutes. Add beans and bake for 1 hour.

Note: May add an extra can of drained beans and a whole pound of bacon and then double or triple the liquid mixture. May also bake the beans for 2 hours rather than 1 hour. Great for barbecue dishes.

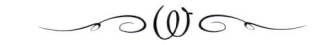

"21~Bean" Casserole

Serves 8 to 10

2	onions, chopped
½	pound bacon, cut in small pieces
1	15¼-ounce can lima beans, drained
1	15½-ounce can kidney beans, drained
1	15½-ounce can butter beans, drained
1	16-ounce can pork and beans
¾	cup brown sugar
1	tablespoon dry mustard
⅓	cup vinegar

Preheat oven to 325 degrees. Sauté onions with bacon until soft. Combine rest of ingredients and pour into 9x12-inch baking pan. Bake for 2 hours.

Texas Beans, Chicago Style

Serves 8 to 10

- 1 1-pound package pork sausage, mild or spicy-hot, crumbled
- 1 15¼-ounce can green lima beans, drained
- 1 14½-ounce can green beans, drained
- 1 14½-ounce can wax beans, drained
- 1 15½-ounce can light red kidney beans, drained
- 2 16-ounce cans pork and beans
- ½ cup catsup
- ¼ cup prepared barbecue sauce, your choice
- 1 cup brown sugar
- 1 medium onion, chopped
- 6 bacon strips

Preheat oven to 325 degrees. Brown and drain crumbled sausage. Combine all ingredients, except bacon strips, in a roasting pan. Mix carefully, being careful not to break beans apart. Lay the bacon strips evenly across the top of the mixture. Cover, and bake for 2 hours. Serve right out of the pan!

Baked Garbanzos

Serves 6

- 4 cups canned garbanzo beans (chickpeas)
- 1 teaspoon salt
- ½ teaspoon pepper
- 3 large tomatoes, peeled, seeded and chopped
- 1 large onion, chopped
- 1 garlic clove, chopped
- 1 teaspoon rosemary
- ½ cup olive oil

Preheat oven to 350 degrees. Combine all ingredients in a greased baking dish. Bake for 1 hour. Adjust seasoning to taste. Serve hot.

Note: Great served with lamb. May also be served with rice pilaf.

Lentil Casserole with Sausage

Serves 6

2 cups lentil beans
1 tablespoon salt
1 whole onion
2 cloves
1 bay leaf
12 Italian sausages
½ cup onion, finely chopped
4 tablespoons butter
salt & pepper, freshly ground, to taste
1 cup red wine

Insert cloves into sides of whole onion. Cover lentils with water; add salt, whole onion with cloves and bay leaf. Bring to a boil and simmer until lentils are tender. While lentils are cooking, poach sausages about 5 minutes in enough water to cover. Preheat oven to 350 degrees. Sauté chopped onion in butter. Arrange half the sausages in the bottom of a greased 2½-quart baking dish. Drain the lentils, removing the whole onion and bay leaf. Add half the lentils, a little sautéed onion, salt and pepper. Layer again with lentils, sausages and onions. Pour in wine. Bake for 25 to 30 minutes, or until sausages have browned.

Mofongo ~ Plantain Pudding

Serves 6 to 8

Adapted for your kitchen... from the original Walgreens recipe!

Walgreen Grills in Puerto Rico, 1960's ~ 1980's

4 green plantains (*platanos*), cut into ½-inch pieces
vegetable oil
1 1-pound bag crispy pork rinds
1 teaspoon salt
garlic butter
chicken broth or stock, heated

Deep-fry plantains in 360-degree oil in an electric skillet or frying pan until tender. Cool. In food processor, combine plantains, pork rinds and salt to make a paste or pudding. Divide mixture into 5-ounce portions. Using a small bowl (*pilōn*), shape portions into rounded mounds (mofongo). Brush each mofongo on top with garlic butter. Serve with hot chicken broth.

Note: To eat mofongo: first sip the hot broth, then, using the same spoon, dip into the mofongo and take a bite!

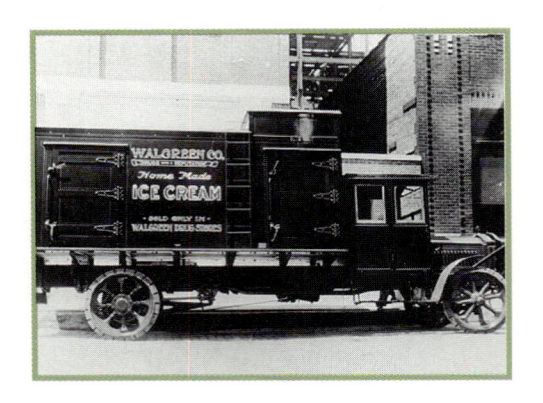

This 1923 refrigerated Packard truck delivered gallons of freshly-made Walgreens ice cream from the Commissary to the stores.

Facing Page: *Tortellini Alfredo Primavera*
Photo: Scott Lanza, 1995
Stylist: F. Lynn Nelson

PASTA, GRAINS & POTATOES

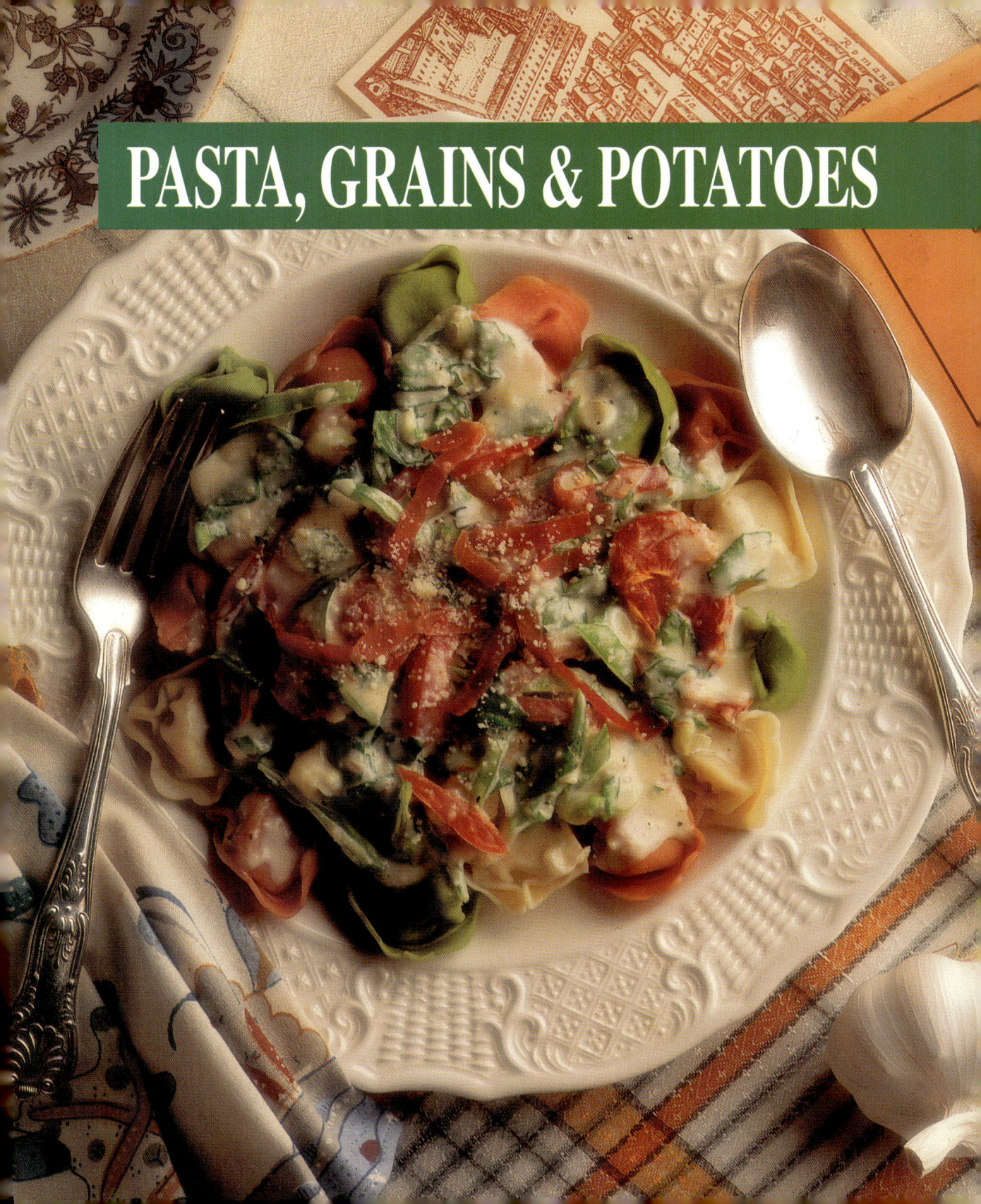

The Commissaries
Welcome to the Kitchens of Walgreens

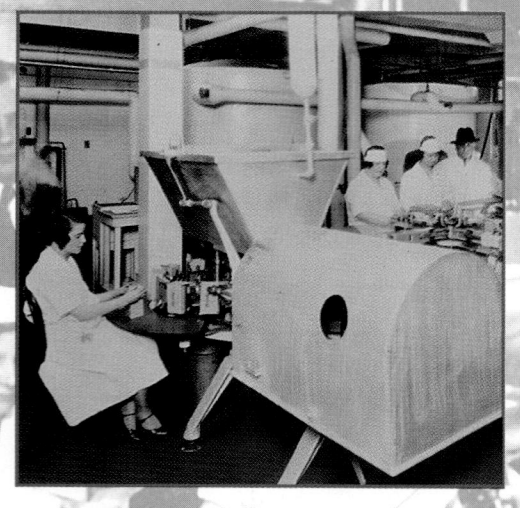

"Charles remarked, 'I think if we served a few good sandwiches and something hot, maybe some soup and a little dessert, we could keep the [soda counter] open all winter.'."
Myrtle R. Walgreen, recounting C. R. Walgreen, Sr.'s plan to expand the soda fountain in her autobiography, Never A Dull Day (1963).

Established in 1916, Walgreens very first Commissary was created in two vacant stores at 3740 Cottage Grove Avenue. Its purpose was to supply and prepare foods for the soda fountains. (A year earlier, in about 1915, Myrtle R. Walgreen prepared the food herself, using her own recipes, in her own kitchen!) Truly a "mom's kitchen," it was here at the Commissary that Walgreens made its very own ice cream and bread, created and tested its food and dessert menus, and ground and roasted its own high-grade Colombian coffee beans. In 1929, Walgreens added a chocolate factory, which ground Colombian cocoa beans and made a line of hand-dipped candies. During the 1930's, Walgreens won the *National Baker's* prize for its cinnamon-raisin bread. In 1922, Walgreens moved the Commissary to 500 East 40th Street.

Later, when the old fountains grew into cafeterias, food was prepared right in restaurant kitchens. Eventually, the Commissaries became warehouses for Walgreens restaurants nationwide.

President Reagan's Favorite ~ Macaroni & Cheese

Serves 4

An authentic recipe from Nancy Reagan!

- 8 ounces elbow macaroni
- 1 teaspoon butter
- 1 egg, beaten
- 1 teaspoon dry mustard
- 1 teaspoon salt
- 1 tablespoon hot water
- 1 cup milk
- 3 cups sharp cheddar cheese, grated

Preheat oven to 350 degrees. Boil macaroni in water until tender and drain thoroughly; stir in butter and egg. Mix mustard and salt in 1 tablespoon hot water, and add to milk. Add cheese, leaving enough to sprinkle on top. Pour macaroni-egg mixture into buttered casserole, add milk-seasoning-cheese mixture and sprinkle with remaining cheese. Bake for about 45 minutes, or until custard is set and top is crusty.

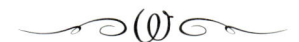

Vegetable & Olive Rotini in Mustard Sauce

Serves 4 to 6

A Note on Cooking Pasta: *Cook pasta rapidly at a rolling boil. Pasta cooked* al dente *is cooked tender, but firm to the bite (with a slight crunch). Pasta should never be limp, soft or mushy; over-cooked pasta loses its taste and nutritional value!*

- 1 pound rotini (spiral-shaped pasta)
- 2 cups broccoli florets
- 2 cups cauliflower florets
- 2 red peppers, diced
- 2 shallots, peeled and diced
- 2 tablespoons parsley, minced
- ⅔ cup dry, cured black olives

Mustard sauce:
- ½ cup olive oil
- 4 teaspoons Dijon mustard
- 1 teaspoon lemon juice
- ¼ teaspoon pepper

salt, to taste

In a large pot, bring 3 quarts of water to a boil. Add broccoli and cauliflower, and cook about 5 minutes until al dente. Remove vegetables with a slotted spoon and reserve water. Cook rotini in vegetable cooking water until tender, but still slightly firm. Drain well. Place vegetables in a serving bowl with rotini, red peppers, shallots, parsley and olives. Combine oil, mustard, lemon juice, pepper and salt in bowl. Stir well. Pour over pasta and toss. Serve warm or at room temperature.

Fusilli with Cottage Cheese Pesto & Broccoli

Serves 4 to 6

1 pound fusilli (thin, spiral-shaped pasta)
1 head (about 1½ to 2 pounds) broccoli, broken into florets

Cottage cheese pesto sauce:
2 to 3 garlic cloves (or to taste), peeled
½ cup fresh basil leaves, washed and dried
1 cup plain nonfat cottage cheese
seas salt, to taste
pepper, freshly ground, to taste
¼ cup plain nonfat yogurt
1 tablespoon olive oil
¼ cup Parmesan cheese, freshly grated

First, prepare pesto sauce. Turn on food processor fitted with steel blade, and drop in garlic. Process until finely chopped. Add basil and chop fine. Add cottage cheese, salt pepper, yogurt, olive oil and Parmesan cheese. Pureé until mixture is creamy and smooth. Bring a large pot of water to a rolling boil. Add salt (about 1 tablespoon) and pasta. Boil 4 minutes and add broccoli. Continue to boil until pasta is cooked al dente (firm to the bite) and broccoli is crisp-tender, about 4 more minutes. Drain, toss with cottage cheese pesto mixture, and serve immediately.

Jorie's Linguine with Pesto

Serves 4 to 6

1 pound linguine, cooked per package directions

Pesto sauce:
2 cups fresh basil
¼ cup Italian parsley
2 tablespoons walnut pieces
1 tablespoon pine nuts
1 garlic clove
3 tablespoons butter, melted
¼ tablespoon white pepper
¼ tablespoon nutmeg
1 cup Italian (Romano) cheese
3 ounces olive oil

To prepare pesto, put all ingredients, except olive oil, in food processor or blender. Pulse until combined, with motor running slowly. Add olive oil. Drain cooked linguine and pour into serving dish. Cover with pesto.

Linguine with Artichoke Sauce

Serves 4

8 ounces linguine, cooked per package directions
green onions, chopped (optional)

Artichoke sauce:
¼ cup olive oil
½ stick butter or margarine
1 teaspoon flour
1 cup chicken broth
1 garlic clove, crushed
2 teaspoons lemon juice
1 teaspoon parsley flakes
salt and pepper, to taste
1 14½-ounce can artichoke hearts, drained and quartered
2 tablespoons Romano cheese

First, prepare sauce. In a saucepan, heat oil and butter. Add flour gradually, stirring and cooking 3 minutes. Stir in broth. Increase heat and cook 1 minute. Add garlic, lemon juice, parsley and seasonings. Stir 5 minutes. Add artichoke hearts and cheese. Cook and stir 8 minutes. Pour over cooked linguine. If desired, add extra cheese and green onions.

Linguine with White Clam Sauce

Serves 4 to 6

1 pound linguine, cooked per package directions
Parmesan cheese, grated

White clam sauce:
1 medium onion, chopped
1 garlic clove, finely chopped
3 tablespoons margarine or butter
1 tablespoon flour
3 6½-ounce cans minced clams, with liquid
½ teaspoon salt
½ teaspoon dried basil
⅛ teaspoon pepper
¼ cup parsley, snipped

First prepare sauce. Cook and stir onion and garlic in margarine in a 2-quart saucepan until onion is tender. Stir in flour. Add clams with liquid, salt, basil and pepper. Heat to boiling; reduce heat and simmer 5 minutes. Drain cooked linguine and put on a serving platter. Add parsley to clam sauce. Pour sauce over hot linguine, sprinkle with Parmesan cheese, and serve.

Nona's Tuscana Sugo with Fettuccine

Serves 2 to 12

1 pound fettuccine, cooked per package directions
½ cup imported Romano cheese, grated

Nona's Tuscana Sugo (meat sauce):

¼ cup extra-virgin olive oil
1 pound sirloin, ground
1 pound veal, ground
1 pound pork, ground
2 cups celery, chopped
1 cup onion, chopped
1 cup carrots, thinly sliced
2 garlic cloves, thinly sliced
¼ teaspoon nutmeg
⅛ teaspoon cinnamon
salt and pepper, to taste
red pepper, to taste (optional)
1 6-ounce can tomato paste
1 14½-ounce can imported Italian plum tomatoes, crushed
½ cup Italian flat-leaf parsley, chopped
½ 16-ounce can (8 ounces) imported Italian tomato pureé
8 ounces water

To make sauce (*sugo*), heat 2 tablespoons olive oil; brown ground meats in a 5-quart saucepan and drain fat. While meat is browning, sauté celery, onion and carrots in remaining olive oil until onions are just translucent. Add garlic and stir. When garlic is golden, add mixture to drained, cooked meat. Mix well, adding nutmeg, cinnamon, salt, pepper and red pepper. Adjust seasoning to taste. Nutmeg and cinnamon should not be overpowering, just subtle enough for nutty flavor. Add tomato paste. Mix well. Add crushed plum tomatoes, chopped Italian parsley and stir. Add tomato pureé and water. Bring to a boil. Sauce should be red-brown in color. May add more tomato pureé, at this point, if you prefer. Stir 1 to 2 minutes; reduce heat to low, add cheese, stir and simmer.

Drain cooked pasta. Using the pan pasta was cooked in, add about 1 cup sauce and all the pasta. Mix well. Place in serving dish; add sauce, to your liking, on top. Sprinkle with cheese and serve.

Note: Serves as few as 2 or as many as 12! Sauce freezes well. For a variation, try with capellini (angel hair pasta) or mostaccioli.

Fettuccine Alfredo Tomaselli

Serves 4 to 6

1 pound fettuccine, cooked per package directions

Alfredo sauce:
- 8 tablespoons sweet butter, softened
- 1 large egg yolk
- ¼ cup heavy cream
- ½ cup Parmesan cheese, grated
- ½ teaspoon salt
- ¼ teaspoon white pepper
- ¼ cup parsley, finely minced

First, prepare sauce. Put butter, egg yolk, heavy cream, Parmesan cheese, salt and pepper in food processor and blend until creamy. (Mixture will have a somewhat lumpy consistency because of the cheese.) Meanwhile, drain cooked pasta. Scoop alfredo sauce out of food processor and add directly to hot, drained pasta. Garnish with parsley and serve immediately.

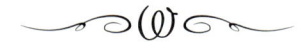

Pesto Francesca Fettuccine

Serves 4 to 6

1 pound fettuccine, cooked per package directions

Pesto Sauce:
- 1½ cup fresh basil (no stems)
- 3 garlic cloves
- 3 tablespoons pine nuts (pignoli)
- ½ teaspoon salt
- ¼ teaspoon black pepper, freshly ground
- ½ cup virgin olive oil
- ½ cup Parmesan cheese

First prepare pesto sauce. Wash basil in cold water; pat dry with paper towel. Put basil, garlic, pine nuts, salt and pepper in food processor. With pulse button, chop until evenly blended. With food processor running, add olive oil through feeder cap. When well-blended, remove top and add cheese. Process until well-blended and creamy. Set aside. Drain cooked fettuccine. Add pesto sauce, and carefully stir in with a rubber spatula. Put fettuccine into serving dish and serve hot, with extra Parmesan cheese.

Spaghetti Carbonara

Serves 4 to 6

- 1 pound spaghetti or linguine, cooked per package directions
- 1 pound bacon, cut into 1-inch pieces
- ½ cup Romano cheese, grated
- 4 egg yolks, beaten
- 1 cup whipping cream
- ½ cup butter, divided

Fry bacon until fully cooked, and set aside. Beat eggs. Beat 1½ cups of cheese with eggs until mixture becomes thick and foamy. Set aside. Put cream in saucepan with ¼-cup butter and cook over high heat until butter is melted and cream is foamy. Put ¼-cup butter in large bowl and mix with cooked linguine. Pour cream and cheese mixtures over linguine, and toss. Add drained bacon and toss again. Serve with remaining cheese on side.

Spectacular Spaghetti & Meatballs

Serves 4 to 6

- 1 pound spaghetti or linguine, cooked per package directions

Marinara sauce:
- 1 46-ounce can tomato juice
- 1 15-ounce can Hunt's special chunky sauce
- 3 garlic cloves, crushed
- 2 tablespoons parsley flakes
- 2 tablespoons celery flakes
- 1 medium Bermuda onion, diced
- 1 tablespoon oregano
- 1 7.3-ounce (4-ounce drained) can (or fresh) mushrooms, chopped

Meatballs:
- 1½ pounds lean ground beef
- 1 egg
- 1 cup bread crumbs
- 1 teaspoon salt
- ½ teaspoon pepper
- 2 tablespoons Parmesan cheese

First prepare sauce. In large pot combine all sauce ingredients. Bring to a boil. Then prepare meatballs. Combine all meatball ingredients; mix well. Roll into small balls and drop into sauce without browning. Reduce heat to a simmer. Continue cooking sauce with meatballs for 1½ hours. Sprinkle more Parmesan cheese into mixture and cook another 15 minutes. Rinse cooked noodles with warm water. Cover noodles with sauce and meatball mixture.

Spaghetti with Tuna & Lemon

Serves 4 to 6

- 1 pound spaghetti, cooked per package directions
- 2 tablespoons olive oil
- 1 garlic clove, finely chopped
- 4 tablespoons parsley, chopped
- 1 6-ounce can tuna, drained and flaked
- juice of ½ of 1 lemon
- ¾ cup Parmesan cheese, freshly grated
- 1 tablespoon butter, divided into small pieces
- salt and pepper, freshly ground, to taste

First, prepare sauce. Heat olive oil, and add garlic and parsley. Stir continually, over low heat, gradually adding tuna. Heat should remain low so ingredients do not change color. Drain pasta and turn into a heated serving dish. Add sauce and stir well. Add lemon juice, Parmesan cheese, butter, salt and pepper. Stir well. Serve at once.

Arrabiata Sauce with Angel Hair Pasta

Serves 4 to 6

- 1 pound angel hair pasta (capellini), cooked al dente

Arrabiata Sauce:

- ¼ cup virgin olive oil
- 4 garlic cloves, minced
- 1 tablespoon crushed red pepper
- 1 cup fresh basil leaves, chopped (no stems)
- 1 28-ounce can crushed Italian plum tomatoes
- 1 teaspoon salt
- ¼ teaspoon black pepper, freshly ground
- ½ cup Parmesan cheese, grated
- ½ cup Romano cheese, grated

First, prepare sauce. In a medium saucepan over low heat, heat olive oil and sauté garlic, red pepper and ½-cup basil leaves. As soon as garlic starts to turn golden, add tomatoes with salt and pepper. Bring to a boil, stirring constantly, then reduce to low heat. Meanwhile, cook pasta al dente. Before serving, add ¼-cup Parmesan cheese and ¼-cup Romano cheese to sauce; stir to blend. To serve, drain pasta, then stir in three-quarters of the sauce and the remaining basil leaves. Put pasta into a large serving bowl and top with remaining sauce and cheeses.

Green Noodle Casserole

Serves 6 to 8

1 pound spinach (green) noodles
1 onion, sliced
12 ounces mozzarella cheese, sliced
1 16-ounce container fresh tomato sauce
oregano, basil, salt and pepper, to taste
½ pound sharp cheddar cheese, grated

Preheat oven to 350 degrees. In 6-quart pot, bring 3 quarts water to rolling boil. Cook noodles with sliced onion. Do not over-cook! Noodles should be just barely al dente. Drain. Layer in greased casserole dish with sliced mozzarella cheese. Pour tomato sauce mixed with spices over top. Sprinkle with grated cheddar cheese. Bake for 45 minutes, or until cheese is lightly browned. Serve with any main course meat. May be made a day or two ahead, refrigerated, then baked before serving.

Spinach~Stuffed Manicotti

Serves 6

1 package Prince manicotti, cooked per package directions
1 quart homemade marinara sauce
     or one 32-ounce jar prepared pasta sauce
Parmesan cheese, grated

Spinach-ricotta filling:
2 tablespoons oil, butter or margarine
1 medium onion, chopped
1 package frozen chopped spinach, thawed and drained
1 cup bread crumbs
5 tablespoons Parmesan cheese, grated
2 eggs
salt and pepper, to taste
½ pound ricotta cheese

Preheat oven to 350 degrees. In saucepan, heat oil and sauté onion in oil and add spinach. Simmer for about 10 minutes. Remove from heat. Add bread crumbs, grated cheese, eggs, salt and pepper. Add ricotta and mix well. Drain manicotti and stuff with filling. Put about ½-cup marinara sauce on bottom of greased 2 quart baking dish. Place filled manicotti in baking dish and cover with 2 cups sauce. Cover with foil and bake for 1 hour. Serve with remaining sauce and grated cheese.

Aunt Netta's Manicotti

Serves 6

Dough:
- 3 eggs, lightly beaten
- ¼ cup lukewarm water
- 1 teaspoon extra-virgin olive oil
- 1 teaspoon salt
- 2 cups all-purpose flour

- 2 tablespoons salt
- 2 tablespoons olive oil
- 3 quarts boiling water
- 6 cups ricotta cheese, drained on paper towel

Nona's Tuscana Sugo *(see recipe, this section)* or prepared pasta sauce
- 1 cup Parmesan or Romano cheese, grated

Begin by making dough. Beat eggs lightly with fork. Add water, extra-virgin olive oil, flour and 1 teaspoon salt, forming a medium-thick dough. Knead, adding only enough additional flour to prevent sticking. Continue kneading until elastic and soft. Cover with a warm bowl and let rest. If still sticky, flour hands and knead a little more, dusting with flour as needed.

To make manicotti, cut dough into 3 equal pieces. Roll each into a 10x10-inch square on floured boards. Cut each square into 4 uniform pieces.

To cook pasta, add 2 tablespoons each salt and olive oil to 3 quarts boiling water. One at a time, at 5-second intervals, drop dough squares into boiling water. Cover pot and cook 5 minutes. Remove pot from stove and add cold water. Remove manicotti noodles one at a time, taking care not to break them. Lay on paper towels to drain. Spread ½-cup drained ricotta on each piece. Roll up, like jelly roll. Rub olive oil into 8x12 or 9x13-inch glass dish. Place manicotti in dish, seam-side down. Pour Tuscana sauce on top. Top with grated cheese. Bake, covered with heavy foil, at 300 degrees for 1 hour. Let sit 10 minutes. If dry, add more sauce.

Spinach~Stuffed Jumbo Shells

Serves 4 to 6

1 pound jumbo pasta shells (conchiglioni), cooked per package directions

Spinach-ricotta filling:
1 15-ounce container ricotta cheese
1¼ cup Parmesan cheese, grated
1 egg, beaten
¼ cup bread crumbs
1 10-ounce package frozen spinach, cooked and drained
salt and pepper, to taste
1 tablespoon olive oil
1 32-ounce jar prepared pasta sauce

8 ounces mozzarella cheese, shredded

Preheat oven to 350 degrees. Prepare filling for shells. Mix ricotta cheese, Parmesan cheese, egg, bread crumbs, spinach and salt and pepper. Coat hands with olive oil and place shell in palm of hand to fill. Cover bottom of pan with part of the sauce; place shells in pan and cover with remaining sauce. Cover and bake for 25 minutes. Sprinkle with mozzarella and bake, uncovered, until cheese bubbles.

Stuffed Shells, The Fast Version

Serves 4 to 6

1 pound medium pasta shells (conchiglie), cooked per package directions
1 15-ounce carton ricotta cheese
1 32-ounce jar prepared pasta meat sauce
¼ pound mozzarella cheese, grated
¼ pound Romano cheese, grated

Drain cooked pasta shells. Mix with ricotta. Layer sauce, shells, then sauce, again. Sprinkle mozzarella and Romano on top. Cover with foil. Bake at 400 degrees for 15 minutes. Remove foil, reduce heat to 350 degrees and bake 30 to 45 minutes.

Ricotta~Stuffed Shells

Serves 6

Ricotta filling:
2½ pounds ricotta cheese (Italian Mancusso or Falbo brand)
salt
6 eggs, beaten
½ cup imported Romano cheese, grated
1 teaspoon white pepper
Italian flat-leaf parsley, chopped

1 pound medium pasta shells (conchiglie), lasagne or manicotti, cooked per package directions
1 tablespoon olive oil
½ cup butter
1 cup heavy cream
1 cup Parmesan cheese, grated

Preheat oven to 350 degrees. Prepare filling. Drain ricotta in sieve. Sprinkle salt over entire top. Put a plate underneath and refrigerate 30 minutes. Pour off water. Pat with paper towels, absorbing excess moisture, until dry. Place in mixing bowl. Add beaten eggs, and mix until blended. Add Romano cheese, white pepper and parsley. Blend with spatula until thoroughly mixed (do not use electric mixer). Taste to determine if more salt is needed; add sparingly.

Prepare pasta shells. Drain cooked pasta. Lightly grease hands with olive oil. Lift shells and stuff with ricotta filling. Put stuffed shells in a lightly greased baking dish. To sauce stuffed shells, dot pasta shells with pieces of butter. Pour over cream and sprinkle with grated Parmesan cheese. Bake for 20 to 30 minutes or until lightly browned.

Note: To serve 12, double the recipe.

Two~Sauce Lasagne ~ Red & White

Serves 6

Spinach-ricotta filling:
- 3 large eggs, mixed
- 6 cups fresh ricotta cheese, drained on paper towels and squeezed dry
- 1½ cups Swiss or mozzarella cheese, grated
- 2 cups Romano cheese, grated
- 1 10-ounce package frozen spinach, thawed & squeezed of excess water
- ½ cup parsley, chopped
- ½ teaspoon nutmeg, grated
- 2 teaspoons salt
- 2 teaspoons pepper

Red sauce:
- ½ cup virgin olive oil
- 2 tablespoons butter
- ½ cup onions, diced and minced
- 2 garlic cloves, chopped
- 3 28-ounce cans crushed plum tomatoes
- ½ cup red wine

salt and pepper, to taste
4 or 5 sprigs of fresh basil

Pasta:
- 1 pound lasagne, cooked per package directions, drained and cooled on a clean cloth

White sauce:
- ¼ pound unsalted butter
- ½ cup all-purpose flour, sifted
- 4 cups milk, heated
- 1 teaspoon salt
- ½ teaspoon nutmeg

Cheese topping:
- 3 cups combination grated Mozzarella and Romano cheeses

Prepare ricotta filling, mix eggs and add to ricotta; mix in all other filling ingredients. Refrigerate. Make sure you start with ricotta that has been drained on paper towels to remove excess water! Prepare the red sauce. In large, heavy saucepan, heat olive oil and butter. Add onion and sauté until soft. Add garlic and sauté until soft. Add tomatoes and stir to blend.

Two-Sauce Lasagne, *continued on next page.*

Two-Sauce Lasagne, continued.

Add wine, salt, pepper and basil. Stir well. Bring to a boil, lower heat, and simmer for 25 minutes. Set aside. Prepare lasagne noodles. Prepare the white sauce. In heavy saucepan, melt butter. Stir in flour with wooden spoon; cook until bubbly, but not brown. Gradually stir in hot milk; add salt and nutmeg. Cook, stirring until mixture thickens; bring to a boil. Continue to cook until mixture thickens, 5 to 8 minutes or less. Cover top with wax paper.

Assemble the lasagne. Preheat oven to 350 degrees. Retain some of each of the sauces for garnish. Place some red sauce on bottom of lightly greased 9x13-inch baking dish. Add one layer of lasagne noodles on top of sauce (lengthwise, in single layer). Spread 2 cups of ricotta filling on noodles. Add some white sauce. Sprinkle with grated cheese. Continue layering sauces and filling with noodles as before until dish is filled (about 3 layers of each). Sprinkle top with grated cheese. Cover with foil and bake until heated-through; about 30 minutes. Uncover and let sit for 15 minutes. To serve, cut into squares and serve with reserved heated sauces.

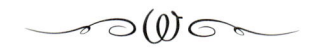

Spinach Lasagne Rolls

Serves 4 to 6

Adapted for your kitchen... from the original Walgreens recipe!

Corporate Cafeteria, Walgreen Company Headquarters

6 lasagne noodles, cooked per package directions
1 tablespoon olive oil
1 10-ounce package frozen, chopped spinach, thawed and drained
1 15-ounce carton ricotta cheese
½ cup Parmesan cheese, grated
1 large, whole egg
1½ tablespoons Italian parsley, chopped
salt and pepper, to taste
2 cups pasta sauce, homemade or prepared
1¼ cups mozzarella cheese, shredded

Preheat oven to 350 degrees. Drain cooked noodles and set aside to cool. Heat oil in skillet and sauté spinach over medium heat until tender, about 4 minutes. Cool spinach; combine with ricotta and Parmesan cheeses, egg and parsley in a large bowl. Season with salt and pepper. Spread 1 cup of the spaghetti sauce over bottom of an 8-inch square baking dish. Pat 1 lasagne noodle dry with a paper towel. Set on a sheet of wax paper. Spread one-sixth of the spinach mixture evenly along the noodle. Carefully roll up noodle to enclose filling. Arrange rolled-up noodle seam-side down in baking dish. Repeat with remaining noodles. Top with remaining sauce. Sprinkle mozzarella cheese over top. Bake until cheese melts, 15 to 20 minutes.

Grandma Katie Romano's Luria Meat Sauce for Pasta

Yield: 4 meals
Serves 4 to 6, each meal

- 2 slabs pork back ribs
- 2 pounds boneless chuck roast
- 1 1 or 2-pound piece pork shoulder
- 2 pounds meatballs (or desired amount) ~ follow recipe below

Meatballs:
- 2 pounds ground chuck
- 1 cup Italian flat-leaf parsley, chopped
- 1 garlic clove, finely chopped
- 4 slices stale bread, covered with enough milk to make crumbly
- 2 eggs, beaten
- ½ cup imported Romano cheese, grated
- 2 tablespoons big onion flakes, to taste
- 1 teaspoon oregano
- 1 teaspoon basil
- 2 teaspoons salt
- 1 teaspoon pepper
- red pepper, to taste (optional)

Marinara sauce:
- ¼ cup olive oil
- 1 or 2 onions, thinly sliced
- 4 garlic cloves, thinly sliced
- 1 10¾-ounce can tomato paste
- 3 14½-ounce cans Italian plum tomatoes
- 3 16-ounce cans Italian tomato pureé
- 1½ cans water (use tomato paste can)

Garnish: (optional)
- 2 cups bread crumbs
- 2 garlic cloves, minced
- 2 tablespoons olive oil
- 1 8-ounce jar Giardiniera mild (optional)

- 1 pound pasta (any kind), cooked per package directions
- garlic bread, on the side

Prepare the meat. Cut pork ribs, chuck roast and pork shoulder in big pieces and broil until cooked, but not browned. Set aside. To make meatballs, mix ground chuck, parsley and garlic; blend well. Add bread, beaten eggs, cheese and onion. Mix well with wet hands. Add oregano and basil, and continue mixing until sticky and thoroughly mixed. Season with salt, pepper and red pepper, to taste. Roll to any size with both hands.

Grandma Katie Romano's Luria Meat Sauce, continued on next page.

Grandma Katie Romano's Luria Meat Sauce, continued.

To make sauce, heata olive oil in 12-quart kettle. Saute onions, then garlic. Add tomato paste and cook, stirring for a few minutes. Add plum tomatoes; breaking them up while stirring. Add tomato puree. Save can, and add 1½ cans water to sauce. Stir sauce until it comes to a rolling boil. Drop in meatballs and stir gently. Boil 2 or 3 minutes. Lower heat to medium-low and add all remaining meat. Remove meatballs after 30 minutes. Simmer for 3 hours. Add meatballs 30 minutes before serving. Meanwhile, prepare pasta. Pour cooked, drained pasta into a large serving platter. Top with meat sauce. Garnish with brown bread crumbs and garlic in olive oil until golden. Sprinkle on top of pasta sauce. May add Giardiniera, hot or mild, depending on taste. Serve with garlic bread on the side. Meatballs and extra sauce may be frozen.

Tortellini Alfredo Primavera

Serves 6

8 ounces spinach tortellini
8 ounces tomato tortellini
8 ounces egg tortellini

Alfredo sauce:
2 tablespoons olive oil
2 garlic cloves, chopped
½ cup green onion, chopped
½ cup sun-dried tomatoes (seeded and dried)
½ cup ripe tomatoes
1 cup fresh spinach, chopped
½ cup julienne snow pea pods
1 cup chicken stock
2½ cups heavy whipping cream
1 cup Parmesan cheese, grated
1 cup prosciutto (optional)
fresh basil leaves
cracked pepper, to taste

First, prepare pasta. Cook spinach, tomato and egg tortellini separately; drain and lightly toss with olive oil. Set aside. Prepare alfredo prima vera sauce. Heat olive oil and chopped garlic in heavy saucepan over medium heat. Add chopped onion, sun-dried and ripe tomatoes, spinach and pea pods. Sauté lightly and remove from heat. In a saucepan over medium heat, reduce chicken stock to half a cup. Add whipping cream and reduce until thickened. Add sautéed vegetables, pepper, basil, Parmesan cheese and prosciutto. Mix well and remove from heat. Portion tortellini to 6 serving plates, covering each portion with vegetables in alfredo, and serve.

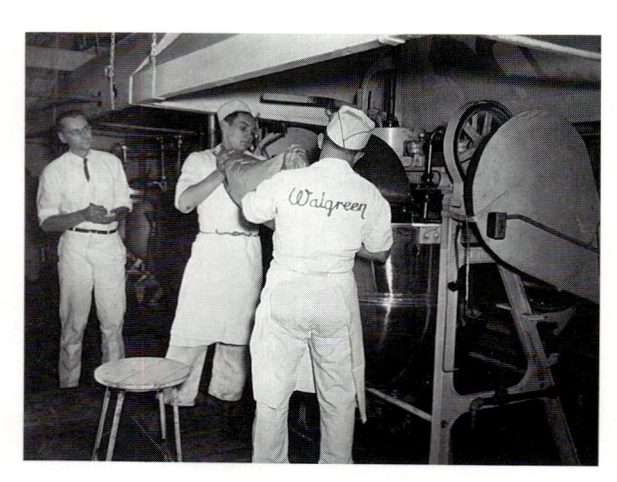

Walgreens at work...making chocolate syrup. The Syrup Department at 4750 South St. Louis Avenue in Chicago, 1950's.

Nutty Barley Bake

Serves 6 to 8

- ¼ cup celery, chopped
- ¼ cup mushrooms, chopped
- ½ cup green onions, chopped
- 5 tablespoons butter
- 1 cup pearled barley
- ½ cup parsley, chopped
- 2 to 3 cups canned or homemade chicken broth
- ½ cup pine nuts
- salt and pepper, to taste

Preheat oven to 350 degrees. Sauté celery, mushrooms and onions in butter until soft. Add barley and cook until golden. In a 2-quart casserole, combine barley mixture, parsley and 1 cup chicken broth. Bake, covered, for 30 minutes. Stir in pine nuts and 1 cup chicken broth. Bake, uncovered, for 45 minutes, or until barley is tender. If necessary, add more broth. Season with salt and pepper.

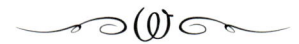

Zesty Spanish Bulgar

Serves 2

- 1 8-ounce can whole tomatoes, coarsely chopped, reserve juice
- water
- 1 cup bulgar wheat or brown rice
- ⅓ cup onion, chopped
- ¼ cup green pepper, chopped
- ¼ cup celery, thinly sliced
- 1 bay leaf, crushed
- 1 garlic clove, minced
- ¼ teaspoon dried red pepper flakes
- ¼ teaspoon thyme
- salt and pepper, to taste

In a measuring cup, add enough water to reserved tomato juice to equal 2¼ cups. Bring to a boil in small saucepan. Stir in remaining ingredients, including tomatoes. Cover tightly and simmer 15 to 20 minutes, or until bulgar is tender. Remove from heat, keep covered and let stand until most of liquid is absorbed, about 5 minutes. Remove bay leaf and serve.

Wild Veggie Brown Rice Bake

Serves 2

1 8-ounce can whole tomatoes, chopped ~ reserve juice
water
1 8¾-ounce can kidney beans, drained
½ cup brown rice
¼ cup wild rice
⅔ cup zucchini, sliced
½ cup onion, chopped
1 teaspoon chili powder
¾ teaspoon cumin
¼ teaspoon garlic salt
⅛ cup green pepper, cut into strips
⅛ cup red pepper, cut into strips
¼ cup mozzarella cheese, shredded
salt and pepper, to taste

Preheat oven to 350 degrees. In a measuring cup, add enough water to reserved tomato juice to equal 1⅔ cups. Combine tomatoes, tomato liquid, kidney beans, rice, zucchini, onion, chili powder, cumin and garlic salt in 8-inch square baking pan; mix well. Cover tightly with foil. Bake for 45 minutes or until most of liquid is absorbed. Uncover and stir. Sprinkle green pepper and cheese on top. Return to oven and bake until cheese is melted, about 5 minutes.

Wild Rice ~ Pecan Casserole

Serves 12

½ cup butter
2 7.3-ounce (4¼-ounce drained) cans sliced mushrooms, drained
1 onion, chopped
2 tablespoons green pepper, chopped
1 garlic clove, minced
1 cup wild rice
1 cup pecans, chopped
3 cups canned or homemade chicken broth
salt and pepper, to taste

Preheat oven to 350 degrees. Heat butter in large pan. Add mushrooms, onions, green pepper and garlic. Cook 5 minutes. Wash rice well and drain. Add rice and pecans to pan, and mix well. Add broth, and salt and pepper. Turn into well-greased, 2-quart casserole. Cover and bake for 1 hour.

Wisconsin Wild Rice Casserole

Serves 6 to 8

- 1 6-ounce package long-grain and wild rice, cooked per package directions
- 1 cup onion, chopped
- ½ cup celery, diced
- 1 green pepper, chopped
- 2 tablespoons butter
- 1 teaspoon salt
- 1 teaspoon sage
- 1 egg, lightly beaten
- 1 10¾-ounce can cream of mushroom soup
- ¼ cup almonds, sliced

Preheat oven to 350 degrees. Prepare rice as directed on package. Sauté onion, celery and green pepper in butter until soft. Remove from heat. Combine all remaining ingredients and pour into casserole. Bake, covered, for 30 minutes.

Basmati Rice Ratatouille

Serves 2

- 2½ cups water
- 1 cup brown basmati or long-grain rice, cooked per package directions
- 2 tablespoons extra-light olive oil
- ⅔ cup onion, chopped
- ⅓ cup yellow summer squash, sliced
- ⅓ cup zucchini, sliced
- ⅛ cup green pepper, coarsely chopped
- ⅛ cup red pepper, coarsely chopped
- 1 garlic clove, minced
- 1 teaspoon basil
- ¼ teaspoon salt
- 1 small tomato, diced
- 2 teaspoons parsley, chopped

Prepare rice, reserving 1 cup. Cover and refrigerate remaining rice. Heat olive oil in skillet. Sauté onion, stirring constantly, for 1 minute. Stir in yellow squash, zucchini, red and green pepper, clove, basil and salt. Cover and cook over low heat, stirring occasionally, until vegetables are tender, about 10 minutes. Stir in tomato and reserved rice. Cook, covered, 10 minutes longer, stirring several times. Sprinkle with parsley.

Rice~Noodle Casserole

Serves 8

- ¼ pound butter
- 4 ounces very fine egg noodles
- 1½ cups fresh mushrooms, sliced
- 1 3-ounce package almonds, slivered
- 1 chicken bouillon cube, dissolved in 1 cup water
- 1 cup medium or long-grain rice, uncooked
- 1 13¾-ounce can chicken broth

salt and pepper, to taste

Melt 4 tablespoons butter; add noodles and brown in large skillet. In separate pan, melt remaining 4 tablespoons butter and brown mushrooms and almonds. Dissolve bouillon cube in cup of hot water. Add all ingredients to skillet with noodles. Simmer about 30 minutes or until liquid is absorbed. Season with salt and pepper.

Note: To reheat, add additional water and bouillon.

Rochester Spanish Rice with Beef

Serves 6 to 8

- 2 tablespoons butter
- 1 medium onion, chopped
- 1 large green pepper, diced
- 2 pounds ground round
- 1 28-ounce can tomatoes, chopped
- 3 tablespoons tomato paste
- 2 teaspoons crushed red pepper (optional)

salt and pepper, to taste

- 2 cups long-grain rice, cooked per package directions
- ½ cup Parmesan or Monterey Jack cheese

Sauté onions and green pepper in butter until golden brown. With a slotted spoon, remove onion and pepper from skillet and add ground beef. Cook over medium heat until lightly browned. Drain skillet to remove grease; then add tomatoes, tomato paste, crushed red pepper (if desired), salt and pepper. Blend in onions and green pepper, and cook over low heat for 15 minutes, stirring occasionally. Add cooked rice; mix well. Stir in ½-cup of either Parmesan or Monterey Jack cheese.

Note: Works well as a side dish with steak fajitas!

Kay's Spanish Rice

Serves 4 to 6

4 green onions, finely chopped
1 green pepper, finely chopped
½ cup olive oil
1 cup long-grain rice
1 cup Italian plum tomatoes
1 cup tomato juice
1 cup water
1 teaspoon salt
1 teaspoon oregano
Parmesan cheese, grated
parsley, chopped

Sauté green onions and green pepper in olive oil for 3 minutes, stirring frequently. Add rice, stir and cook until rice takes on color. Add tomatoes, tomato juice, water and seasonings. Cover and cook over low heat until rice is tender and liquid is absorbed. Additional liquid may be needed. Sprinkle with Parmesan cheese and chopped parsley.

Note: May be served with pork or ham.

Southern Paint Yellow Rice

Serves 4 to 6

1 cup medium-grain rice
½ stick butter
3 cups rich, homemade or canned chicken stock, heated
1 medium onion, cut in half
1 teaspoon saffron, ground (or 6 to 8 threads, crushed)
½ cup dry white white
¾ cup Parmesan cheese, freshly grated
salt and pepper, to taste

Combine rice and 2 tablespoons butter in heavy saucepan. Stir over medium heat until grains of rice are coated with butter. Add 1 cup of stock, and stir well. Add onion and simmer, adding more stock as rice dries out. Stir constantly with a wooden spoon, scraping bottom of pan so rice doesn't stick. Dissolve saffron in ¼-cup of remaining stock, and add it and the white wine to rice. Continue stirring, adding remaining stock a little at a time. Stir constantly until rice is cooked, about 20 to 25 minutes. When rice is tender, discard onion. Stir in remaining butter and ½-cup Parmesan cheese with a fork. Add salt and pepper. Garnish with remaining Parmesan cheese.

Rice Pilaf ~ Three Ways

Serves 4 to 6

1 ~ Traditional Pilaf

1 cup long-grain rice
4 tablespoons butter or olive oil
1 small onion, finely chopped
1 teaspoon salt
½ teaspoon pepper, freshly ground
1 teaspoon thyme
2½ cups water, heated to boiling
butter, melted
parsley, chopped

Preheat oven to 350 degrees. Heat butter in a covered 1½-quart casserole; sauté onions until soft. Add rice and sauté 5 minutes over medium heat. Add salt, pepper and thyme. Add boiling water, and stir. Cover and bake for 20 minutes, or until all liquid is absorbed and rice is tender. Add melted butter to taste and a sprinkling of chopped parsley.

2 ~ Pilaf with Mint and Peas

2 cups small green peas, fresh or frozen, cooked with salt
3 tablespoons butter, melted
fresh mint leaves, chopped

Prepare rice as indicated above for *Traditional Pilaf*. Toss peas, butter and mint into rice with fork; mix well.

Note: May be served with veal, chicken or lamb.

3 ~ Pilaf with Almonds and Raisins

1 pinch saffron
¾ cup almonds, toasted
1 tablespoon olive oil
½ cup raisins, puffed

Prepare rice as indicated above for *Traditional Pilaf*; but add saffron before baking. Sauté toasted almond s in olive oil. Soak raisins in hot water until puffed. Toss almonds and raisins with rice. Sprinkle with fresh coriander.

Note: May be served with lamb kebabs or curried dishes.

Risotto Milanese

Serves 4

	2	carrots, diced
	2	small zucchini, diced
	1	small yellow squash, diced
	2	cups short-grain brown rice, uncooked
	1	pinch saffron threads
	½	pound mushrooms, sliced
	½	cup Marsala wine
	¼	cup olive oil
	2	garlic cloves, minced
	1	small red onion, chopped
	1	red pepper, seeded and diced
	salt and pepper, to taste	
	¼	cup flat-leaf parsley, chopped
	1	10-ounce box frozen green peas, thawed
	¼	cup Parmesan cheese, grated
	¼	cup walnuts, chopped
	4	ounces mozzarella cheese, shredded (optional)

Boil carrots, zucchini and yellow squash in enough water to cover by 2 inches. Cook about 5 minutes, or until crisp-tender. Drain vegetables, reserving cooking liquid. Add enough water to cooking liquid to measure 5 cups. Pour into large pot. Add rice and saffron. Cover and bring to boil over medium-high heat. Lower heat and simmer, covered, about 35 minutes, or until rice is tender and water is absorbed.

Meanwhile, preheat oven to 350 degrees. Place mushrooms and Marsala wine in a bowl. Toss lightly to coat. Set aside. Heat olive oil in a skillet over medium-low heat. Add garlic, onion and bell pepper. Sprinkle lightly with salt and pepper. Cook for 10 minutes, stirring frequently, until crisp-tender.

Stir in parsley and peas. Cook for 5 minutes, stirring frequently. Put into large bowl. Add cooked rice, vegetables, mushrooms (including mushroom liquid), Parmesan cheese, walnuts and mozzarella (if using). Stir to mix well. Put into a well-greased baking dish. Bake for 20 minutes.

Risotto Erbacci

Serves 8

1 onion, finely diced
6 tablespoons olive oil
1 pound ground beef
1 6-ounce can tomato paste
2 cups long grain rice or arribito (Italian rice)
12 cups chicken broth, warmed
1 cup Parmesan cheese, grated
salt and pepper, to taste

In large pot, sauté onion in olive oil. Add ground beef and cook until beef is browned. Stir in tomato paste and simmer for about 5 minutes. Add rice. Mix well. Start adding broth a ladle at a time, stirring constantly until rice starts to expand. Keep adding rice until rice is cooked and broth is absorbed. Mix in half the Parmesan cheese, salt and pepper to taste. Garnish with remaining cheese.

Parmesan Polenta

Serves 6

3½ cups chicken stock
1 garlic clove, finely chopped
salt and pepper, to taste
1 cup coarse, yellow cornmeal
½ cup Parmesan cheese, grated (more, if desired)
¼ cup fresh basil, chopped

Bring chicken stock to boil and add garlic, salt and pepper. Turn burner to simmer and slowly add cornmeal (about ¼-cup at a time), stirring constantly. Cook until cornmeal comes off sides of the pot. Then add cheese and basil. Stir until cheese is melted. Serve in individual bowls.

Note: Makes a great side dish!

Cornmeal Spoon Bread

Serves 4 to 6

- 2 cups milk
- ½ teaspoon salt
- ¾ cup cornmeal
- 4 tablespoons butter
- 4 eggs, separated

Preheat oven to 375 degrees. Bring milk and salt to a boil; reduce heat and simmer. Stir in cornmeal; cook until thickened, stirring constantly. Remove from heat. Beat egg yolks slightly, then beat them into the cornmeal. Cool slightly. Stiffly beat egg whites. Fold into cornmeal mixture. Bake in a butter-greased 1½-quart casserole dish for about 40 minutes.

Note: This is a heavy soufflé. May eat with butter or serve with the sauces from chicken dishes.

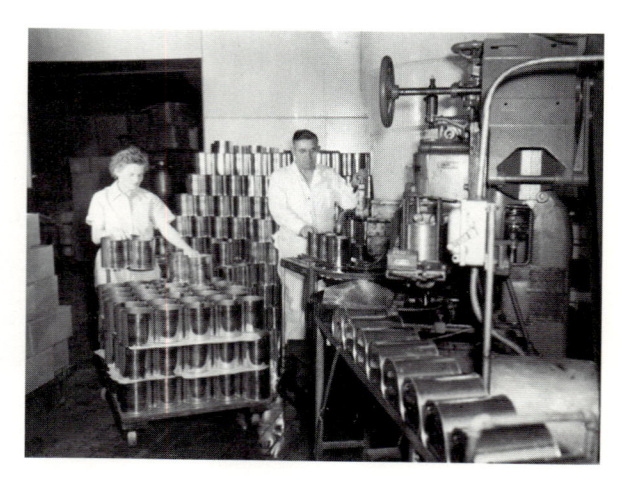

Walgreen made its own syrup for the famous and delicious ice cream specialties. Here are some cans, ready for the soda fountains, Chicago, 1950's.

Cheese & Bacon Potato Skins

Serves 2 to 4

Adapted for your kitchen… from the original Walgreens recipe!

Wags & Humpty Dumpty Restaurants, 1970's ~ 1980's

4 potato skins
2 tablespoons Italian salad dressing
½ cup Tostitos Salsa Con Queso, restaurant style, heated
¼ cup sour cream
McCormick's Real Bacon Bits
fresh parsley

Preheat oven to 450 degrees. Brush inside of scooped-out potato skins with Italian salad dressing. Put in baking dish and roast for 10 minutes or until crisp. To serve, pour hot Salsa Con Queso in skins. Top with sour cream and bacon bits. Garnish with parsley.

Potatoes & Sweet Onions Au Gratin

Serves 8

½ cup (1 stick) butter
3 tablespoons all-purpose flour
2 cups heavy cream or whole milk, heated
2½ pounds potatoes, peeled and sliced
2½ cups sweet onions, peeled and sliced
salt and pepper, to taste
⅓ cup parsley, chopped
3 ounces Parmesan cheese, grated
6 ounces provolone cheese, shredded

Preheat oven to 350 degrees. Melt butter in saucepan. Whisk in flour and stir until smooth. Add hot cream or milk and stir constantly until mixture starts to thicken. Set aside. Place half the potatoes in deep, well-greased baking dish and top with half the onions. Season with salt and pepper, and sprinkle with half the parsley. Top with two-thirds the Parmesan and provolone cheese. Cover with half the sauce. Repeat layering process with remaining potatoes, onion, seasoning, parsley and sauce; and finish with remaining cheese. Bake, covered, for 2 to 2½ hours, removing lid for final 15 minutes to brown top.

Penn Dutch Potatoes

Serves 4

5 medium to large potatoes
1 medium onion, chopped
1 small sprig parsley
1 stick butter

Peel potatoes and cook in boiling water for 30 minutes; mash potatoes. Add all but 1 tablespoon butter. In frying pan, heat 1 tablespoon butter and sauté onion and parsley until soft. Add onion mixture to potatoes; mix well and serve immediately.

Boiled New Potatoes

Serves 4

12 new potatoes, scrubbed
3 to 6 tablespoons butter
salt, to taste
2 tablespoons parsley, chopped

Drop potatoes in boiling water to cover. Cook covered until tender, about 20 to 30 minutes. Remove skins. Melt butter in skillet. Add potatoes and shake gently over low heat until they are well coated. Serve sprinkled with salt and chopped parsley.

Creamy Mashed Potato Casserole

Serves 8 to 10

4½ pounds potatoes, scrubbed
⅓ cup milk, heated
1 8-ounce package Philadelphia cream cheese, softened
2 eggs
½ cup butter, softened
1 small onion, grated (or garlic powder, to taste)
paprika (optional)

Preheat oven to 350 degrees. Cover potatoes with water and boil slowly for 30 minutes or until tender. Drain and peel. Mash potatoes; add milk, cream cheese, eggs and ⅓-cup butter. Add grated onion or garlic powder to taste. Place in lightly-greased 3-quart casserole. Bake for 20 to 30 minutes to warm. Garnish top with remaining butter and paprika.

Potato Casserole Boldt

Serves 12

- 2 pounds frozen hash browns, thawed
- ½ cup margarine, melted
- 1 teaspoon salt
- 1 pint sour cream
- 2 tablespoons onions, minced (optional)
- 1 10¾-ounce can cream of celery or cream of mushroom soup
- 2 cups Velveeta cheese, grated

Topping:
- ¼ cup margarine, melted
- 2 cups corn flakes, crushed

Preheat oven to 350 degrees. Mix thawed hash browns with margarine, salt, sour cream, onions, soup and cheese. Place in greased 9x14-inch casserole dish. Combine melted margarine and corn flakes. Sprinkle over top of casserole. Bake 45 minutes to 1 hour.

Note: May mix and freeze ahead of time; baking time will be longer.

Peggy's Potato Casserole

Serves 8

- 1 pound frozen hash browns (Ore Ida southern-style), thawed
- 1 10¾-ounce can cream of chicken or cream of celery soup
- 1 8-ounce container sour cream
- 1 16-ounce bag shredded cheddar cheese
- ¼ cup onion, chopped
- ½ teaspoon salt
- ¼ teaspoon pepper

Topping:
- ¼ cup butter, melted
- 3 cups Rice Chex, crushed

Preheat oven to 350 degrees. Grease 1½-quart, 12x7-inch shallow pan. Break up potatoes. Combine soup, sour cream, cheese, onion, salt and pepper. Add to potatoes and mix thoroughly. Put in pan. Combine cereal and butter and mix well. Spread over potatoes. Bake for 50 minutes.

Note: May be made day before and refrigerated. Bring to room temperature before baking. Serve with any meat or poultry dish.

Baked Potatoes with Bacon & Scallions

Serves 8

8 medium red potatoes
salt and pepper, to taste
1 bunch scallions (green onions), chopped
6 to 8 slices bacon, cooked, drained and crumbled
1 stick butter
½ pint whipping cream

Preheat oven to 375 degrees. Peel and slice potatoes ¼-inch thick; add salt and pepper to taste. Line potatoes in a greased baking dish. Sprinkle chopped scallions on top of potatoes. Top with crumbled bacon and dots of butter. Pour cream in corner of baking dish. Cover with foil; bake 45 minutes to 1 hour. Test to see if potatoes are thoroughly cooked.

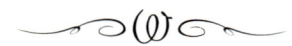

Baked Paprika Potato Fans

Serves 8

8 large baking potatoes
½ cup margarine, melted
1 teaspoon garlic salt or powder
1 teaspoon pepper, freshly ground
¾ cup Parmesan cheese, grated
4 tablespoons dry bread crumbs
paprika

Preheat oven to 375 degrees. Cut potatoes crosswise into ⅛-inch partial slices; cut only three-quarters of the way through (to make a "fan"). Place cut side up in a greased casserole dish. Brush each potato with melted margarine (save some for basting); sprinkle each with garlic salt and pepper. Bake for 45 minutes, basting with remaining margarine occasionally. Combine cheese and bread crumbs; sprinkle over potatoes. Garnish with paprika. Bake for 20 to 30 minutes more, or until tender.

Twice~Baked Potatoes

Serves 6

6 large baking potatoes
1 16-ounce container sour cream
1 stick butter
2 tablespoons frozen chives
salt and pepper, to taste
paprika

Preheat oven to 425 degrees. Bake potatoes for 1 hour or until tender. Cut out hole in top of potato and scoop out inner portion. Put scooped potatoes in mixing bowl. While hot, mash in mixer with butter, sour cream, chives, salt and pepper to taste. Spoon back into potato skins and sprinkle with paprika. When ready to serve, heat in 350 degree oven for 25 minutes.

Note: Watch potatoes; when they puff up, remove from oven. If left in too long, they will run over.

Cream Cheese Potato Bake

Serves 6

2 cups water
½ teaspoon salt
¾ cup milk
2 cups instant mashed potato flakes
1 4-ounce container whipped cream cheese
1 egg, beaten
2 tablespoons onion, finely chopped
1 tablespoon parsley, finely snipped
2 tablespoons butter or margarine
paprika, to taste

Preheat oven to 400 degrees. Prepare instant mashed potatoes per package directions (omitting butter). Add cream cheese, beat well. Stir in egg, onion and parsley. Blend thoroughly. Transfer to well-greased, 1-quart baking dish. Dot with butter. Sprinkle with paprika. Bake for 30 minutes.

Adeline's Cheesy Potato Bake

Serves 6 to 8

6 to 8 medium potatoes, boiled in skins and sliced into bite-size pieces
2 cups cheddar cheese, shredded
⅓ bunch green onions, chopped
¼ cup margarine, melted
8 ounces sour cream and onion (or chives) dip
6 slices bacon, fried crisp and crumbled into tiny pieces

Preheat oven to 350 degrees. In a 9x13-inch baking dish, combine potatoes, 1½ cups cheddar cheese, green onions, margarine, and sour cream and onion (or chives) dip. Spread remaining ½-cup cheddar cheese and bacon on top of mixture. Bake for 30 minutes (or microwave for 10 minutes.)

Note: This recipe can be prepared and refrigerated for up to a day before it is needed. To increase recipe, add a potato for each additional person; increase other ingredients proportionately.

Party Potatoes

Serves 8 to 10

8 to 10 medium potatoes
1 8-ounce package cream cheese
1 8-ounce container sour cream
garlic salt, to taste
2 tablespoons chives
2 tablespoons butter, melted
paprika, to taste

Preheat oven to 350 degrees. Peel potatoes and cook in boiling water for 30 minutes; mash potatoes. Beat cream cheese and sour cream until well blended. Add hot potatoes, gradually beating until light and fluffy. Season with garlic sauce to taste. Add chives. Put into 9x13-inch greased casserole dish. Brush with melted butter and sprinkle with paprika. Brown for 30 minutes in oven.

Note: May be prepared a day ahead of time.

Cheese & Bacon Potato Bake

Serves 6

- 6 medium potatoes
- 1 large onion, chopped
- 1 pound cheese, cheddar or Velveeta, grated
- 1 cup mayonnaise
- 5 pieces bacon, cooked, drained and crumbled

Preheat oven to 350 degrees. Peel and dice potatoes. Cover with water and boil for 20 minutes. Drain. Mix potatoes with onion, grated cheese and mayonnaise. Put in greased 9x12-inch glass pan. Sprinkle bacon on top. Bake for 30 minutes.

Grandma's Crunchy Potato Slices

Serves 4

- 4 baking potatoes, cut into ¼-inch slices
- ½ cup butter, melted
- ½ cup cheddar cheese, grated
- ½ cup Rice Chex, crumbled
- 1 teaspoon seasoned salt

Preheat oven to 350 degrees. Coat both sides of sliced potatoes with melted butter. Place potato slices in pan. Top with grated cheese, Rice Chex and seasoned salt. Bake 30 minutes or until tender.

Colcannon

Serves 4 to 6

- 8 medium potatoes, scrubbed
- 1 medium green cabbage head, shredded
- 1 onion, chopped
- 1¼ cups milk
- 8 tablespoons butter or margarine
- salt and pepper, freshly ground, to taste

Simmer potatoes and cabbage separately, 20 to 30 minutes each, until tender; drain. Remove skin from potatoes. Cook onion in milk at low to medium heat until tender. Mash potatoes with warm milk and onion. Add cabbage and butter; mash well. Season with salt and pepper; serve.

Potatoes Hashed in Cream

Serves 6

6 medium baking potatoes, freshly baked
¼ pound butter
1 teaspoon salt
1 teaspoon pepper
¾ cup heavy cream
½ cup Parmesan cheese, freshly grated

Slit potatoes right from the oven; squeeze insides into a mixing bowl. Add butter and toss; do not mash. Cover a 10x15-inch, butter-greased baking dish with foil. Make a firm ring of foil, 10-inches in diameter. Set ring in center of pan. Place potatoes in ring; slowly pour cream over them. Let stand for 15 minutes. Meanwhile, preheat oven to 375 degrees. Sprinkle potatoes with Parmesan cheese. Bake for 20 minutes, or until golden brown.

Grandmother's French~Style Potatoes

Serves 8

8 large potatoes with skins, scrubbed
2 tablespoons onion flakes
1 teaspoon Lawry's salt
½ pint whipping cream (do not whip)
1 pint half-and-half
4 ounces cheddar cheese, grated

Cover unpeeled potatoes with water; bring to boil. Cook potatoes for about 20 minutes. Remove from heat and drain. Cool and refrigerate for 8 hours or overnight. Grease a 2½-quart casserole. Grate potatoes. Make a layer of potatoes, then sprinkle with onion and salt. Make several layers until all potatoes are used. Then pour whipping cream and half-and-half over potatoes. Top with cheddar cheese. Cover and refrigerate until 1 hour before baking (may be done evening before). Preheat oven to 350 degrees. Bake for 1 hour, or until golden brown.

New~Style Potato Pancakes

Serves 4

- 3 eggs
- 2 tablespoons flour
- 1 teaspoon salt
- 1 dash white pepper
- 1 tablespoon onion, minced
- ⅛ teaspoon nutmeg
- 1 pound frozen hash browns, thawed
- 8 slices bacon, fried crisp ~ reserve fat
- applesauce

Combine eggs, flour, salt, pepper, onion and nutmeg; mix thoroughly. Stir in potatoes. Heat reserved bacon fat in large skillet until hot. To each pancake, spoon ¼-cup potato mixture into skillet. Flatten pancakes and cook over medium heat until golden brown on both sides. Use more fat as needed. Serve with bacon and applesauce.

Mama Kozol's Polish Potato Dumplings

Serves 6

- 2 cups potatoes, grated
- 2 eggs
- 1 teaspoon salt
- ½ cup dry bread crumbs, finely crushed
- 1½ cups all-purpose flour
- boiling water, salted

Rinse grated potatoes in cold water; drain well. In large bowl, mix potatoes, eggs, salt, bread crumbs and enough flour to make stiff dough. In a large soup pot or Dutch oven bring salted water to boil. Using wet spoon, drop tablespoons of dough into boiling water. Cook about 20 minutes, until dumplings float to top of water.

Note: Dumplings measure approximately 1½x½-inch when fully cooked. May be served with fresh cabbage soup.

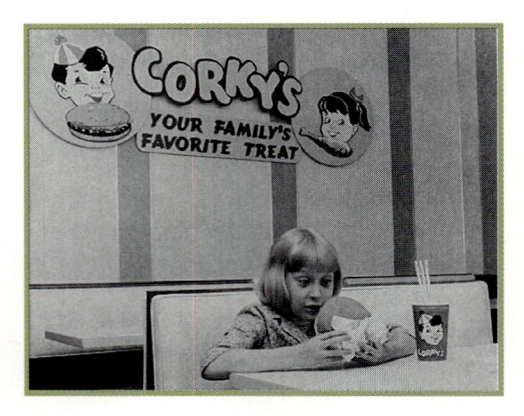

Corky's represented the newest trend in food service in 1969...fast food! Consequently, it was a very popular tour stop for classrooms and scout troops. The girl shown here, made her own Corker Burger!

Facing Page: *Sandra's Blueberry Oat Scones*
Photo: Scott Lanza, 1995
Stylist: F. Lynn Nelson

BREADS

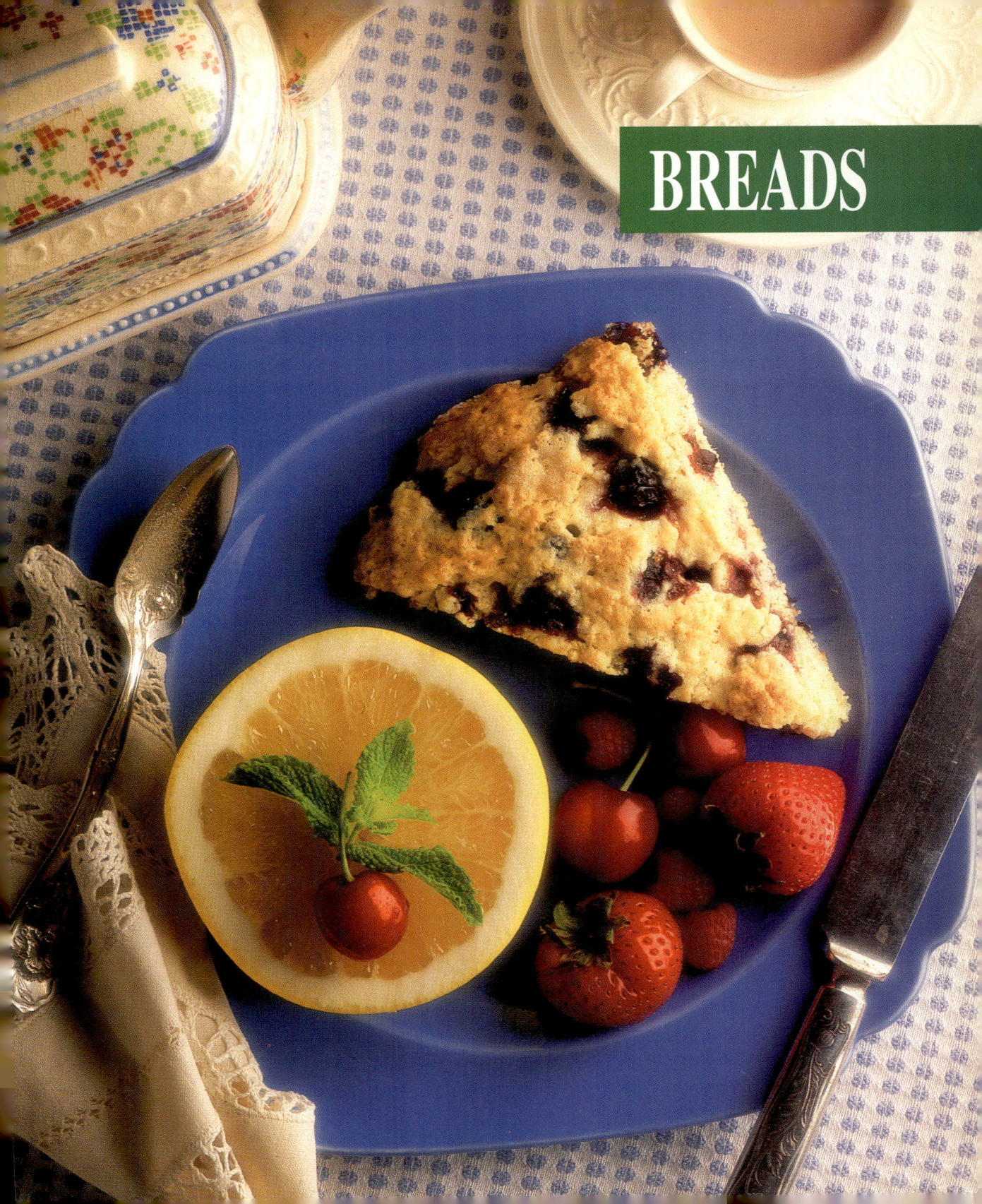

Corky's, Plaza Grill & Wigwam Grill
Three "Firsts" in the Food Service

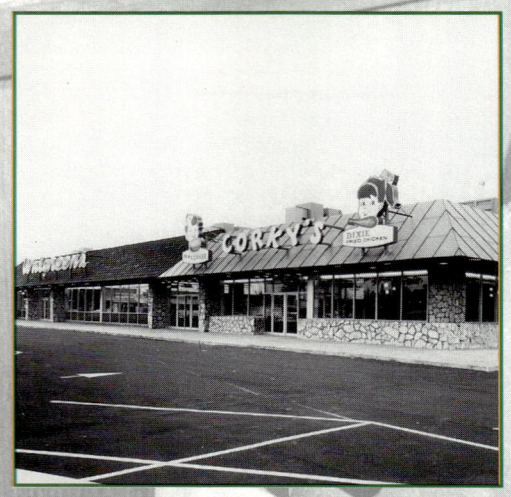

Bob Schmitt, a vice president at the time, suggested naming the fast food restaurant "Corky's," after Charles R. Walgreen, III.

First automated operation...*Corky's*, was a feat for 1969! A new idea in food service, Corky's featured quick-service dine-in or carry-out, and a menu that included the Corker Burger, Dixie-Fried Chicken, shakes and fries. Originally built adjacent to existing Walgreens, Corky's biggest competitors were McDonald's and Burger King.

First carving bar...business at the *Plaza Grill* in St. Louis was a little sluggish prior to receiving the largest of these new additions in the early 1970's. But business really boomed after adding the carving bar, which enveloped the entire center of the restaurant! The Plaza Grill served roast and corned beef, and turkey ~ carved fresh and hot from standing stacks.

First Walgreens Super Center...*Wigwam Grill* opened in the late 1960's, as a part of this giant Sioux City, Iowa store ~ which also had a huge snack bar and delicatessen running the length of its front. Wigwam was also once Walgreens largest grill with seating for 200 diners. A legend within the company, Wigwam sported elaborate Native American decor ~ right down to the uniforms of its wait staff!

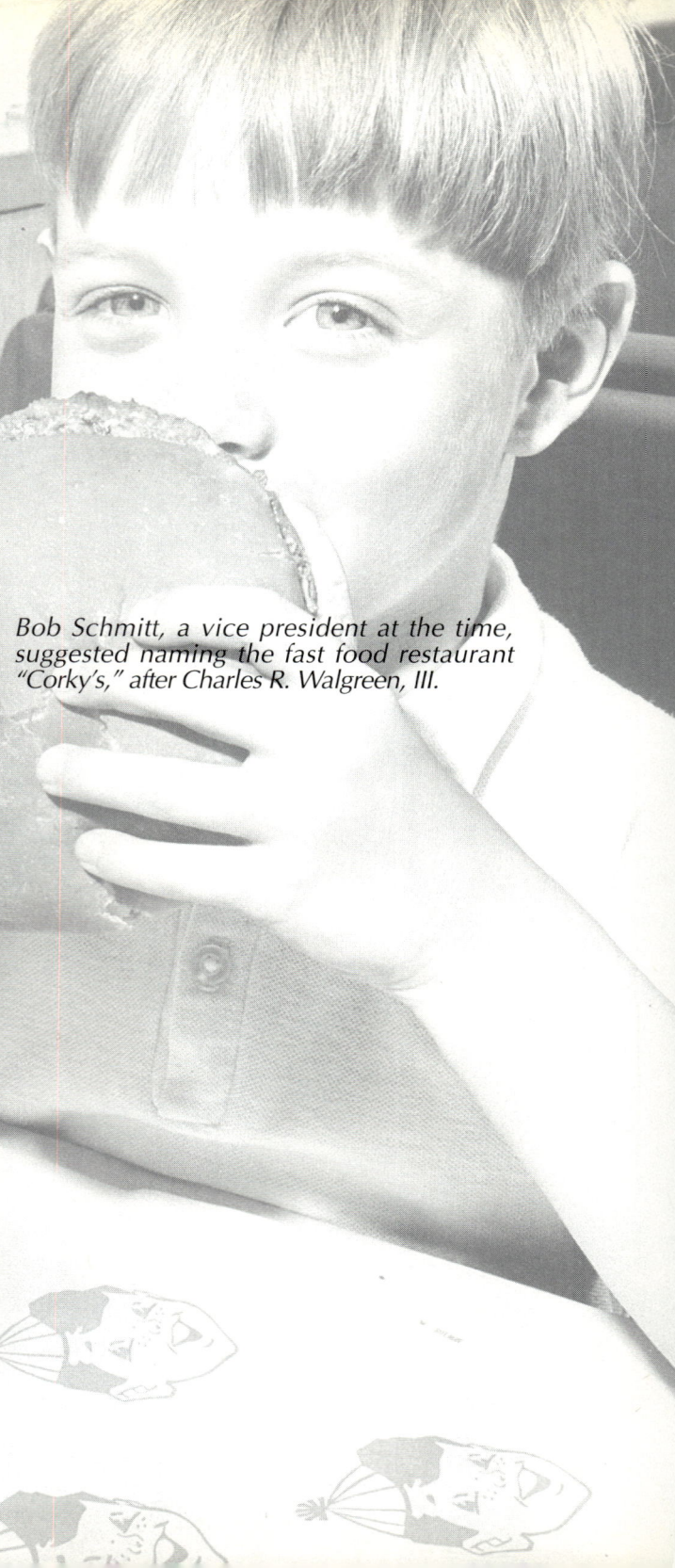

Sweet Roll Dough for Pecan Twists

Yield: 2 dozen rolls

Created by a group of U.S. soldiers in the Philippines during World War II, 1944!

This dough may be used for any type of sweet roll.

Dough:
- 2 packages active dry yeast
- ½ cup warm water
- 1½ cups lukewarm milk
- 1 cup butter, softened
- 3 eggs, beaten
- ⅓ cup sugar
- 1 teaspoon salt
- 2 teaspoons lemon rind, grated
- 6 cups all-purpose flour, sifted

Glaze:
- ½ cup butter
- ¾ cup brown sugar, firmly packed
- 2 tablespoons dark corn syrup
- 1½ cup pecans, chopped

Filling:
- 4 tablespoons butter, melted
- ¼ cup dark brown sugar
- 2 teaspoons cinnamon

To make dough, sprinkle yeast in warm water and let sit for 5 minutes. Combine activated yeast with lukewarm milk, 1 cup softened butter, beaten eggs, sugar, salt, grated lemon rind and sifted flour in mixing bowl. Mix with a dough hook until smooth, about 1 minute. Dough will be very soft. Remove dough hook. Cover dough with a damp cloth and refrigerate for at least 2 hours, or overnight.

To prepare pecan twists, combine ½-cup butter, firmly-packed brown sugar and corn syrup in a saucepan. Bring to a boil. Pour immediately into two, greased 15x10x1-inch jelly roll pans. Sprinkle each pan with ¼-cup chopped pecans. Divide dough in half. Roll each half into a 12x12-inch square; brush each with 2 tablespoons melted butter. Combine dark brown sugar and cinnamon and sprinkle center third of each square with 2 tablespoons of the mixture. Fold the bottom third up over the other third, like a business letter. Sprinkle with 2 tablespoons cinnamon mixture, then fold the remaining top third over the two layers. Pinch edges together. With a sharp knife cut widthwise into 1-inch wide strips. Take hold of each end of strip and twist in opposite directions. Pinch ends to seal firmly. Place in prepared pans about 1½ inches apart. Cover and let rise in warm place (free from draft) until double in size, about 1 hour. Bake in a 400-degree, preheated oven for about 20 minutes. Invert pan and serve rolls warm.

Sour Cream Twists

Yield: 4 dozen rolls

- 1 package Fleischmann's active dry yeast
- ¼ cup very warm water
- 1 teaspoon sugar
- 4 cups flour, sifted
- 1 cup (2 sticks) margarine, melted
- 1 cup sour cream
- 2 eggs, slightly beaten
- 1 teaspoon salt
- 1 teaspoon vanilla extract

Filling:
- 1 cup sugar
- 1 teaspoon cinnamon

Sprinkle Fleischmann's yeast and 1 teaspoon sugar into very warm water; stir until dissolved. Combine flour, margarine, sour cream, eggs, salt and vanilla extract in large bowl. Stir in dissolved yeast; beat until smooth. Cover with damp cloth. Refrigerate at least 2 hours or up to 2 days. Preheat oven to 375 degrees. Combine sugar and cinnamon. Sprinkle on board. Roll dough into rectangle, about 15x18 inches; turn so both sides are coated to prevent sticking. Fold over three times, as you would a business letter. Roll into ¼-inch thick rectangle, using up all sugar. Cut into 1x4-inch strips. Twist and place on greased baking sheet. Bake for 15 minutes.

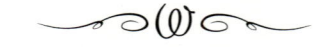

Cinnamon Twists

Yield: 16 rolls

- 1 8-ounce package crescent rolls

Filling:
- 2 tablespoons butter, softened
- 2 teaspoons cinnamon
- ¼ cup brown sugar

Glaze:
- ¾ cup powdered sugar
- 1 tablespoon butter, melted
- 1 to 2 tablespoons hot water

Preheat oven to 375 degrees. Unroll crescent dough into 2 large rectangles. Mix soft butter, cinnamon and brown sugar; spread on half the crescent dough. Place the second half of the dough on top like a sandwich and cut into 16 strips (parallel with the short end). Twist and seal ends. Bake for 10 to 15 minutes. Mix glaze ingredients and drizzle over the warm rolls.

Cheese Danish

Yield: 1 dozen rolls

- 2 packages crescent rolls
- 1 egg yolk
- 1 teaspoon vanilla
- 2 8-ounce packages cream cheese
- 1 cup sugar

Glaze:
½ cup powdered sugar
1 to 2 tablespoons warm milk

Preheat oven to 350 degrees. Remove dough from package; do not separate. Press entire sheet of dough into a 9x13-inch greased pan, smoothing out perforated lines. Mix egg yolk, vanilla, cream cheese and sugar and spread on top. Remove entire piece of dough from second package and cover the cheese mixture. Pinch dough together along all four sides. Bake for 25 to 30 minutes. Remove. Combine powdered sugar and milk to make glaze; drizzle immediately over the hot danish.

Variation: Instead of making glaze, sprinkle powdered confectioner's sugar on top and garnish with a few raspberries.

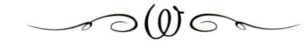

Swedish Cinnamon Rolls

Yield: 3 dozen rolls

- 2 cups milk, scalded
- ½ cup Crisco vegetable shortening
- 1 teaspoon salt
- 1 cup sugar
- 12 cardamom seeds, shelled and crushed
- 1 yeast cake, dissolved in ½-cup warm water
- 1 egg, unbeaten
- 4 to 6 cups flour

Filling:
- 1 tablespoon cinnamon
- 1½ cups sugar
- ½ cup butter, melted

Dissolve Crisco in scalded milk. Let cool. Add salt, sugar, unbeaten egg, crushed cardamom, yeast and 4 cups flour. Pour mixture in large bowl and let rise to top. Add more flour, enough to make dough easy to knead. Mix together cinnamon and sugar in separate bowl. Roll out dough and brush with melted butter, then cinnamon and sugar mixture. Roll up and cut into 1-inch sections. Arrange on buttered cookie sheet. Bake at 375 degrees for 20 minutes.

Nutty Scotsburn Butterscotch Rolls

Yield: 15 to 20 rolls

- 2 cups flour
- ½ cups white sugar
- 2 teaspoons cream of tartar
- 1 teaspoon baking soda
- ½ teaspoon salt
- ½ cup vegetable shortening
- 1 egg, beaten
- ½ cup milk

Filling:
- ¼ cup butter, softened
- ¾ cup brown sugar
- ¼ cup pecans or walnuts, chopped

Preheat oven to 450 degrees. In a small bowl, add milk to beaten egg. In a large bowl, combine milk-egg mixture with flour, sugar, cream of tartar, baking soda, salt and sugar. Knead into dough. Do not overwork. Dust working surface with flour and roll out dough. Spread a layer of softened butter on dough. Sprinkle a layer of brown sugar over butter. Sprinkle with pecans. Roll up dough like a jelly roll. Slice into sections and arrange on butter-greased cookie sheet. Bake for about 14 minutes, or until dough is just golden brown.

Bev's Easy Butterscotch Rolls

Yield: 15 to 20 rolls

- 2¼ cups Bisquick
- ⅔ cup milk

Filling:
- ¼ cup butter, softened
- ¾ cup brown sugar

Preheat oven to 450 degrees. Mix Bisquick and milk to form dough. Dust hands and work surface with flour. Place dough on floured surface; knead about 10 times. Do not overwork. Roll out dough to ½-inch thickness. Spread a layer of butter on top of dough. Sprinkle brown sugar over butter and spread evenly. Roll up dough into long tube. Cut tube into ½ to 1-inch sections and arrange sections on butter-greased cookie sheet. Bake for 10 to 12 minutes, or until dough is just golden brown.

Pumpkin Roll

Serves 12

- 3 eggs
- 1 cup white sugar
- ⅔ cup pumpkin
- ¾ cup flour
- 1 teaspoon baking soda
- 1½ teaspoons cinnamon
- ½ teaspoon nutmeg
- ½ teaspoon salt
- 1 teaspoon lemon juice
- ½ cup pecans, chopped

Filling:
- 2 3-ounce packages cream cheese
- ½ cup butter
- 1 cup powdered sugar
- ½ teaspoon vanilla extract

Preheat oven to 375 degrees. Beat eggs and sugar at high speed for 5 minutes. Fold in pumpkin. Sift together flour, baking soda, cinnamon, nutmeg and salt and fold into pumpkin mixture with lemon juice. Grease a 10x15-inch jelly roll pan and spread in batter. Sprinkle with chopped pecans. Bake 15 minutes. Let set 5 minutes. With knife, loosen sides and turn cake onto damp cloth. Roll cake in cloth and let cool. While cooling, make filling. Mix cream cheese and butter together, then beat in sugar and vanilla extract. Unroll cake and spread on filling. Reroll cake and wrap tightly in foil. Keep refrigerated.

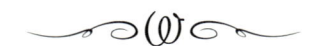

English Tea Scones

Yield: 16 to 20 scones

- 2 cups flour
- ½ teaspoon baking soda
- ½ teaspoon salt
- 1 teaspoon baking powder
- ½ cup sugar
- ½ cup margarine
- 1 egg
- buttermilk, enough to fill 1 cup with egg

Preheat oven to 400 degrees. Mix flour, baking soda, salt, baking powder and sugar; cut in margarine. Beat egg in a cup and fill with buttermilk. Add to dry ingredients and mix well. Drop, with teaspoon onto greased baking sheet. Bake for 10 to 12 minutes, until lightly browned.

Sandra's Blueberry Oat Scones

Yield: 8 scones

Scones:
- 1½ cups all-purpose flour
- ¾ cup quick-cooking rolled oats
- ⅓ cup sugar
- 2 teaspoons baking powder
- ¼ teaspoon salt
- ¼ teaspoon nutmeg
- ⅓ cup margarine or butter
- 1 egg, beaten slightly
- ½ cup orange juice
- ½ teaspoon orange peel, grated
- 1 cup fresh or frozen blueberries

Topping:
- 1 tablespoon butter or margarine
- 2 tablespoons sugar

Preheat oven to 375 degrees. Grease cookie sheet. In medium bowl, combine flour, oats, sugar, baking powder, salt and nutmeg; mix well. Using pastry blender or fork, cut in margarine until mixture resembles coarse crumbs. In small bowl, beat egg; beat in orange juice and orange peel. Add egg mixture to flour mixture. Stir until blended. Stir in blueberries.

On a floured surface, gently knead dough to make a smooth ball. Place on greased cookie sheet. With floured hands, press dough into one 8-inch circle. Cut into 8 wedges; do not separate. Brush top of dough with melted margarine; sprinkle with sugar. Bake for 20 to 25 minutes or until golden brown. Serve warm.

Pecan Corn Muffins

Yield: 12 to 16 muffins

- 1¼ cup yellow cornmeal
- 1 cup sugar
- ¾ cup flour
- 2 teaspoons baking powder
- ¼ teaspoon salt
- 1 cup chopped pecans
- 1 cup milk
- ½ cup oil
- 2 eggs or substitute

Pecan Corn Muffins, continued on next page.

Pecan Corn Muffins, *continued.*

Preheat oven to 425 degrees. In medium bowl, mix cornmeal, sugar, flour, baking powder, salt and pecans. In small bowl, beat milk, oil and eggs with fork. Add dry ingredients. Stir briefly. Pour ¼-cup batter into greased or paper-lined 2½-inch muffin cups. Bake for 15 minutes.

Blueberry Buttermilk Muffins

Yield: 2 dozen small or 12 large muffins

- 2½ cups all-purpose flour
- 2½ teaspoons baking powder
- 1 cup sugar
- ¼ teaspoon salt
- 1 cup buttermilk
- 2 eggs, beaten
- ½ cup (1 stick) butter, melted and browned slightly
- 1½ cups fresh or dry-pack frozen blueberries, rinsed and drained
- sugar (optional)

Preheat oven to 400 degrees. Sift flour, baking powder, sugar, and salt together into large bowl. Make a well, add buttermilk, eggs, and melted butter. Mix well. Fold in blueberries. Fill greased or paper-lined muffin pans three-quarters full. Sprinkle generously with sugar. Bake for 20 minutes, or until puffed and golden brown. May substitute blueberries with other fruit.

Cranberry ~ Nut Muffins

Yield: 1 dozen muffins

- 2 cups all-purpose flour
- ¾ cup brown sugar, packed
- 2 teaspoons baking powder
- 2 eggs, beaten
- ⅔ cup orange juice
- ⅓ cup vegetable oil
- 1 cup cranberries, coarsely chopped
- 1 cup pecans, chopped

Preheat oven to 375 degrees. In a large bowl, combine flour, brown sugar and baking powder. In another bowl, beat eggs. Add orange juice and oil to eggs. Stir into the dry ingredients until just moistened; batter will be lumpy. Fold in cranberries and pecans. Fill 12 greased or paper-lined muffin pans three-quarters full. Bake for 20 minutes, or until golden brown. Remove from pan and cool on a wire rack.

Lemon Muffins

Yield: 2 dozen muffins

- 1 cup butter
- 1 cup sugar
- 4 eggs, separated
- 2 cups flour
- 2 teaspoons baking powder
- 1 teaspoon salt
- ½ cup lemon juice
- 2 teaspoons lemon peel, grated

Preheat oven to 375 degrees. Cream butter and sugar until smooth. Add egg yolks, one at a time; beat until light. Sift flour with baking powder and salt. Add alternately with lemon juice, mixing thoroughly after each addition. Do not over mix. In a separate bowl, beat egg whites until stiff peaks form. Fold in egg whites and lemon peel. Fill butter-greased or paper-lined muffin pans three-quarters full. Bake for about 20 minutes.

Pear Bran Muffins

Yield: 1 dozen muffins

- 1 cup flour
- ½ cup sugar
- 2½ teaspoons baking powder
- ½ teaspoon salt
- 1 16-ounce can Bartlett pears, drained and diced
- 1¼ cups whole bran cereal
- ½ cup milk
- ¼ cup oil
- 1 egg, beaten (or egg substitute)

Preheat oven to 400 degrees. Combine flour, sugar, baking powder and salt. Combine pears with bran and milk. Let stand 5 minutes. Add oil and egg to pear mixture. Add all at once to dry ingredients. Stir only until dry ingredients are moistened. Fill greased or paper-lined muffin pans three-quarters full. Bake for 18 to 20 minutes.

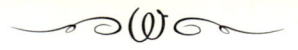

Refrigerator Bran Muffins

Yield: 10 to 12 muffins

- 1 cup boiling water
- 1 cup Nabisco 100% Bran
- ½ cup butter
- 1 cup sugar
- 2 eggs
- 2½ teaspoons baking soda
- ½ teaspoon salt
- 2½ cups flour
- 2 cups buttermilk
- 2 cups Kellogg's Bran Flakes

Preheat oven to 400 degrees. Mix boiling water and 100% Bran together. Cool. Except for Bran Flakes, mix all remaining ingredients together (butter, sugar, eggs, baking soda, salt, flour and buttermilk). Add to bran mixture. Fold in 2 cups Bran Flakes. Refrigerate. Fill greased or paper-lined muffin pans three-quarters full. Bake for 20 to 30 minutes.

Note: Muffins will keep for 6 weeks refrigerated.

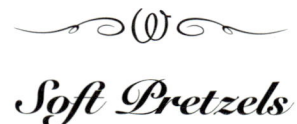

Soft Pretzels

Serves 8 to 10

- ½ cup warm water
- 1 package yeast
- 1 teaspoon salt
- 1 tablespoon sugar
- 4 cups flour
- 1 egg, beaten
- coarse salt

Preheat oven to 425 degrees. Pour warm water into large mixing bowl; sprinkle on yeast and stir until soft. Add salt, sugar and flour. Mix and knead dough. Take a small ball of dough; roll and twist into shapes like letters, numbers or snakes. Lay twisted pretzels on greased cookie sheets. Brush with beaten egg; sprinkle with coarse salt. Bake for 12 to 15 minutes.

Pull~Apart Cheese Loaf

Yield: One 8x4-inch loaf or 9x1½-inch round

- 1 package Pillsbury hot roll mix
- 1 cup hot water
- 1 tablespoon Good Season's Italian salad dressing mix
- 1 egg
- ⅓ cup butter or margarine
- ½ teaspoon paprika
- ¼ teaspoon garlic powder
- ⅓ cup Romano cheese, grated
- ⅓ cup Parmesan cheese, grated

Dissolve yeast from roll mix in warm water. In a large bowl, stir in dry salad dressing mix and egg. Add flour mixture from Pillsbury package and blend well. Cover and let rise until light and doubled in size (45 to 60 minutes). In a small skillet, melt butter and stir in paprika and garlic powder. In a small bowl, combine the two cheeses. On a floured surface, toss dough until it is no longer sticky. Then, cut into 16 equal pieces. Dip each piece in butter mixture; then, lightly, in cheese mixture. Arrange randomly on a greased baking pan (can be a round cake pan or loaf pan). Preheat oven to 350 degrees. Sprinkle with any remaining butter and cheese. Cover and let rise again in a warm place, until doubled in size, about 25 to 30 minutes. Bake for 25 to 30 minutes, or until golden brown. Serve warm.

Saint John Banana Bread

Yield: One 9x5x3-inch loaf

- ½ cup butter
- 1 cup sugar
- 2 eggs
- 2 cups flour, sifted
- 1 teaspoon baking soda
- ½ teaspoon salt
- 3 large bananas, mashed
- 1 teaspoon vanilla
- ½ cup nuts (optional)

Preheat oven to 350 degrees. Cream together butter and sugar. Beat in eggs one at a time. Mix in flour, baking soda and salt. Beat in bananas and add vanilla and nuts. Pour batter into greased 9x5x3-inch loaf pan and bake for 50 minutes to 1 hour. Let cool completely in pan; turn out loaf and shake powdered sugar over top.

Bonanza Bread

Yield: Two 7⅜x3⅝ x2¼-inch loaves

- 1 cup flour, sifted
- ½ teaspoon salt
- 2 teaspoons baking powder
- ⅓ cup wheat germ
- 1 cup whole wheat flour
- ½ teaspoon baking soda
- ⅔ cup nonfat dry milk powder
- ½ cup brown sugar, packed
- ¼ cup walnuts, chopped
- ½ cup peanuts, chopped
- ½ cup raisins
- 3 eggs or egg substitute
- ½ cup oil
- ½ cup molasses
- ¾ cup orange juice
- 2 medium bananas, mashed
- ⅓ cup dried apricots

Preheat oven to 325 degrees. Combine flour, salt, baking powder, wheat germ, wheat flour, baking soda, nonfat dry milk and brown sugar with walnuts, peanuts and raisins. Mix thoroughly. Mix eggs in blender until foamy. Add oil, molasses, orange juice and bananas, blending after each addition. Add apricots and blend just to chop coarsely.

Pour mixture into bowl with dry ingredients. Stir until flour is moistened. Pour batter into two greased 7⅜x3⅝x2¼-inch loaf pans or use greased muffin pans. Bake loaf pans for 1 hour; muffins at 350 degrees for about 20 minutes. Remove from pans, cool completely. Slice and serve as is, or spread with cream cheese.

Variations: Try using other nuts in place of walnuts. May also substitute bananas with chopped apples (raw), grated carrots, applesauce, peaches, pears or grated zucchini. Note: Freezes well.

Pineapple Date~Nut Bread

Yield: One 9x5-inch loaf

- 1 egg
- ⅓ cup milk
- ⅓ cup oil
- 1 cup pineapple, crushed, with juice
- 2¾ cups flour
- ¾ cup sugar
- 1 tablespoon baking powder
- ¼ teaspoon baking soda
- 1 cup walnuts, chopped
- 1 cup dates, chopped

Preheat oven to 350 degrees. Mix all ingredients together. Pour into greased 9x5-inch loaf pan and bake for 1 hour and 15 minutes.

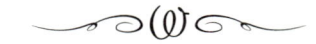

One~Bowl Applesauce Nut Bread

Yield: Two 9x5x3-inch loaves

- 2 cups fruit ~ candied fruit, chopped dates, raisins, or raw, chopped cranberries
- 2 cups walnuts chopped
- 4 cups flour, sifted
- 4 teaspoons baking powder
- 2 teaspoons salt
- 2 teaspoons baking soda
- 1 cup sugar (add 1 cup more sugar, if using cranberries)
- 2 teaspoons cinnamon
- 1 teaspoon nutmeg
- 2½ cups applesauce
- 2 eggs, slightly beaten (or egg substitute)
- ¼ cup vegetable oil

Preheat oven to 350 degrees. Line two 9x5x3-inch loaf pans with aluminum foil with extra foil extending over top of pan. Grease bottom and part way up sides. Combine fruit and nuts in a large mixing bowl. Sift flour, baking powder, salt, baking soda, sugar, cinnamon and nutmeg together over fruit. Mix. Add applesauce, eggs and oil. Stir until just blended. Divide into lined pans. Bake 1 hour or until tests done. Cool in pan 10 minutes. Lift out by foil. Cool thoroughly. Refrigerate for easiest slicing.

Amarillo Armenian Bread

Yield: Three 15-inch rounds

- 2 envelopes active dry yeast
- 2¼ cups water, very warm
- ¾ cup non-fat dry milk
- 3 tablespoons sugar
- 2 teaspoons salt
- 3 tablespoons olive or vegetable oil
- 6½ cups all-purpose flour, sifted
- 1 egg, beaten
- ¼ cup sesame seeds

Pour very warm water into a large bowl and sprinkle in yeast. (Water should feel comfortably warm when dropped on wrist.) Stir until yeast dissolves; then stir in dry milk, sugar, salt and oil. Beat in 2 cups of the flour, until smooth. Beat in enough of the remaining flour to make a soft dough. Turn dough out onto a lightly-floured pastry board. Knead until smooth and elastic, about 10 minutes, using as much flour as needed to keep dough smooth and pliant. Invert large bowl over dough; allow to rest for 20 minutes.

Divide dough into 4 pieces. Divide one of these pieces into 3 smaller pieces. There will be 3 large pieces and 3 small pieces of dough. Grease 3 cookie sheets with oil. Pat out one of the large pieces of dough into a 9-inch round on a cookie sheet. Make a 3-inch hole in center of round by pulling dough back with fingers. Pat one of the small pieces of dough into a 3-inch round, and place in center. Repeat twice with remaining pieces of dough to make two more loaves. Wrap each of the cookie sheets, with the 3 loaves, in plastic, and chill from 2 to a maximum of 6 hours.

Preheat oven to 350 degrees. Remove loaves from refrigerator and remove plastic. Allow to stand at room temperature for 10 minutes. Brush with beaten egg and sprinkle with sesame seeds. Bake for about 30 minutes, or until loaves are golden and give a hollow sound when tapped.

Eve's Zucchini Bread

Yield: Two 9x5-inch loaves or seven 5x3-inch loaves

4 cups zucchini, coarsely grated
1¼ cups vegetable oil
3 cups flour
2½ cups sugar
4 eggs, beaten
1 tablespoon vanilla extract
1 tablespoon cinnamon
1½ teaspoons salt
1½ teaspoons baking soda
½ teaspoon baking powder
1 cup pecans, chopped

Preheat oven to 325 degrees. Mix all ingredients together. Pour evenly into two greased 9x5-inch loaf pans; or seven greased 5⅝x3⅛-inch loaf pans. Bake large loaves for 1 hour and small loaves for 45 minutes; or until loaves are lightly browned and pull away from sides of pans. Cool on cookie racks.

Deluxe Zucchini Bread

Yield: Two 9x5-inch loaves

1 cup vegetable oil
3 eggs
2 cups sugar
2 teaspoons vanilla extract
2 cups zucchini, unpeeled and shredded
½ cup applesauce
½ cup orange juice
3 cups flour
2 teaspoons baking soda
½ teaspoon cinnamon
1 teaspoon salt
¾ teaspoon nutmeg
¼ teaspoon baking soda
2 teaspoons baking powder
1 cup pecans or walnuts, chopped

Preheat oven to 350 degrees. Beat eggs, oil, sugar and vanilla until thick. Stir in remaining ingredients, mixing well. Pour mixture into two greased 9x5-inch loaf pans. Bake for about 1 hour, or until a wooden toothpick inserted in the center, comes out clean.

Lydia's Poppy Seed Bread, Circa 1950

Yield: Two 9x5-inch loaves

- 2 cups vegetable oil (preferably Mazola)
- 4 eggs
- 1 cup Pet evaporated milk
- 2 cups sugar
- 4 cups flour, sifted
- 4 teaspoons baking powder
- 1 teaspoon salt
- ½ cup poppy seeds
- 1 teaspoon vanilla extract

Preheat oven to 350 degrees. Beat vegetable oil, eggs, evaporated milk, and sugar until creamy. Sift sugar, flour, baking powder and salt. Add to creamy mixture in 1-cup intervals. Beat until smooth. Add poppy seeds and vanilla. Pour into two greased and floured 9x5-inch bread pans. Bake for 1 hour, or until a toothpick comes out clean. Serve slices toasted, with butter.

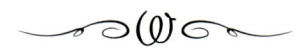

Conway's Almond Poppy Seed Bread

Yield: Two 8x4-inch loaves

- 3 cups all-purpose flour
- 1¼ cups sugar
- 1½ teaspoons poppy seeds
- 1½ teaspoons baking powder
- ½ teaspoon salt
- 2 eggs, lightly beaten
- 1½ cups skim milk
- ½ cup light corn syrup
- ½ cup vegetable oil
- 1½ teaspoons vanilla extract
- 1½ teaspoons almond extract

Preheat oven to 350 degrees. Spray two 8x4-inch loaf pans with a non-stick vegetable coating. Combine dry ingredients in large bowl. Add eggs, milk, corn syrup, oil and extracts. Mix until dry ingredients are just moistened. Pour into coated pans. Bake until edges are browned and toothpick inserted in center comes out clean, about 55 minutes. Cool completely in pans before turning out loaves.

Oatmeal Molasses Bread

Yield: Two 8x4-inch loaves

- 1 cup oatmeal
- 2 tablespoons margarine, at room temperature
- 2 cups boiling water
- 1 package active dry yeast
- ¼ cup lukewarm water
- ½ cup molasses
- 1½ teaspoons salt (optional)
- 5 cups flour

In a large mixing bowl, combine oatmeal, margarine and boiling water; let stand for 1 hour. Dissolve yeast in lukewarm water; let sit for 5 to 10 minutes. Add molasses and salt with yeast mixture to oatmeal mixture. Stir in enough flour to make a stiff, sticky dough. Turn into greased bowl; cover. Let rise in warm place until double in bulk. Punch down; allow to rest. Divide in half, shape into loaves. Place in two, greased, 8x4-inch loaf pans. Let rise for 45 minutes, or until almost to top of pan. Preheat oven to 350 degrees. Bake for 45 to 50 minutes, or until loaves sound hollow when thumped with finger.

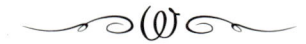

Mandel Bread

Yield: 70 to 80 pieces

- ¼ pound butter
- 1 cup Wesson oil
- 2 cups sugar
- 6 eggs
- 2 teaspoons vanilla extract
- 2 teaspoons lemon extract
- 1 cup slivered almonds

Sift together:
- 6 cups flour
- 2 teaspoons baking powder
- ¼ teaspoon salt

Preheat oven to 350 degrees. Cream butter and oil. Add sugar. Add eggs one at a time; beat well. Add extracts, flour sifted with baking powder and salt, and almonds. Chill in refrigerator 2 hours or overnight. Flour hands. Divide into parts and form into rolls, 1½-inch in diameter. Bake on greased cookie sheet for 20 to 25 minutes. Remove from oven; slice each roll diagonally. Place slices face up on same cookie sheet and bake an additional 10 minutes each side.

Irish Soda Bread

Yield: One 9 to 10-inch round loaf

4 cups all-purpose flour
1 cup sugar
1 teaspoon baking soda
1 teaspoon baking powder
¼ teaspoon salt
⅓ cup unsalted butter, melted
1⅓ cups buttermilk
1 egg, lightly beaten
1 cup raisins

Preheat oven to 350 degrees. Grease a 9 or 10-inch cast iron skillet or large baking sheet. Combine flour, sugar, baking soda, baking powder and salt in large bowl; make a well in center. In smaller bowl combine butter, buttermilk and egg. Add liquids to dry ingredients, pouring into well and stirring to make soft dough. Add raisins and mix lightly. Transfer batter to skillet or baking sheet, shaping into a ball. Slash an "X" on top. Bake until set, 50 to 60 minutes. Thump bottom to test for hollow sound.

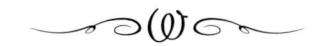

Cheese Caraway Batter Bread

Yield: One 9x5-inch loaf

1 cup warm water
1 package dry yeast
1 4-ounce package grated cheddar cheese
1 teaspoon caraway seeds, crushed
2 tablespoons margarine, at room temperature
2 tablespoons sugar
2 tablespoons salt
2½ cups flour

Grease a 9x5-inch loaf pan. Pour warm water into large bowl and sprinkle the yeast on top; stir with a whisk. When the yeast mixture starts to bubble (about 5 minutes), add the cheese, crushed caraway seeds, margarine, sugar, salt and 1½-cups flour. Beat 2 minutes in an electric mixer. By hand, stir in the remaining flour. Work dough with a wooden spoon until smooth. Cover the bowl tightly with plastic wrap and let dough rise until double in bulk (about 45 minutes). Stir down batter and pour into the prepared loaf pan. Spread batter evenly over pan with a rubber spatula. Cover with wax paper; allow to rise again in a warm place until it has doubled (about 45 minutes). Preheat oven to 375 degrees. Bake for 45 minutes or until loaf sounds hollow on bottom when tapped with fingers. Turn out of pan immediately and cool on wire rack before slicing.

Apricot Refrigerator Coffee Cake

Serves 20
Yield: 2 coffee cakes

- 1 package dry yeast
- ¼ cup warm water
- 1 teaspoon sugar
- 4 egg yolks, well beaten
- 3 tablespoons sugar
- 1 teaspoon salt
- 1 teaspoon lemon extract
- 1 cup milk, scalded
- 1 cup butter or margarine, melted
- 4½ cups flour (approximately)
- 1 12-ounce can Solo apricot filling

Dissolve yeast in warm water. Sprinkle with 1 teaspoon sugar. Set aside. In a large mixing bowl, combine egg yolks, 3 tablespoons sugar, salt, lemon extract, milk and melted butter. Cool. Add yeast mixture. Add flour gradually; beat until smooth. Dough will be soft and moist. Place in bowl, cover with wax paper, and store in refrigerator 4 hours or overnight. Preheat oven to 350 degrees. Divide dough in half. Roll each half out on a floured surface into a 12x16-inch rectangle. Spread each with filling. Fold dough over; pinch sides to seal. Cover with towel; let sit until doubled in bulk. Bake for 30 minutes.

Cowboy Coffeecake

Serves 12
Yield: One 9x13-inch coffee cake

- 2½ cups flour, sifted
- ½ teaspoon salt
- 2 cups brown sugar
- ⅔ cup butter or margarine
- 2 teaspoons baking powder
- ½ teaspoon baking soda
- ½ teaspoon cinnamon
- ½ teaspoon nutmeg
- 1 cup sour milk* or buttermilk or plain yogurt
- 2 beaten eggs

Cowboy Coffeecake, continued on next page.

Cowboy Coffeecake, *continued.*

Preheat oven to 375 degrees. In a large mixing bowl, combine flour, salt, sugar and butter. Mix until crumbly. Reserve ½-cup to sprinkle over batter. To remaining crumbly mixture, add baking powder, baking soda, cinnamon and nutmeg. Mix thoroughly. Add milk and eggs, mixing well. Pour batter into greased 9x13-inch pan. Sprinkle with reserved crumbs. Chopped nuts and cinnamon may also be sprinkled over batter at this time if desired. Bake for 25 to 30 minutes. Serve warm.

Note: *Sour milk is unpasteurized milk that has been allowed to sour naturally. (Pasteurized milk allowed to sour will spoil.)

Lola's Sour Cream Coffee Cake

Serves 12
Yield: One 9x13-inch coffee cake

Dough:
- 2 teaspoons baking soda
- 1 16-ounce carton sour cream
- ½ pound butter (2 sticks)
- 2 cups sugar
- 4 eggs
- 2 teaspoons vanilla
- 3 cups flour
- 2 teaspoons baking powder

Topping:
- ½ cup sugar
- 2 teaspoons cinnamon
- 1 cup walnuts or pecans, chopped

Preheat oven to 350 degrees. First, make topping by blending ingredients together; set aside. Then make dough. Mix baking soda and sour cream; set aside. In a large mixing bowl, cream butter, sugar, eggs and vanilla. Add flour and baking powder. Fold in sour cream mixture. Pour half of the batter into greased 9x13-inch glass baking dish. Layer half the topping, then the rest of the batter and finally, the rest of the topping. Using a knife, cut a zigzag pattern through the batter. Bake for 45 minutes.

Day~Before French Toast

Serves 4

6 slices of Italian bread, ¾-inch thick
4 eggs
1 cup milk
3 tablespoons sugar
¼ teaspoon salt
1 teaspoon vanilla
3 tablespoons butter
powdered sugar
syrup, sour cream or preserves

Arrange bread in single layer in 9x13-inch baking pan. In small bowl, beat eggs, milk, sugar, salt and vanilla until blended. Pour over bread, turn slices to coat evenly. Refrigerate covered overnight. Heat butter in skillet and sauté bread until golden, 4 to 5 minutes, on each side. Sprinkle with powdered sugar; serve with sour cream, syrup or preserves.

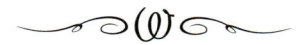

Zygmun Inn Apple Pancake

Serves 2

½ cup milk
½ cup flour, sifted
3 eggs
1 teaspoon sugar
1 dash of salt
2 large apples, peeled and sliced
1 tablespoon butter
sugar and cinnamon

Preheat oven to 500 degrees. Combine milk, flour, eggs, sugar and salt; mix well. Sauté sliced apples in butter in a large frying pan. Pour batter over apples in frying pan and bake until pancake starts to brown and puff. Dot pancake with butter and sprinkle generously with sugar and cinnamon.

Zina's "Russian" Pancakes

Yield: 12 to 16 pancakes

- 2 eggs
- 1 tablespoon Wesson oil
- 1 tablespoon mayonnaise
- ½ cup water
- 1 cup milk
- ½ teaspoon baking soda
- ½ teaspoon vinegar
- 1½ to 2 cups flour (add more to get thin consistency)

Whisk together all ingredients; batter consistency should be thin. Let batter stand for 30 minutes before cooking. At this point, if batter is too thick, thin with milk or water. Heat a lightly oiled, small frying pan over low heat. Pour small amount of batter, just to cover pan. Cook on one side. Turn when bubbly and lightly cook on other side. Serve with butter, jellies, jams or syrup.

Peach Popover Pancake

Serves 2 to 4

- 3 eggs
- ¾ cup milk
- ½ cup flour, sifted
- ½ teaspoon salt
- 1 teaspoon melted butter or oil
- 1 pound canned sliced peaches or apricots, with syrup
- 1 tablespoon cornstarch
- ¼ cup water
- ¼ teaspoon salt
- 2 tablespoons sugar
- ½ teaspoon cinnamon
- ½ stick butter or margarine, melted

Preheat oven to 450 degrees. Grease and flour 13x9-inch baking pan. Make batter. Beat eggs until light. Add ¼-cup of milk plus flour, salt and 1-teaspoon butter. Beat for 1 minute. Add remaining ½-cup milk and beat another minute. Set batter aside for at least 15 minutes. For topping, cook peaches with syrup, cornstarch and salt together until clear and slightly thickened. Set aside and keep warm. Pour egg batter into greased baking pan. Bake for 15 minutes; reduce heat to 350 degrees; bake for 5 more minutes, or until golden brown. To serve, sprinkle with sugar, cinnamon and melted butter. Pour on peach topping and serve.

Baton Rouge Hushpuppies

Yield: 30 hushpuppies

- 1 cup cornmeal
- ½ cup white flour
- ½ cup corn flour
- 1 tablespoon baking powder
- ¾ teaspoon cayenne pepper
- ½ teaspoon salt
- ½ teaspoon black pepper
- ½ teaspoon thyme leaves, dried
- ¼ teaspoon white pepper
- ⅛ teaspoon oregano leaves, dried
- ¼ cup green onion tops, finely chopped
- 1½ teaspoons garlic, minced
- 2 eggs, beaten
- 1 cup milk
- 2 tablespoons vegetable oil
- **vegetable oil, for deep frying**

In a large bowl, combine cornmeal, white flour, corn flour, baking powder, and the six seasonings and spices; break any lumps. Stir in green onions and garlic. Add eggs and blend well. In a saucepan, bring the milk and 2 tablespoons vegetable oil to a boil. Remove from heat and add to flour mixture, half at a time, stirring well after each addition. Refrigerate one hour. In a large skillet, or deep fryer, heat 4 inches of oil to 350 degrees. Drop batter, by tablespoons, into the hot oil. Be careful not to crowd them. Cook until dark golden brown on each side and cooked-through, about 1 minute on each side. Drain on paper towels. Try serving with batter-fried fish.

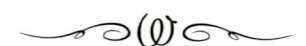

Nana's Popovers

Yield: 11 popovers

- 2 large eggs
- 1 cup milk
- 1 cup all-purpose flour, sifted
- ¼ teaspoon salt
- 2 tablespoons butter, melted, plus 1 tablespoon butter, melted for greasing pans

Place the oven rack on the rungs just below center. Preheat oven to 450 degrees. Place black iron popover pans (11-cups, ½-cup each) in oven

Nana's Popovers, *continued on next page.*

Nana's Popovers, continued.

while preheating, so they will become very hot. In electric blender whirl eggs, milk, flour, salt and butter, scraping down once or twice until smooth. Generously brush the hot popover cups with extra melted butter. Pour in the batter, filling each cup about half full. Bake for 15 minutes; reduce heat to 350 degrees and continue baking until popovers are high, crisp and golden brown, about 20 to 25 minutes longer. Serve at once with butter.

London Yorkshire Puddings

Serves 4 to 6

2 extra-large eggs
1 cup milk
1 cup flour, sifted
¼ teaspoon salt
½ cup vegetable oil, or ½-cup meat drippings from roast beef

Preheat oven to 450 degrees. Make sure all ingredients are at room temperature; this ensures that puddings will puff. Beat eggs with milk. Thoroughly whisk in flour and salt. (You may blend all ingredients in food processor.) Pour meat drippings or oil into muffin pan (1 tablespoon per muffin cup). Place in oven until grease begins to smoke. Remove pan and fill each cup two-thirds full. Bake for 20 minutes, or until browned and puffed.

Peggy's Yorkshire Pudding

Serves 6

2 small or 1 large egg
1 teaspoon salt
2 tablespoons water
1 cup flour
1⅓ cups milk
1 to 2 tablespoons oil (may be combined with drippings from roast)

Preheat oven to 450 degrees. Mix and beat eggs, salt and water in mixing bowl. Add flour and milk alternately, ending with flour. Continue to beat until batter is smooth and creamy; adjust amounts of milk and flour as needed. Leave to rest 1 to 2 hours at room temperature. Heat enough oil just to cover bottom of 13x9-inch pan. Heat pan in oven. Pull pan from oven and pour in batter. Bake for 8 minutes without opening oven door. Reduce heat to 400 degrees and bake 15 minutes longer until well-browned and crisp. Cut in large squares.

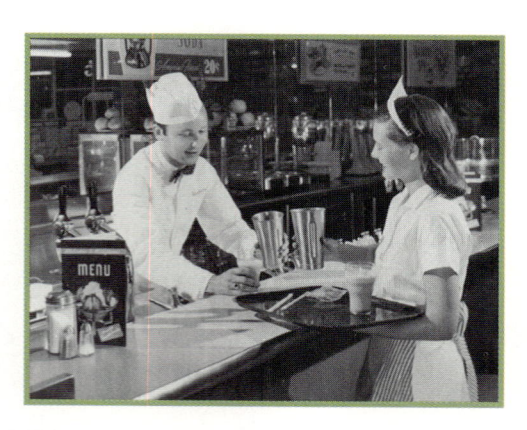

The Walgreens fountain in New York's Paramount Building was such a popular place for aspiring actors and actresses to work, that Columbia Pictures recreated it for the 1955 movie, My Sister Eileen. *Lucille Ball worked there in the 1930's.*

Facing Page: *Orange Chocolate Chip Cake, 1945*
Photo: Scott Lanza, 1995
Stylist: F. Lynn Nelson

DESSERTS & TREATS

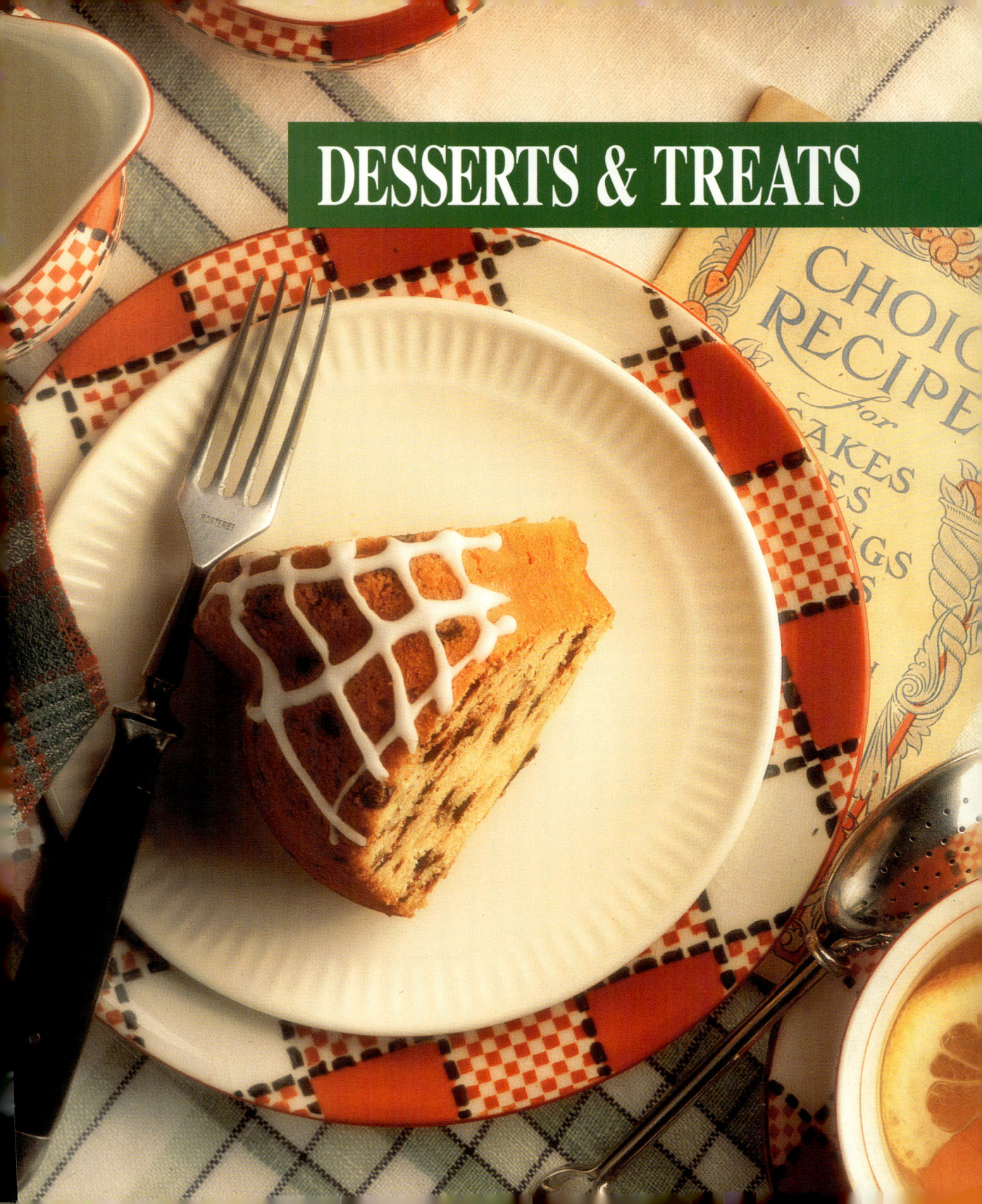

The Soda Fountains
Serving the Rich & Famous... the Walgreens Malted

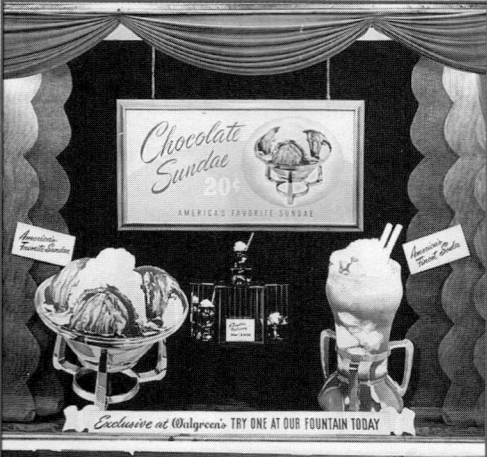

"[Soda] fountains are the magnets drawing customers into the store."
Charles R. Walgreen, Sr.
Chain Store Age, 1925

As American icons go, "nothin'" could top the soda fountain, especially at Walgreens, where the "rich & famous" ate ~ and were eaten. The latter, of course, refers to Walgreens legendary double-rich chocolate malted milk. Invented by fountain manager Ivar "Pop" Coulsen one hot summer day in Chicago, 1922, its fame spread all over the nation, and Walgreen soda fountains ~ always clean and well-maintained ~ became a mainstay. Walgreens own handmade, extra-rich ice cream was the malted's secret ingredient, and the company opened its own creamery in the mid-1920's to fill the demand!

In 1955, a Walgreens soda fountain "starred" in the Hollywood movie, *My Sister Eileen*, with Jack Lemmon and Janet Leigh! Columbia Pictures reproduced the Walgreens in the Paramount Building in New York, and was famous as a haven of employment for aspiring actors and actresses ~ including Lucille Ball. But the soda fountain's real fame came from its endurance. Evolving through the years as a lunch counter, it was absorbed into Walgreens cafeterias in the 1960's. But its famous ice cream treats remained on Walgreens menus.

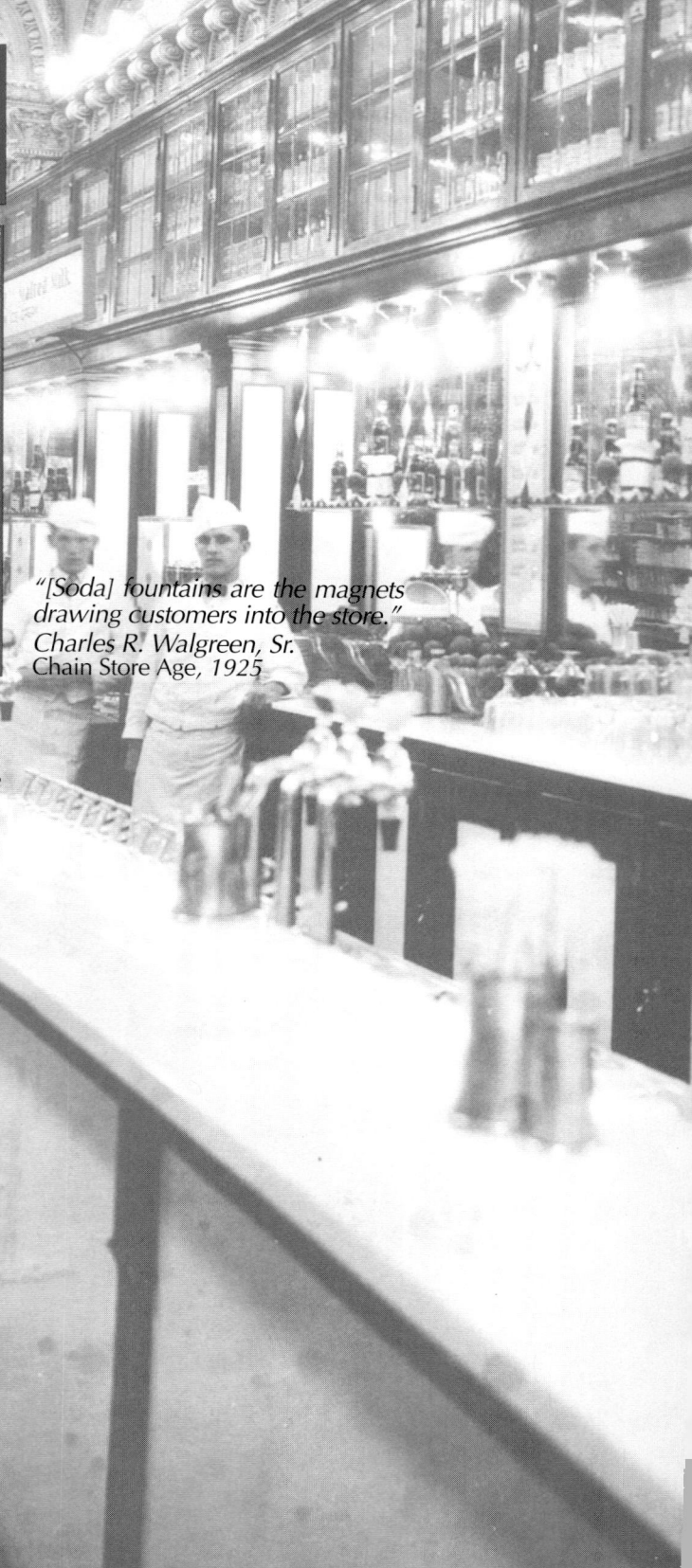

Old~Fashioned Banana Split

Serves 1

The original Walgreens recipe!

Walgreens Soda Fountains, 1920's ~ 1960's

Wag's "Old-Fashioned Ice Cream Favorites", 1970's ~ 1980's

1 banana, split in half lengthwise
1 rounded scoop chocolate ice cream
1 rounded scoop vanilla ice cream
1 rounded scoop strawberry ice cream
1 ounce chocolate syrup
1 ounce strawberry preserves, pie filling or fresh sauce
1 ounce crushed pineapple
whipped topping
1 teaspoon nuts, chopped
1 teaspoon chocolate shavings
1 cookie treat
3 maraschino cherries, with stem
1 metal banana split dish

Place banana halves in bottom of dish with cut sides facing up. Place chocolate ice cream in middle and vanilla and strawberry ice cream on either end. Top chocolate ice cream with chocolate syrup, strawberry ice cream with strawberry preserves and vanilla ice cream with crushed pineapple. Place a mound of whipped topping (equal to ice cream scoop) on each scoop of ice cream. Sprinkle chopped nuts and chocolate shavings over whipped topping. Place a cookie treat at one end of dish and top whipped topping with maraschino cherries. Serve on a small, doily-lined platter with a teaspoon.

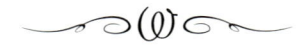

Hot Fudge Sundae

Serves 1

The original Walgreens recipe!

Walgreens Soda Fountains, 1920's ~ 1960's

Wag's "Old-Fashioned Ice Cream Favorites", 1970's ~ 1980's

2 rounded scoops vanilla ice cream
1½ ounces hot fudge
1 teaspoon nuts, chopped
1 teaspoon chocolate shavings
1 maraschino cherry, with stem
whipped topping
1 lily tulip sundae dish

Place 1 teaspoon of whipped topping in bottom of sundae dish. Add 2 scoops of ice cream. Cover with hot fudge. Top with a generous amount of whipped topping and maraschino cherry. Sprinkle chopped nuts and chocolate shavings over topping. Serve sundae on an underliner with ice tea spoon.

Blueberry Torte Pie

Serves 6 to 8

Crust:
1½ cups graham cracker crumbs
½ cup sugar
½ cup butter, melted

1 8-ounce package cream cheese
½ cup sugar
2 eggs
1 teaspoon vanilla extract
2 21-ounce cans blueberries
2 tablespoons powdered sugar
¼ cup cornstarch
2 tablespoons lemon juice
1 cup whipped cream

Preheat oven to 350 degrees. To make crust, mix graham cracker crumbs, ½-cup sugar and melted butter together; press into round, 10-inch pie plate. Whip together cream cheese, ½-cup sugar, eggs and vanilla extract. Put cheese mixture into unbaked pie shell. Bake until firm. In saucepan, blend blueberries, powdered sugar, cornstarch and lemon juice; cook until thickened. Cool. Cover with cooled blueberry mixture. Top with whipped cream.

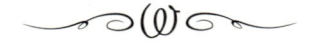

Cherry Pie Raaber

Serves 6 to 8

2 cups sour cherries, fresh or frozen
1 cup sugar
2 tablespoons flour
1 egg, beaten
3 drops almond extract
1 tablespoon butter
1 8-inch pastry for two-crust pie, unbaked

Preheat oven to 400 degrees. Line 8-inch pie dish with 1 unbaked pastry. Mix together: cherries, sugar, flour, egg and almond extract. Pour into piecrust and dot with butter. Put on top crust, flute edges and cut air vents in top. Bake for 35 minutes.

Rhubarb~Strawberry Pie

Serves 6 to 8

4 cups rhubarb, diced
1 pint strawberries, sliced
⅓ cup flour
1¼ cups sugar
⅛ teaspoon salt
⅛ teaspoon nutmeg
2 teaspoons quick-cooking tapioca
2 tablespoons butter or margarine
2 tablespoons cold water
1 8-inch pastry for two-crust pie, unbaked

Preheat oven to 425 degrees. Prepare fruits. Mix flour, sugar, salt, nutmeg and tapioca. Coat rhubarb with mixture. Let mixture stand for 15 minutes before putting it into pastry shell. Turn into unbaked piecrust and cover with strawberries. Dot fruit with bits of butter. Brush rim of pastry with cold water. Add top crust, trim, seal and crimp edges; vent top. A more decorative top is to cover pie with lattice of pastry strips. Bake for about 40 minutes, or until done. Line oven rack underneath with foil to catch drippings; pie will bubble and drip over as it bakes.

Ethel's Peach Pie Supreme

Serves 6 to 8

Crust:
½ cup butter
1 3-ounce package cream cheese
1 cup flour, sifted
½ teaspoon salt

8 peaches, peeled and sliced
1 tablespoon butter, melted
1 cup sugar
2 eggs, well beaten
1 tablespoon flour

Preheat oven to 400 degrees. Cream butter and cream cheese. Blend in flour and salt. Turn out on wax paper, cover dough and refrigerate for short time. Press into bottom and sides of 10-inch pie tin. Arrange peeled, sliced peaches in pie pan. Mix butter, sugar, eggs and flour. Pour over peaches. Bake for 5 minutes; lower heat to 325 degrees and bake 45 minutes longer, or until custard is set. Serve hot or if served cold, top with whipped cream.

Sugar~Free Apple Pie

Serves 6 to 8

6 to 7 Jonathan or Rome apples, pared and thinly sliced
½ cup raisins
1 cup water (or less)
1 12-ounce can frozen, unsweetened apple juice concentrate, thawed
2 tablespoons cornstarch
1 teaspoon cinnamon
2 tablespoons margarine
1 8-inch pastry for two-crust pie, unbaked

Preheat oven to 375 degrees. In bowl mix sliced apples with raisins and water. Cook until just tender. Drain water, reserving ¼-cup. Place apples and raisins in piecrust. Boil apple juice. Mix cornstarch with ¼-cup reserved, cooled water. Add cinnamon and margarine. Apple juice should be thick. Pour over apples and raisins. Add top crust or pastry lattice strips. Bake until crust is golden brown, approximately 50 to 60 minutes. Line oven rack with foil; apple mixture will bubble during baking.

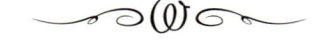

Apple Slices Pie

Serves 12 to 15

3 pounds tart apples
1 cup water
1½ cups sugar
1 teaspoon cinnamon
¼ teaspoon salt
2 tablespoons cornstarch
¼ cup cold water

Crust:
2 cups flour
½ teaspoon baking powder
¼ teaspoon salt
¾ cup shortening
1 teaspoon lemon juice
2 egg yolks, beaten
½ cup water

Apple Slices Pie, *continued on next page.*

Apple Slices Pie, continued.

Icing:
- 2 cups powdered sugar
- 4 tablespoons water
- ½ teaspoon vanilla extract

Preheat oven to 450 degrees. Cut apples into 8 pieces each. Bring water, sugar, cinnamon and salt to boiling point. Add apples and cook slowly for 10 minutes. Blend corn starch in cold water and add to hot mixture. Cook additional 5 minutes, stirring gently. To make crust, sift together flour, baking powder and salt. Cut shortening into sifted flour mixture. Mix lemon juice, egg yolk and water together and sprinkle over flour mixture. Blend it in lightly. Divide into two parts. Roll first piece to fit bottom and sides of a shallow 9x13-inch pan. Fill with apple mixture. Roll remaining dough to fit top. Seal edges and cut design for steam vents. Bake for 20 minutes; reduce heat to 350 degrees and bake additional 30 minutes. When cool, combine icing ingredients, mixing well, and drizzle over top.

Mother's Ice Box Pie, Circa 1935

Serves 6 to 8

Crust:
- 15 graham crackers, crumbled
- 3 tablespoons butter, softened
- 3 tablespoons brown sugar

- ½ cup sugar
- 2 egg yolks
- ¾ cup milk
- 1 envelope Knox gelatin
- ½ cup cold water
- 1 teaspoon vanilla extract
- ¼ teaspoon salt
- 1 cup whipped cream
- 2 egg whites

In blender or food processor, grind graham crackers with sugar; blend with butter until mixture forms into a ball. Line pie pan with crust ingredients. Save enough crumb mixture to sprinkle on top of filling. Mix sugar and egg yolks in top of double boiler and add milk. Cook until it thickens a little. Dissolve Knox gelatin in ½-cup cold water. Add to hot mixture. Add vanilla extract and salt. When cool, add 1 cup whipped cream and 2 stiffly-beaten egg whites. Pour into pie shell. Top with remaining crumbs. Refrigerate until firm.

Banana Split Pie

Serves 10 to 12

Crust:
40 graham crackers
½ cup sugar
½ cup butter, melted

2 cups powdered sugar
1 cup butter
2 eggs
5 bananas, sliced
1 20-ounce can crushed pineapple, drained
1 12-ounce container Cool Whip
¼ cup cherries, chopped
¼ cup nuts, chopped

To prepare crust, crush graham crackers with sugar in small batches in blender or food processor. Add margarine. Press into two 8-inch pie pans or in one 9x13-inch pan. Freeze until ready to use. In large bowl of food processor or blender, mix powdered sugar, butter and eggs at high speed until well-blended and spread on chilled graham cracker crust. Pour sliced bananas and crushed pineapple over mixture. Top with Cool Whip, cherries and nuts. Chill well, 4 to 6 hours.

Oreo~Lovers' Chocolate Mousse Pie

Serves 8 to 10

An original Hazelwood recipe!

Crust:
¼ cup margarine, melted
20 to 30 Oreo cookies, finely crushed
¼ cup sugar

1 4-ounce package Bakers German sweet chocolate
⅓ cup milk
2 tablespoons sugar
1 3-ounce package cream cheese, softened
1 8-ounce container Cool Whip, thawed
1 cup whipped cream
chocolate curls

Chocolate Mousse Pie, *continued on next page.*

Chocolate Mousse Pie, continued.

To prepare crust, add sugar to Oreo cookie crumbs and mix well with melted margarine. Press crust into bottom and sides of a lightly greased 10-inch pie tin. To prepare filling, heat chocolate and 2 tablespoons milk in saucepan over low heat, stirring until chocolate is melted. Beat sugar into cream cheese. Add remaining milk and chocolate mixture, and beat until smooth. Fold Cool Whip into chocolate mixture; blend until smooth. Spoon filling into crust. Freeze until firm, about 4 hours. Garnish with whipped cream and chocolate curls.

Chocolate Cream Pie

Serves 8 to 10

- 3 eggs, with whites reserved
- 1 cup sugar
- 3 cups milk
- 3 tablespoons cornstarch
- 4 tablespoons flour
- 2 ounces chocolate
- 1 teaspoon vanilla extract
- 1 tablespoon butter
- 1 9-inch piecrust, baked

Meringue topping:
- 3 reserved egg whites
- ⅓ teaspoon cream of tartar
- 4 tablespoons sugar
- ½ teaspoon vanilla

Separate eggs and set aside whites for meringue. Beat egg yolks in bowl. Add sugar and enough milk to make a paste. Sift together flour, cornstarch and enough milk to make a smooth, thin paste. Set aside. Preheat oven to 325 or 350 degrees. Scald the remaining milk and add some to each of the two paste mixtures. Slowly stir the two mixtures into the remaining scalded milk. Melt the chocolate squares in the microwave and add to custard mixture. Cook and stir until thickened. Add vanilla extract and butter, stirring well. Pour into a baked 9-inch pastry shell. To prepare meringue, whip three reserved egg whites until they are frothy. Add cream of tartar. Whip until stiff, but not dry. Beat in sugar, ½-teaspoon at a time. Do not over-beat. Beat in vanilla. Top pie with meringue, covering completely. Bake 10 to 15 minutes at 325 or 350 degrees so meringue will set and dry. Cool pie in a warm place away from draft to avoid shrinkage.

Cream Cheese Pie

Serves 6 to 8

- 2 8-ounce packages cream cheese
- 3 eggs
- ⅔ cup sugar
- ½ teaspoon almond extract
- 1 9-inch pastry crust, uncooked and chilled or 9-inch crumb crust, uncooked

Topping:
- 1 8-ounce container sour cream
- 3 tablespoons sugar
- 1 tablespoon vanilla extract

Preheat oven to 350 degrees. Mix pie ingredients together, blending well. Pour into 9-inch pastry or crumb crust (if using crumb crust, press into bottom and sides of dish). Bake for 25 minutes; cool 20 minutes. Combine topping ingredients and beat. Pour onto cooled pie. Bake pie for 10 more minutes. Cool, and serve.

Ritz Cracker Pie

Serves 6 to 8

- 4 egg whites
- 1 cup sugar
- ¾ cup pecans or walnuts, chopped
- 16 Ritz crackers, broken into small pieces
- 1 teaspoon baking powder
- 1 teaspoon vanilla extract
- whipped cream

Preheat oven to 350 degrees. Beat egg whites until they peak. Add sugar a little at a time, beat after each addition. Fold in nuts, crackers, baking powder and vanilla extract. Bake in 9-inch pie tin (do not grease) for 30 to 35 minutes. Serve with ice cream. Top with whipped cream. May also be served with fruit such as strawberries or raspberries.

Butterscotch Cream Cheese Pie

Serves 6 to 8

Crust:
⅓ cup butter or margarine, melted
1½ cups graham cracker crumbs
⅓ cup brown sugar, firmly packed

1 14-ounce can Eagle Brand sweetened condensed milk
¾ cup cold water
1 3⅝-ounce package butterscotch pudding and pie filling mix
3 8-ounce packages cream cheese, softened
3 eggs
1 teaspoon vanilla extract
½ pint whipped cream
10 pieces butterscotch candy, crushed

Preheat oven to 375 degrees. Combine margarine, crumbs and brown sugar. Press firmly on bottom of 9-inch springform pan. In medium saucepan, combine Eagle Brand Milk and water. Mix well. Stir in pudding mix over medium heat. Cook and stir until thickened and bubbly. In large mixer bowl, beat cheese until fluffy. Beat in eggs and vanilla extract, then add pudding mix. Pour into prepared pan and bake 50 minutes or until golden brown around the edges. Center will be soft. Cool at room temperature; chill thoroughly. Garnish with whipped cream; sprinkle with butterscotch pieces.

New Orleans Café Peanut Butter Pie

Yield: 2 pies
Serves 6 to 8, per pie

1 cup peanut butter, crunchy or smooth
1 14-ounce can Eagle Brand sweetened condensed milk
8 ounces softened cream cheese
1 cup powdered sugar
1 8 to 12-ounce container Cool Whip
2 9-inch graham cracker pie crusts
peanuts or chocolate curls

In large bowl, cream peanut butter, Eagle Brand milk and cream cheese. Add powdered sugar. Gently fold in Cool Whip. Pour into prepared pie crusts. May frost with more Cool Whip. Garnish with peanuts or chocolate curls. Freeze. Remove from freezer 5 to 10 minutes before cutting.

Never~Fail Piecrust

Yield: 2 double-crust pie shells

- 3 cups flour
- 1 teaspoon salt
- 1½ cups shortening or 1¼ cups lard ~ do not use oil
- 1 egg, beaten
- 5 tablespoons water
- 1 tablespoon vinegar

In a large mixing bowl, sift flour with salt. With a pastry blender or fork, cut shortening in half, working lightly with fingertips until mixture resembles grain of corn meal. Cut in remaining shortening, once again working lightly until mixture resembles size of a pea. Blend egg with water and vinegar. Pour over mixture, lifting lightly with fork. Gather dough up in hands to form a ball. Wrap in wax paper. Refrigerate until ready to use. Dough can also be frozen. Defrost in refrigerator when ready to use.

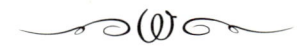

No~Bake Chocolate Eclair Cake

Serves 8 to 10

- 1 box graham crackers (do not use honey grahams), left whole
- 1 6-ounce package instant vanilla pudding
- 3½ cups cold milk
- 1 8-ounce container Cool Whip
- 1 can chocolate frosting, or homemade chocolate frosting

Butter and line bottom of a 13x9-inch pan with *whole* graham crackers. Mix milk with pudding for 2 minutes, using electric mixer on medium speed. Blend in cool whip. Spread half the mixture over the crackers. Cover mixture with another layer of whole graham crackers. Repeat with mixture, then finish with crackers. Refrigerate 2 hours or overnight. Frost before serving, when mixture has set.

Note: A very rich dessert; servings can be small!

Chocolate~Covered Cherry Cake

Serves 15 to 20

- 1 22¼-ounce package chocolate or fudge cake mix
- 1 22-ounce can cherry pie filling
- 1 12-ounce package chocolate chips
- 3 eggs
- ¼ cup oil

Cool Whip

Preheat oven to 350 degrees. Stir all ingredients (except Cool Whip) together with spoon. Grease a 9x13-inch pan, and pour mixture into pan. Bake for 30 to 35 minutes; let cool. Top with Cool Whip.

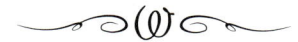

Auntie Netta's Every~Party Chocolate Cake

Serves 12 to 15

- 2 cups flour
- 2 cups sugar
- ½ teaspoon salt
- 1 teaspoon baking soda
- 2 eggs, beaten
- ½ cup sour cream
- 2 sticks butter
- 1 cup water
- 4 tablespoons cocoa

Icing:
- 2 cups powdered sugar
- 1 teaspoon vanilla extract
- 1 stick butter
- 4 tablespoons cocoa
- 6 tablespoons milk

pecan halves

Preheat oven to 350 degrees. To make cake, place flour, sugar, salt, baking soda, eggs and sour cream in bowl; mix. In a saucepan, combine 2 sticks butter, water and 4 tablespoons cocoa; bring to a boil. Immediately add boiled ingredients to flour mix. Cream well. Pour into a greased 11¾x17-inch pan. Bake for 20 minutes. To make icing, place powdered sugar and vanilla extract in a bowl; mix. In a saucepan, combine 1 stick butter, 4 tablespoons cocoa and milk; bring to a boil. Immediately, add boiled ingredients to sugar mixture and stir. Ice cake as soon as it is removed from the oven. Garnish with pecan halves.

"Killer" Chocolate Chip Fudge Cake

Serves 8 to 10

6 ounces unsalted butter
6 ounces unsweetened chocolate, chopped
6 eggs
3 cups sugar
½ teaspoon salt
1 tablespoon vanilla extract
1½ cups flour
1½ cups chocolate chips

Frosting:

1¼ cups sugar
2 tablespoons instant coffee
1 cup heavy cream
5 ounces unsweetened chocolate, finely chopped
4 ounces unsalted butter
1½ teaspoons vanilla extract

Preheat oven to 350 degrees. To make cake, grease two 9x1½-inch cake tins; line bottoms with wax paper. Melt butter and chocolate together over simmering water. Cool to lukewarm. In large bowl, whisk together for 1 minute: eggs, sugar, salt and vanilla extract. Whisk in butter-chocolate mixture. Stir in flour and chocolate chips. Beat gently, by hand. Pour batter into pans and bake for 30 to 35 minutes. Do not over bake; cake tester should come out clean. Cool on racks and remove from pans. Wrap layers well if not using same day.

To make frosting, combine sugar, coffee and cream in a small, deep saucepan. Stirring, bring to a boil. Reduce heat and simmer without stirring for 6 minutes or until candy thermometer reaches 234 degrees. Remove from heat. Add chopped chocolate and stir until melted and blended. Add butter and vanilla extract. Whisk well. Cool until mixture reaches 120 degrees. Mixture will begin to thicken. Beat by hand or mixer until thick and of good spreading consistency. If frosting seems too thick, add a little cream; if too thin, sift in some confectioner's sugar. (If made day before, bring back to room temperature and beat until of spreading consistency before using.)

To assemble, put one cake layer bottom-side up on cake plate. Spread with a third of the frosting. Top with second layer, also bottom-side up. Trim circumference of cake to remove excess crusty protrusions, so it is smooth for even frosting. Pour all but ½-cup of frosting on top of cake, spreading it over top and then sides. Put reserved icing into a pastry bag fitted with a small star tip and pipe 16 rosettes around top of cake. May serve with lightly-sweetened whipped cream. Refrigerate if not serving immediately.

Fudge~Drenched Chocolate Cake

Serves 10 to 12

- ½ cup vegetable oil
- 1 tablespoon vegetable oil
- 4 eggs
- 1 cup sugar
- 1 cup cake flour, sifted
- ½ cup cocoa
- 2 teaspoons baking powder
- ⅛ teaspoon baking soda
- ½ cup milk
- 1 teaspoon vanilla extract

Hot fudge sauce:

- 4 1-ounce squares unsweetened baking chocolate
- 2 tablespoons (¼-stick) butter
- ⅓ cup strong, black coffee, brewed
- ⅓ cup boiling water
- 2 cups sugar
- ¼ cup corn syrup
- 1 tablespoon rum

whipped cream

Preheat oven to 350 degrees. To make cake, flour a 9-inch tube or bundt pan. Shake out excess flour. Beat oil, eggs and sugar with an electric mixer on medium speed until mixture is light and lemon-colored. Resift flour with cocoa, baking powder and soda. Add flour mixture, milk and vanilla extract to egg mixture. Beat at low speed until blended. Pour into prepared pan. Bake until toothpick inserted in center of cake comes out clean, about 1 hour. Cool 10 to 20 minutes in pan. Invert onto platter.

While cake is cooling, make hot fudge sauce. Melt chocolate in top of double boiler set over gently-simmering water. Add butter and stir until melted. Pour in coffee and water, stirring constantly until well-combined. Blend in sugar and corn syrup. Transfer mixture to a small saucepan. Cover and boil, without stirring, for 3 minutes. Reduce heat and cook uncovered, without stirring, for 2 minutes. Remove from heat and stir in rum. Serve immediately with warm cake, garnished with whipped cream.

Chocolate~Deluxe Zucchini Cake

Serves 15 to 20

- 3 cups flour
- 1¼ teaspoons baking soda
- 1¼ teaspoons baking powder
- 1 teaspoon salt
- ¼ teaspoon cinnamon
- ⅔ cup cocoa
- 4 eggs
- 2 cups sugar
- 1½ cups vegetable oil
- 1½ teaspoons vanilla extract
- ½ teaspoon almond extract
- 3 cups zucchini, washed (but not peeled) and coarsely grated
- 1 cup nuts, chopped
- ½ cup dates (optional)

Glaze:
- 4 1-ounce squares unsweetened chocolate
- 2 teaspoons butter or margarine
- 2 cups confectioner's sugar, sifted
- 6 tablespoons warm water

Preheat oven to 350 degrees. To make cake, sift together flour, baking soda, baking powder, salt, cinnamon and cocoa; set aside. Beat eggs in large bowl until frothy. Gradually beat in sugar and oil. Add flavorings. Add flour gradually. Squeeze excess moisture from zucchini and fold into batter along with nuts and dates. Pour into greased and floured 10-inch tube pan. Bake 1 hour and 15 minutes. After 50 to 60 minutes, test with toothpick to prevent overbaking. When done, cake appears moist. Let stand inverted, for 20 minutes, on a wire rack. Remove cake from pan and cool on wire rack.

While cake is cooling, make the glaze. Melt chocolate in top of double boiler over simmering water; stir to blend well. Remove from heat. Stir in 1 cup confectioner's sugar and 2 tablespoons water; beat until smooth. Add remaining sugar and water; beat until glossy. Frost cake with chocolate glaze.

Note: Try serving with vanilla ice cream.

Iced Spice Cake

Serves 15 to 20

- 1 cup shortening
- 2 cups sugar
- 2 eggs
- 3 cups all-purpose flour
- 4 teaspoons powdered cocoa
- ¼ teaspoon cloves, ground
- 1 teaspoon cinnamon
- 1 teaspoon allspice
- 2 teaspoons baking soda
- 2 cups buttermilk

Icing:
- 6 tablespoons butter or margarine
- ½ cup brown sugar
- ⅓ cup milk
- 1 3-ounce package cream cheese, softened
- 1½ cups confectioner's sugar
- ½ teaspoon vanilla extract
- ¼ teaspoon salt

Preheat oven to 350 degrees. To make cake, cream shortening and sugar until light and fluffy. Add eggs and beat until thoroughly blended. Sift flour with cocoa and spices. Add baking soda to buttermilk. Blend dry ingredients and buttermilk alternately to shortening mixture. Beat only until ingredients are well-blended. Do not over-beat. Pour mixture into a well-greased and floured 9x13-inch pan or 10-inch tube pan. Bake for 45 to 50 minutes. Remove cake from pan and cool on wire racks.

While cake is cooling, make the icing. In a saucepan, melt butter or margarine. Add brown sugar and milk. Bring mixture to a boil and cook for 2 minutes. Remove from heat and cool. Add cream cheese and beat until smooth; then, beat in confectioner's sugar, vanilla extract and salt until of good spreading consistency. May use electric blender for smoother consistency. Frost cake with icing when cool.

Pecan~Filled Carrot Cake

Serves 15 to 20

1¼ cups corn oil
2 cups sugar
2 cups flour
2 teaspoons cinnamon
2 teaspoons baking powder
1 teaspoon baking soda
1 teaspoon salt
4 eggs
4 cups carrots, grated (about a 1-pound bag)
1 cup raisins
1 cup pecans, chopped

Filling:

1½ cups sugar
¼ cup flour
¾ teaspoon salt
1½ cups heavy cream
6 ounces (¾-cup) unsalted butter
1¼ cups pecans, chopped
2 teaspoons vanilla extract

Frosting:

8 ounces unsalted butter, softened
1 8-ounce package cream cheese, softened
1 1-pound package powdered sugar
1 teaspoon vanilla extract
4 ounces (1½ cups) coconut, shredded and sweetened

First, make filling. In a saucepan, blend sugar, flour and salt. Gradually stir in cream; add butter. Cook and stir over low heat until butter is melted. Simmer 20 to 30 minutes, until golden brown; stir occasionally. Cool down until lukewarm. Stir in nuts and vanilla extract. Let cool completely. Refrigerate overnight. If too thick to spread, bring to room temperature before using.

Preheat oven to 350 degrees. To make cake, grease and flour a 10-inch tube cake pan. In a large bowl, whisk together corn oil and sugar. Sift together flour, cinnamon, baking powder, baking soda and salt. Sift half the dry ingredient mixture into oil mixture; blend. Alternately sift in rest of the dry ingredients, while adding eggs, one at a time. Combine well. Add carrots, raisins and pecans. Pour into prepared tube pan. Bake for 70 minutes.

Pecan-Filled Carrot Cake, *continued on next page.*

Pecan-Filled Carrot Cake, *continued.*

Cool upright in pan, on a cooling rack. If not using cake that day, remove from pan, wrap well in plastic wrap and store at room temperature. To make frosting, cream butter well. Add cream cheese; beat until blended. Sift in sugar and add vanilla extract. If too soft to spread, chill a while. If not using immediately, refrigerate and bring to spreadable temperature before using.

Preheat oven to 300 degrees. To assemble, spread coconut on a baking sheet; bake for 10 to 15 minutes, until it colors lightly. Toss coconut occasionally while it is baking so it browns evenly. Cool completely. Have filling and frosting ready at a spreadable consistency. Loosen cake in its pan and invert onto a serving plate. With a long, serrated knife, carefully split cake into 3 horizontal layers. Spread filling between layers. Re-stack layers. Spread frosting over top and sides. Pat toasted coconut onto sides of cake. If desired, reserve ½-cup frosting. Color ¼-cup with orange food coloring and ¼-cup with green. Decorate top of cake with frosting to resemble little carrots; use 1/16-inch wide pastry tube to pipe frosting. Serve cake at room temperature.

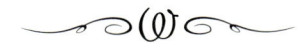

Helen's Hazelwood Carrot Cake

Serves 15 to 20

An original Hazelwood recipe!

- 2 cups flour
- 2 cups sugar
- 2 teaspoons baking powder
- 2 teaspoons cinnamon
- 1 teaspoon salt
- 1½ cups vegetable oil
- 4 eggs, beaten
- 3 cups (about 8 large) carrots, peeled and shredded
- 1 cup nuts, chopped

Frosting:
- 1 stick butter, softened
- 1 pound powdered sugar
- 1 8-ounce package cream cheese
- 2 teaspoons vanilla extract

Preheat oven to 350 degrees. First prepare frosting. Beat together butter and cream cheese. Gradually add powdered sugar, beating until smooth. Add vanilla and beat to good spreading consistency. Next, prepare cake. Grease and flour a 10-inch tube pan. Blend flour, sugar, baking powder, cinnamon and salt into eggs; add vegetable oil and beat. Add carrots and nuts, blending well; do not over-beat. Pour into prepared tube pan. Bake for 30 to 35 minutes, or until toothpick inserted in center of cake comes out clean. Allow cake to cool in pan. When cool, remove and frost.

Mother's Favorite Fresh Orange Cake

Serves 6 to 8

1 cup butter or shortening
2 cups sugar
2 eggs, well-beaten
4 cups flour
2 teaspoons baking soda
2 cups buttermilk
rind of 1 large orange or 2 small oranges, grated
1½ cups raisins and nuts, chopped together
juice of 1 large orange or 2 small oranges

Buttercream icing:

4 tablespoons butter
2 cups confectioner's sugar
1 dash salt
1 teaspoon vanilla extract
3 tablespoons milk

Preheat oven to 350 degrees. Grease and flour 10-inch tube pan. Cream butter and sugar. Add eggs. Combine flour and baking soda and alternate adding this with buttermilk to butter-sugar-egg mixture. Add orange rind, raisins and nuts. Pour batter into pan and bake for 1 hour. After cake is baked and while still hot, pour juice of one large or two small oranges over cake. Ice with butter cream icing when cold. To prepare icing, cream butter; add confectioner's sugar and salt. Add milk and whip until smooth. Finally, add vanilla. Buttercream will be good spreading consistency.

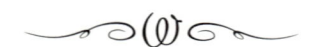

Orange Candy Cake

Serves 20 to 24

2 sticks butter or margarine, softened
2 cups sugar
4 eggs
2 teaspoons baking soda
1½ cups buttermilk
4 cups flour
¼ teaspoon salt
1 pound orange slice candy, chopped
1 pound dates, chopped
2 cups nuts, chopped

Orange Candy Cake, *continued on next page.*

Orange Candy Cake, continued.

¾ cups brown sugar
1 6-ounce can frozen orange juice concentrate

Preheat oven to 275 degrees. Grease and flour one 10-inch tube pan or two 8-inch loaf pans. Cream butter and sugar. Add eggs, one at a time, beating well after each addition. Mix baking soda in ½-cup buttermilk and add to egg mixture. Mix well. Combine flour and salt. Add flour and salt and remaining buttermilk alternately, mixing well after each addition. Add chopped orange slices, dates and nuts. Mix well. Line pan(s) with brown paper and grease paper. Bake 2½ to 3 hours or until toothpick comes out clean. (Loaf pans bake faster.) While cake is baking, mix brown sugar and frozen orange juice concentrate. Let set and pour over cake as soon as it is removed from oven. Poke holes in cake to allow glaze to soak through.

Orange~Chocolate Chip Cake, 1945

Serves 10 to 12

½ cup butter or margarine
½ cup granulated sugar
½ cup brown sugar
1 teaspoon vanilla extract
3 eggs, beaten
1 small package chocolate chips
rind from one orange
½ cup nuts, chopped
2¼ cups enriched flour
¼ teaspoon salt
2 teaspoons baking soda
1 cup sour milk (may substitute buttermilk or add 1 teaspoon vinegar to 1 cup sweet milk to achieve sour effect)

Preheat oven to 350 degrees. Grease and flour 10-inch bundt or 9x13x2-inch pan. Thoroughly cream butter and sugars. Add vanilla extract, then eggs. Mix well. Stir in chocolate chips and orange rind. Add nuts. Sift together flour, salt and baking soda. Stir in sifted dry ingredients alternately with sour milk. Mix just until smooth. Pour into prepared pan. Bake for 50 minutes, or until done.

Conjurer's Pecan Rum Cake

Serves 10 to 12

- ½ cup pecans, chopped
- 1 8¼-ounce package yellow cake mix
- 1 3¾-ounce package instant vanilla pudding
- 4 eggs
- ½ cup water
- ½ cup vegetable oil
- ½ cup light rum

Glaze:
- 1 cup sugar
- ¼ pound butter
- ¼ cup rum
- ¼ cup water

Preheat oven to 350 degrees. Sprinkle nuts evenly into bottom of greased and floured 10-inch tube or bundt pan. Set aside. Blend cake mix, pudding, eggs, water, oil and rum in large bowl until moistened. Beat at medium speed for 2 minutes. Pour batter into prepared pan. Bake for 1 hour.

Fifteen minutes before cake has finished baking, prepare glaze. In a saucepan, mix sugar, butter, rum and water. Bring to a full boil, stirring frequently. Then simmer 5 minutes. Cool slightly. Remove cake from oven and pierce top of cake with fork or ice pick. Pour warm glaze over cake. Cool completely. Turn out onto a serving platter.

Chicago Pistachio Cake, 1970

Serves 8 to 10

- 1 8¼-ounce package yellow cake mix
- 2 3¾-ounce boxes pistachio pudding
- ½ cup water
- ½ cup milk
- ½ cup vegetable oil
- 5 eggs

walnuts, ground (optional)

Preheat oven to 350 degrees. Grease a 9x13-inch pan or line bottom with wax paper. Combine cake mix, puddings, water, milk and oil in a mixing bowl, and mix well. Add 1 egg at a time, mixing well after each addition. Continue to mix for another 2 minutes. If desired, add ground walnuts. Pour mixture into prepared pan. Bake for 50 minutes. Cake is done when toothpick comes out clean.

Dark Rum Cake

Serves 12 to 15

1½ cups butter, softened
rind of one lemon, grated
1 cup sugar
5 eggs
3 cups all-purpose flour
1 teaspoon cinnamon
2 teaspoons baking powder
1 pinch salt
2 tablespoons dark rum
1 cup milk
½ cup almonds, slivered
confectioner's sugar

Preheat oven to 325 degrees. Generously grease 10-inch spring-form cake pan. Place butter and lemon rind in large bowl. Work butter until soft. Add sugar and cream together, using spatula. Add 1 egg and 3 tablespoons flour and cinnamon. Beat together with mixer. Add remaining eggs and beat until completely incorporated. Place remaining flour with baking powder and salt in small bowl. Mix together. Sift half into egg batter and mix very well. Add rum and mix with spatula. Add remaining flour and continue mixing. Pour in milk and almonds, and fold into batter. Pour batter into prepared pan. Bake 45 minutes to 1 hour or until toothpick comes out clean. Test after 45 minutes. Remove pan from oven; allow cake to cool completely in pan. When cool, turn out onto cake rack. Dust cake with icing sugar.

Rhoda's Wacky Cake

Serves 6 to 8

1½ cups flour
1 cup sugar
1 teaspoon baking soda
¼ cup cocoa
3 teaspoons vinegar
3 teaspoons vanilla extract
6 tablespoons margarine, melted
1 cup water

Preheat oven to 350 degrees. Mix flour, sugar, baking soda and cocoa in an 8x11-inch pan. Make three wells in the dry mixture, and pour 1-teaspoon vinegar, 1-teaspoon vanilla extract and 2 tablespoons margarine into each well. Pour water over all, and mix very well. Bake for 30 minutes in the same pan.

Earthquake Cake

Serves 20 to 24

- 2 tablespoons margarine
- 1 cup coconut
- 1 cup nuts, chopped
- 1 stick margarine, softened
- 1 8-ounce package cream cheese, softened
- 1 pound powdered sugar
- 1 teaspoon vanilla extract
- 1 package German chocolate cake mix

Preheat oven to 350 degrees. Melt 2 tablespoons margarine in 9x13-inch pan in oven, being careful not to brown. Brush sides with melted margarine. Sprinkle coconut over bottom of pan. Sprinkle chopped nuts on top. Prepare topping. Mix together stick of margarine, cream cheese, powdered sugar and vanilla extract. Drop cream cheese mixture by teaspoon over coconut and nut mixture. Use all of it. Prepare cake mix according to package directions. Pour over topping mixture. Bake cake for 50 to 55 minutes. Cool in pan no more than 5 or 10 minutes. Turn cake upside down with serving plate over cake. Cake will end up with a German chocolate cake frosting.

Note: A very moist, all-in-one pan dessert.

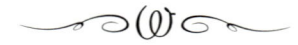

Grandmother's Cake

Serves 10 to 12

- 1 18¼-ounce package yellow cake mix
- 1 3¼-ounce package instant butterscotch pudding
- 1 3¼-ounce package instant vanilla pudding
- 1 cup vegetable oil
- 1 cup water
- 4 eggs

Topping:
- 1 cup brown sugar
- 1 cup nuts, chopped

Preheat oven to 350 degrees. Mix cake mix, puddings, oil, water and eggs together. Pour half of batter into a 9x13-inch greased pan. Mix brown sugar and nuts together and sprinkle 1 cup mixture over batter. Pour rest of batter over nuts and sugar; sprinkle rest of hot mixture on top. Bake for 40 to 45 minutes.

Heavenly Raspberry Cake

Serves 10 to 12

1 package angel food cake mix
1 16-ounce container whipping cream
2 10-ounce packages frozen red raspberries, well drained

Mix, bake and cool cake as directed on cake mix package. Whip cream until soft peaks form. Be careful to not over-beat, or cream will turn to butter. Fold in well-drained red raspberries. Ice cake with whipping cream mixture and refrigerate several hours or overnight.

Sunshine Cake

Serves 10 to 12

9 egg yolks
¾ cup sugar
¾ cup flour
1 teaspoon vanilla extract
9 egg whites
¾ teaspoon cream of tartar
1 pinch salt

Frosting:
½ cup milk
3 egg yolks, lightly beaten
½ cup powdered sugar
¼ pound margarine
1 4-ounce can coconut, toasted

Preheat oven to 350 degrees. Beat egg yolks until light and lemon colored. Add sugar gradually, then add vanilla extract. Fold in flour and salt. Beat egg whites and cream of tartar and fold in lightly. Pour in bundt pan and bake 45 minutes to 1 hour. Remove from oven and invert cake. Allow inverted pan to rest on a funnel or soda bottle. Let cake hang for 1½ hours; this allows the cake to thoroughly set. Remove cake from pan. Meanwhile, make frosting. Scald milk in top of double boiler. Remove a small amount of milk and whisk into egg yolks. Add this to rest of milk in double boiler; add powdered sugar. Cook until mixture thickens to a custard consistency and coats a spoon. Beat well. Set pot in cold water to cool. Add margarine and beat well. Preheat oven to 300 degrees. Spread coconut on baking sheet and toast in oven for 10 to 15 minutes. Then frost cake and sprinkle toasted coconut over top and sides of cake.

"Rave About It" Cake

Serves 10 to 12

- 1   18¼-ounce package yellow cake mix
- 1½ cups cold water
- 1   3¼-ounce package instant vanilla pudding mix
- 4   eggs
- ¼   cup vegetable oil
- 2   cups coconut, shredded
- ½   cup nuts

Frosting:
- 4   tablespoons butter
- 1   8-ounce package cream cheese, softened
- 2   teaspoons milk
- 3   cups confectioner's sugar
- ½   teaspoon vanilla extract
- 2   cups coconut, toasted
- ½   cup nuts

Preheat oven to 350 degrees. Beat cake mix, water, pudding, eggs and oil for 4 minutes in mixer. Stir in shredded coconut and nuts. Pour into 3 greased and floured 9-inch cake pans. Bake for 35 minutes. Meanwhile, toast coconut in 300-degree oven for 10 to 15 minutes, until golden brown. Let cool before blending in frosting. To make frosting: cream butter and cream cheese together. Add milk, sugar, vanilla extract and blend. Stir in 1¾ cups toasted coconut and nuts. Spread frosting on cooled cake layers, stack and spread over whole cake. Sprinkle remaining coconut on top.

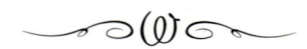

Esther's Imperial Cake

Serves 10 to 12

- ¾   pound Imperial margarine (do not use diet)
- 1   pound powdered sugar
- 6   eggs
- 3   cups cake flour, sifted
- 1   teaspoon lemon rind, grated
- 1½ teaspoons vanilla

Preheat oven to 350 degrees. Cream margarine and sugar well. Add eggs, one at a time, beating well after each addition. Add flour a little at a time, along with the lemon and vanilla; blend well. Pour batter in greased, 10-inch angel food pan. Smooth top. Bake 1 hour to 1 hour, 15 minutes.

Best~Ever Cake

Serves 12 to 15

- 1 cup nuts, chopped
- 2 cups sugar
- 2 cups unsifted flour
- 1 20-ounce can crushed pineapple, with most of juice drained
- 2 teaspoons baking soda
- ½ cup butter, melted
- 2 eggs
- 1 teaspoon vanilla extract
- 1 dash of salt

Frosting:
- 1 stick butter
- 1 8-ounce package cream cheese
- 1⅓ cups powdered sugar
- 1 teaspoon vanilla extract

nuts, chopped

Preheat oven to 350 degrees. Combine cake ingredients in bowl as listed above, stirring well. Place in greased and floured 9x13-inch pan. Bake 40 to 45 minutes. Meanwhile, prepare frosting. Cream together butter and cream cheese. Gradually add powdered sugar until all blended. Add vanilla; beat well. Spread on hot cake, right out of the oven. Sprinkle with nuts.

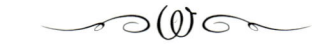

Cherry Streusel Cake

Serves 12 to 15

- 1½ cups butter, softened
- 2 cups sugar
- 2 eggs
- 3 cups flour, sifted
- 2 teaspoons baking powder
- ½ teaspoon salt
- 1 21-ounce can cherry pie filling

Preheat oven to 350 degrees. Cream butter and sugar until light and fluffy. Add eggs and beat thoroughly. Sift together flour, baking powder and salt. Add sifted dry ingredients; mix well. Batter will be heavy. Spread about three-quarters of batter in greased 9x13x2-inch pan. Pour cherry pie filling on top of batter and spread gently. Drop remaining batter over filling. Swirl. To prepare crumb topping, combine ½-cup butter, 1 cup sugar and 1 cup flour; sprinkle on cake. Bake for 45 minutes.

Old~Fashioned Fruit Cake

Yield: 2 cakes

- 1 pound butter or margarine
- 3 cups brown sugar
- 1 cup dark molasses or syrup of preserves
- 4 cups cake flour, plus 1 cup for rolling fruits
- 12 eggs, separated
- 2 teaspoons cinnamon
- 2 teaspoons allspice
- ½ teaspoon cloves
- ½ teaspoon nutmeg
- 2 teaspoons mace
- 1½ pounds nuts ~ mixed pecans and walnuts
- 2 pounds seedless white raisins
- 1 pound candied pineapple
- 1 pound candied cherries
- 1 pound dates
- 1 cup whiskey or wine
- 1 pint peach preserves
- 1 pint fig preserves
- 1 pint pear preserves
- 1 pint watermelon rind preserves

Preheat oven to 350 degrees. Cream butter and sugar; add molasses or syrup and flour. Beat yolks well and then in a separate bowl, beat egg whites until stiff but not dry; add to above mixture. Add cinnamon, allspice, cloves, nutmeg and mace; then add nuts and fruit rolled in flour. Blend in whiskey and peach, fig, pear and watermelon rind preserves. To bake, prepare 2 10-inch tube pans; line bottoms with rounds of wax paper or aluminum foil. Cut a round for the sides. Grease both well. Divide batter between 2 pans, filling to about 2½ inches (if there is extra batter, grease and line an 8x4-inch loaf pan). Place a shallow pan filled with water on lower rack in oven. Bake a 5 pound cake for at least 5 hours, removing pan of water the last 30 minutes of cooking. Cool cakes in pans for 20 to 30 minutes on rack. Remove from pans and remove wax paper or foil. To store, moisten cakes in whiskey; cover with cloths moistened in whiskey; then cover with aluminum foil and place in tin container for about 10 days. Sliver and eat.

Note: Will keep well. Can also be frozen for a long time.

"Coco~Nutty" Oatmeal~Raisin Cake

Serves 20 to 24

- 1 cup quick oatmeal
- 1¼ cups boiling water
- 1 cup brown sugar
- 1 cup white sugar
- ¼ pound butter, softened
- 2 eggs
- 1½ cups flour
- 1 teaspoon baking soda
- 1 teaspoon cinnamon
- 1 cup raisins
- 1 cup walnuts, chopped

Topping:
- ¼ pound butter, melted
- 1 cup brown sugar
- ¼ cup milk
- 1 teaspoon vanilla extract
- 1 cup coconut
- 1 cup nuts, chopped

Preheat oven to 350 degrees. Combine oatmeal and water. Mix other ingredients. Add oatmeal and mix well. Bake in greased 9x13-inch pan for 35 to 40 minutes. Mix topping ingredients by hand and spread on baked cake. Set under broiler for 3 to 5 minutes.

Gudrun's Danish Apple Cake

Serves 8 to 10

- 2 cups very dry French (or Zwieback) bread crumbs, finely crushed
- 2 tablespoons sugar
- ½ cup butter or margarine
- 3 cups apple sauce, cooked and very thick
- ½ pint whipping cream, whipped

Raspberry-strawberry sauce
- 1 10-ounce package frozen raspberries, thawed
- ½ cup sugar
- 1 tablespoon lemon juice
- 2 pints fresh strawberries, thinly sliced

Gudrun's Danish Apple Cake, *continued on next page.*

Gudrun's Danish Apple Cake, continued.

Combine bread crumbs and sugar. Melt butter in skillet. Add crumbs and sugar to butter. Heat on low temperature until light brown. Alternate layers of ½-cup crumbs and ¾-cup apple sauce in glass bowl. Top with whipped cream and decorate with raspberry sauce. To prepare raspberry-strawberry sauce, purée raspberries in electric blender at high speed; add ¼-cup sugar and lemon juice. Add remaining ¼-cup sugar to sliced strawberries. Stir puréed raspberries into strawberries.

Kathy's Apple Cake

Serves 10 to 12

- 3 cups flour
- 2 teaspoons cinnamon
- ½ teaspoon baking soda
- 2 teaspoons baking powder
- 1 teaspoon salt
- 1 cup unsalted butter, room temperature
- ¼ cup vegetable oil
- 2 cups sugar
- 2 teaspoons vanilla extract
- 3 large eggs, room temperature
- 4 cups apples, peeled, cored and cut into ½-inch cubes

Topping:
- 1 teaspoon cinnamon
- 1 tablespoon sugar

Preheat oven to 350 degrees. Sift together flour, cinnamon, baking soda, baking powder and salt. Cream butter, oil, sugar and vanilla extract at medium speed until ingredients are blended (about 2 minutes). Stop to scrape bowl twice. Add eggs one at a time, mixing after each addition. Add half of dry ingredients. Mix at low speed for 15 seconds. Add second half of dry ingredients until blended. Add apples and fold with wooden spoon. Spoon batter into lightly greased 10-inch tube pan. Sprinkle cinnamon and sugar topping over cake. Bake for 1 hour to 1 hour and 5 minutes.

Roberta's Fresh Apple Cake

Serves 8 to 10

- 8 cups cooking apples (Golden Delicious), peeled and sliced
- 2 cups sugar
- 4 cups flour
- 3 teaspoons baking soda
- 2 teaspoons salt
- 4 teaspoons cinnamon
- 2 scant cups Crisco oil
- 4 eggs, beaten
- 4 teaspoons vanilla extract
- 2 cups nuts, chopped

Preheat oven to 350 degrees. Cover sliced apples with sugar. Sift together flour, baking soda, salt and cinnamon. Mix sugar and apples together. Add oil and beaten eggs. Add sifted, dry ingredients; then add vanilla extract and nuts. Do not over-beat. Mix only until all ingredients are well-blended. Grease and flour 12x18-inch pan. Pour mix into pan and bake 45 to 50 minutes, or until toothpick comes out clean. May be served with ice cream or whipped cream.

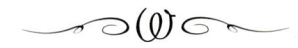

One~Bowl Apple Cake

Serves 8 to 10

- 2 cups flour
- 2 cups sugar
- ½ cup oil
- 2 eggs
- 2 teaspoons cinnamon
- 2 teaspoons baking soda
- 1 teaspoon salt
- 1 21-ounce can Thank You Brand apple pie filling

Frosting:
- 1 8-ounce package cream cheese
- 1 1-pound package confectioner's sugar
- 1 teaspoon vanilla
- 1 to 2 tablespoons milk

Preheat oven to 350 degrees. Butter 9x13-inch dish. Combine all ingredients (except pie filling) and blend well. Gently stir in pie filling. (Adding the pie filling earlier will break up the apples too much.) Turn into dish and bake for about 50 minutes to 1 hour. To make frosting, beat cream cheese until soft. Add confectioner's sugar gradually. Then add vanilla and milk. Mix until frosting is a good spreading consistency. Top cake with frosting.

Ricotta Cheese Cake

Serves 10 to 12

- 1 18¼-ounce package Duncan Hines Golden cake mix
- 3 eggs
- ⅔ cup water
- ½ cup butter, room temperature

Topping:
- 1½ pounds ricotta cheese
- ¼ cup sugar
- 3 eggs
- 1 teaspoon vanilla extract

Preheat oven to 350 degrees. Blend cake mix, water, 3 eggs and butter in large bowl at low speed until moistened. Beat at medium speed for 4 minutes. Pour batter into a greased 9x13-inch pan. Mix ricotta cheese, sugar, 3 eggs and vanilla extract together and gently spoon over the cake evenly. Cheese mixture will settle to bottom of pan while baking. Bake for 1 hour or until toothpick inserted into cake comes out clean. When cool, dust with powdered sugar.

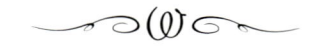

Sour Cream Pound Cake

Serves 15 to 20

- 3 cups sugar
- 2 sticks butter
- 6 eggs, separated
- ¼ teaspoon baking soda
- 1 cup sour cream
- 3 cups cake flour, sifted
- 1 pinch salt
- 1 teaspoon vanilla extract

Preheat oven to 300 degrees. Grease and flour angel food cake pan. Cream sugar and butter, add egg yolks one at a time. Beat egg whites until stiff but not dry. Dissolve soda in sour cream and add alternately with flour mixed with salt. Add vanilla extract. Fold in stiffly beaten egg whites. Bake for 2 hours or until toothpick comes out clean.

Cream Cheese Pound Cake

Serves 12 to 16

3 cups sugar
1 8-ounce package cream cheese
3 sticks butter
6 eggs
3 cups flour
1 teaspoon vanilla extract

Preheat oven to 325 degrees. Cream together sugar, butter and cream cheese. Add eggs, beating well after each one. Then gradually add all the flour and vanilla extract. Beat with electric mixer at least 5 minutes. Bake in greased angel food cake pan for about 1 hour and 15 minutes.

Cherry~Nut Pound Cake

Serves 12 to 16

½ pound butter
½ pound margarine
1 1-pound package confectioner's sugar
6 eggs
1 teaspoon vanilla extract
1 teaspoon salt
3 cups all-purpose flour
1 cup candied cherries, sliced and dusted with flour
½ cup nuts, finely chopped

Preheat oven to 350 degrees. Cream butter and margarine. Add sugar and cream until fluffy. Add eggs, 1 at a time, beating well after each addition. Stir in vanilla extract. Mix salt with flour and blend into batter. Stir in fruit and nuts which have been dusted with flour (prevents sinking). Pour batter into well-greased and floured 10-inch tube pan. Bake 1 hour to 1 hour and 15 minutes. Remove from oven and cool on rack for 10 minutes.

Note: This cake improves with standing and also freezes well. For a variation, try icing the cake with a glaze of powdered sugar and maraschino cherry juice.

Sophie's Pound Cake, 1929

Serves 10 to 12

½ pound butter
1 cup sugar
4 eggs
2 cups flour
½ teaspoon salt
1 teaspoon baking powder
¼ cup milk
1 teaspoon vanilla extract

Preheat oven to 350 degrees. Cream sugar and butter. Add 1 egg at a time, beating well after each. Mix flour, salt and baking powder. Add milk and flour alternately. Add vanilla extract. Mix well. Bake in greased 9x5-inch loaf pan for 1 hour and 10 minutes.

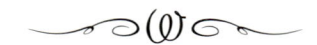

Gloria's Excellent Cheesecake

Serves 8 to 10

Crust:
24 graham crackers, rolled into fine crumbs
½ stick butter, melted

4 8-ounce packages cream cheese, softened
2 cups sugar
5 eggs
1 21-ounce can blueberry or cherry pie filling

Preheat oven to 325 degrees. Mix graham crackers and butter together until well blended. Press into bottom and up sides (as high as possible) of a 10 to 12-inch springform pan. Beat cream cheese with eggs until smooth. Add sugar and beat. Pour batter into springform pan and bake 1 hour. Check to see if cake is done by inserting tester. If tester is wet, continue baking until done, checking every 10 minutes. Cake will be slightly brown on top and top may crack. Remove from oven when done and cool completely. Pour pie filling over cooled cake and spread evenly almost to edge of cake. Refrigerate. To serve, place on cake plate and remove sides of springform.

Cocoa Cheesecake

Serves 10 to 12

Crust:
1½ cups graham cracker crumbs
⅓ cup sugar
⅓ cup butter or margarine, melted

2   8-ounce packages cream cheese, softened
¼   cup plus 2 tablespoons sugar
½   cup Hershey's cocoa
2   teaspoons vanilla extract
2   eggs
1   cup sour cream

Preheat oven to 375 degrees. Mix graham cracker crumbs, butter and sugar together. Press on bottom of 9-inch springform pan, and halfway up sides. Set aside. Beat cream cheese, ¼-cup sugar, cocoa and 1 teaspoon vanilla extract in large mixing bowl until light and fluffy. Add eggs; blend well. Pour into prepared crust. Bake for 20 minutes. Remove from oven; cool 15 minutes. Combine sour cream, 2 tablespoons sugar and 1 teaspoon vanilla extract. Stir until smooth. Spread evenly over baked filling. Bake at 425 degrees for 10 minutes. Cool. Chill several hours or overnight before serving.

Des Plaines Cheesecake

Serves 15 to 20

Crust:
1¾ cups graham cracker crumbs
⅓ cup margarine, melted
¼ cup sugar

1   cup sugar
2   8-ounce packages cream cheese, softened
3   eggs
2   teaspoons vanilla extract
1   pint sour cream

Preheat oven to 375 degrees. Blend graham cracker crumbs, margarine and sugar together. Press in bottom of 8-inch springform pan, and up to 2½ inches of sides. Set aside. Cream sugar and cream cheese. Add eggs, vanilla extract and sour cream. Mix thoroughly. Fill crust with cream cheese mixture. Bake for 35 minutes. Make cake 24 hours before serving. Keep in refrigerator.

Rubly Cheesecake

Serves 10 to 12

Crust:
3 cups graham crackers, crushed
4 slices rusk, crushed
3 tablespoons sugar
1½ teaspoons cinnamon
¾ cup butter or margarine, melted

Cheesecake:
4 eggs, separated
1 8-ounce and one 3-ounce package cream cheese, softened
½ cup sugar
1 teaspoon vanilla extract

Topping:
1 pint sour cream
6 tablespoons sugar
1 teaspoon vanilla extract

Preheat oven to 350 degrees. Combine graham crackers and rusk. Add sugar, cinnamon and butter. Mix and pack sides and bottom of 8x12-inch baking dish. The crust will be thick. Separate eggs and beat yolks. Cream the cheese and mix with egg yolks. In separate bowl, beat egg whites until stiff. Add sugar and vanilla extract. Fold into cream cheese and yolk mixture. Pour into prepared crust and bake for 30 minutes. Cool for 20 minutes. Mix sour cream, sugar and vanilla extract. Spread slowly over top of cake. Bake for 10 to 15 minutes more. Cool completely. Chill.

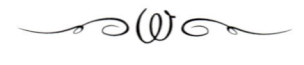

Cheesecake Tarts

Yield: 3 dozen

36 vanilla wafers
2 8-ounce packages cream cheese, softened
3 eggs
⅔ cup sugar
1 teaspoon vanilla extract
1 21-ounce can cherry or blueberry pie filling

Preheat oven to 350 degrees. Line small muffin tins with cupcake papers. Place one wafer in each. Mix cream cheese, eggs, sugar and vanilla extract. Fill lined muffin tins two-thirds full. Bake for 15 to 20 minutes. Cool. Spoon cherry or blueberry pie filling onto each tart.

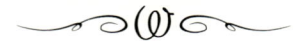

Cheesecake Squares

Serves 10 to 12

Crust:
1 cup butter or margarine
2 cups flour
2 tablespoons sugar

2 8-ounce packages cream cheese, softened
2 cups confectioner's sugar (do not sift)
1 8-ounce container Cool Whip
1 21-ounce can of cherry or strawberry pie filling

Preheat oven to 350 degrees. Mix butter, flour and sugar with pie blender until crumbly. Press evenly into a 10x15-inch pan. Bake for 15 minutes or until slightly brown. In a large bowl, mix cream cheese and confectioner's sugar until creamy. Fold in Cool Whip. Spread over cooled crust. Cover with pie filling. Chill.

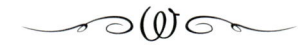

Lemon Cheesecake Bars

Serves 8 to 10

Crust:
½ cup margarine
2 teaspoons sugar
1 cup flour

1 8-ounce package cream cheese, softened
1 cup powdered sugar
1 cup Cool Whip
2 3-ounce packages lemon pudding (do not use instant)
1 12-ounce container Cool Whip, thawed

Preheat oven to 325 degrees. Melt margarine; add sugar and flour. Mix well and pat in bottom of a 9x13-inch pan. Bake for 30 minutes. Combine cream cheese, powdered sugar and fold in Cool Whip. Spread over cooled crust. Cook lemon pudding according to directions on package. Cool and spread over cream cheese mixture. Spread Cool Whip over pudding.

Coconut Dream Bars

Yield: 35 to 40 bars

Crust:
- 2 cups flour
- ½ teaspoon salt
- 1 cup butter

Filling:
- 4 eggs
- 2 teaspoons vanilla extract
- 3 cups brown sugar
- 4 tablespoons flour
- 1 teaspoon salt
- 1 teaspoon baking powder
- 1 cup walnuts, chopped
- 1 cup coconut

Icing:
- 1 cup confectioner's sugar
- ½ cup butter, softened
- 1 teaspoon vanilla extract

Preheat oven to 350 degrees. For crust, mix flour and salt. Cut in butter as for piecrust and spread in bottom of 9x13-inch pan. Bake for 20 to 25 minutes. For filling, beat eggs, add vanilla extract and dry ingredients. Stir in nuts and coconut. Spread over crust. Bake for 25 minutes. When bars have cooled, beat together icing ingredients. Spread over top. Cut into bars.

Magic Cookie Bars

Yield: 40 squares

Crust:
- 1½ cups graham cracker crumbs
- ¼ pound butter, melted

- 1¼ cups chocolate chips
- 1 cup coconut, shredded
- 1½ cups walnuts, chopped
- 1 14-ounce can Eagle Brand sweetened condensed milk

Preheat oven to 350 degrees. Grease or spray 11¼x7¼x¾-inch aluminum foil pan with Pam cooking spray. Mix melted butter and graham cracker crumbs. Pat mixture on bottom of pan. Sprinkle first layer with chocolate chips, second layer with coconut, third layer with nuts. Pour Eagle brand milk over top. Bake for 30 minutes. Remove from oven; cool. Cut into squares.

Cherry~Coconut Bars, 1950

Serves 8 to 10

Crust:
- ½ cup butter
- 1 cup flour
- 3 tablespoons confectioner's sugar

- 2 eggs
- 1 cup sugar
- ¼ cup flour
- ½ teaspoon baking powder
- ¼ teaspoon salt
- 1 teaspoon vanilla extract
- ¾ cup nuts, chopped
- ½ cup coconut
- ½ cup maraschino cherries, quartered

Heat oven to 350 degrees. With hands, mix flour, butter and confectioner's sugar until smooth. Spread thin with fingers in 8-inch square pan. Bake for 25 minutes. Stir rest of ingredients into eggs and spread over top of pastry. Bake for another 25 minutes. Cool and cut into bars.

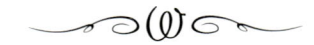

Chocolate~Cherry Bars

Yield: 24 bars

- 1 18½-ounce package Pillsbury fudge cake mix
- 1 teaspoon Almond Extract
- 2 eggs, beaten
- 1 21-ounce can cherry pie filling

Frosting:
- 1 cup sugar
- 5 tablespoons butter or margarine
- ⅓ cup milk
- 1 6-ounce package semi-sweet chocolate pieces

In large bowl combine cake mix, almond extract and eggs. After this is mixed, add filling and stir by hand until mixed. Pour into greased 9x13-inch baking pan. Bake 20 to 30 minutes. To make frosting, combine sugar, butter and milk in a small saucepan. Bring to a boil and cook, stirring constantly for 1 minute. Remove from heat and stir in chocolate pieces until smooth. Frost cake. Cut into 24 bars when cool.

Butter Pecan Turtle Bars

Yield: 48 bars

- 2 cups flour
- ¾ cup light brown sugar, packed
- ½ cup butter, softened
- 1½ cups pecan halves
- ½ cup light brown sugar, packed
- ⅔ cup butter
- 1½ cups milk chocolate chips

Preheat oven to 350 degrees. Combine first three ingredients. Blend until crumbly. Pat firmly onto bottom of 9x13-inch pan (do not grease). Sprinkle pecan halves over unbaked crust. Set aside. In a small saucepan, combine ½-cup brown sugar and ⅔-cup butter. Cook over medium heat, stirring constantly until mixture begins to boil. Boil 1 minute, stirring constantly. Drizzle over pecans and crust. Bake for 18 to 20 minutes, or until caramel layer is bubbly and crust is light brown. Remove from oven and immediately sprinkle with chocolate chips, spreading chips evenly as they melt. Cool completely before cutting.

Easy Toffee Bars

Yield: 35 bars

- 35 unsalted soda crackers
- 1 cup butter or regular margarine
- 1 cup brown sugar, packed
- 1 6-ounce package semisweet chocolate chips
- pistachio or macadamia nuts, chopped

Preheat oven to 350 degrees. Lightly butter 15½x10½x1-inch jelly roll pan. Line bottom of pan evenly with crackers. Cut crackers to fit empty spaces, as needed. Combine butter and brown sugar in 2-quart heavy saucepan. Cook over medium heat, stirring constantly, until mixture comes to a boil. Continue cooking 3 more minutes, stirring constantly. Pour mixture evenly over crackers. Bake for 15 minutes. Remove from oven. Sprinkle with chocolate chips, and let stand for 5 minutes. Then, spread melted chocolate over crackers with metal spatula. Sprinkle chopped nuts over top. While still warm, cut between crackers, making 35 squares. Chill in refrigerator until set.

Note: *These taste like Heath bars; no one will believe you start with saltines, until they turn the bar upside down!*

Mississippi Mud Bars

Yield: 40 bars or brownies

- 1 cup butter or regular margarine
- 2 cups sugar
- ¼ cup baking cocoa
- 4 eggs
- 1 teaspoon vanilla extract
- 1½ cups flour, sifted
- 1 3½-ounce can flaked coconut
- 1½ cups pecans, chopped
- 1 7½-ounce jar marshmallow cream

Frosting:
- ½ cup butter
- ½ cup baking cocoa
- 4 cups confectioner's sugar
- ½ cup evaporated milk
- 1 teaspoon vanilla extract

Preheat oven to 350 degrees. In bowl, using electric mixer, cream together butter, sugar and cocoa until light and fluffy. Add eggs and vanilla. Beat twice more at medium speed. Blend in flour. Stir in coconut and pecans. Spread mixture into greased 15½x10½x1-inch jelly roll pan. Bake for 30 minutes, or until done. Remove from oven. Spoon marshmallow cream over all. Let stand 5 minutes. Spread carefully with spatula. To make frosting, combine butter and baking cocoa in saucepan. Place over low heat until butter melts. Cool slightly. Combine confectioner's sugar, evaporated milk and vanilla in bowl. Add cooled cocoa mixture. Beat with electric mixer until smooth. Frost brownies while still warm. Cool completely. Cut into 4x1-inch bars.

One~Bowl Brownies

Serves 8 to 10

- 2 sticks butter or margarine
- 4 squares unsweetened chocolate
- 2 cups sugar (may use 1 cup white and 1 cup brown)
- 1 cup flour
- 4 eggs, lightly-beaten
- 1 teaspoon vanilla extract
- ¼ teaspoon salt
- 1 3.4-ounce package chopped walnuts or pecans (optional)

Preheat oven to 350 degrees. Melt butter and chocolate together in bowl. Remove from heat. Add sugar, flour, salt, eggs and vanilla extract. Mix well, but do not beat. Add nuts. Bake in greased 9x13-inch pan for 18 to 20 minutes. Do not over-bake.

Nutty Chocolate Chip Brownies

Serves 16

- ⅓ cup butter
- 2 squares chocolate
- 1 cup sugar
- 2 eggs
- ⅔ cup sifted flour
- ½ teaspoon baking powder
- ¼ teaspoon salt
- ½ cup nuts, chopped

Topping:
- 6 ounces chocolate chips
- ½ cup nuts, chopped

Preheat oven to 350 degrees. Melt butter and chocolate squares together and stir. Remove from heat. Add sugar and eggs, one at a time and beat until well blended. In a separate bowl, sift together flour, baking powder and salt. Add dry ingredients and nuts to chocolate mixture. Pour into greased 8-inch square pan. Bake for 30 minutes. Remove from oven and sprinkle with chocolate chips. Spread when melted and sprinkle with nuts. Cool completely. Chill.

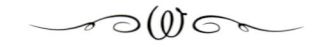

Brownie Drops

Yield: 36 cookies

- 2 4-ounce packages German's Sweet Chocolate
- 1 tablespoon butter
- 2 eggs
- ¾ cup sugar
- ¼ cup all-purpose flour, sifted
- ¼ teaspoon baking powder
- ¼ teaspoon cinnamon
- ⅛ teaspoon salt
- ½ teaspoon vanilla extract
- ¾ cup pecans, finely chopped

Preheat oven to 350 degrees. Melt chocolate and butter in double boiler over hot water. Stir. Cool. Beat eggs until foamy; add sugar, 2 tablespoons at a time and beat until thickened (5 minutes with an electric mixer). Blend in chocolate. Add flour, baking powder, cinnamon and salt; blend. Stir in vanilla extract and nuts. Drop by teaspoon onto greased baking sheet. Bake until cookies feel "set" when very lightly touched, about 8 to 10 minutes.

Grandma's Seven~Layer Cookies

Yield: 3 dozen

- ¼ pound butter or margarine
- 1⅔ cups graham cracker crumbs
- 1 3½-ounce can shredded coconut
- 1 6-ounce package butterscotch chips
- 1 6-ounce package chocolate chips
- 1 14-ounce can sweetened, condensed milk
- 1 cup walnuts, chopped

Preheat oven to 350 degrees. Melt butter in 9x13-inch pan. Do not mix. Add ingredients in order given. Bake for 30 minutes. Cool before cutting. Cookies are rich; cut in small squares.

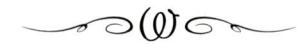

Zucchini Cookies

Yield: 3 dozen

- 1 cup white sugar
- ½ cup margarine
- 1 egg, beaten
- 2 cups flour
- 1 teaspoon baking soda
- ½ teaspoon salt
- ½ teaspoon cloves
- 1 cup zucchini, unpeeled and grated
- 1 cup nuts, chopped
- 1 cup raisins
- ½ apple, peeled and chopped

Frosting:
- ½ cup powdered sugar
- 1 pat of butter
- 1 teaspoon vanilla extract

warm water to thin

Preheat oven to 375 degrees. Mix sugar, margarine and egg well. Sift flour with baking soda, salt and cloves. Add flour mixture alternately with grated zucchini. Fold in nuts, raisins and apple. Drop by teaspoon on greased cookie sheet. Bake for 12 to 15 minutes. Combine frosting ingredients. Mix and brush on baked cookies.

Cape Breton Oat Cakes or Cookies

Serves lots!

A traditional recipe for Scottish oat cakes.

- 1 teaspoon baking soda
- ¾ cup warm water
- 2 cups rolled quick oats (do not use instant oats)
- 2 cups bran flakes or 100% Bran cereal
- 2 cups flour
- 1 teaspoon salt
- 1 cup white sugar (may mix in brown sugar)
- 1 cup vegetable shortening (may mix in a little butter)

Preheat oven to 375 degrees. Dissolve baking soda into water. Mix rolled oats, bran flakes, flour, salt and sugar; then work in shortening and water (with baking soda). Since result will be sticky, dust fingers with flour. Do not overwork or dough will get too stiff. Roll in ball and divide into 4 parts. Refrigerate 4 balls at least 2 hours; remove 1 at a time to roll. Flour pastry cloth and roll out fairly thin for cookies or pat down and cut with saucer in wedges for thicker cake (the Scottish way). For a sweeter cookie, sprinkle with a little sugar in pan before baking. Bake for 8 to 12 minutes, depending on thickness.

Note: The Nova Scotian inventor of these cookies lived to be 105!

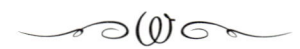

Oatmeal~Chocolate Chip Cookies

Yield: 3 dozen

- 1 cup butter or margarine
- 1 cup brown sugar
- 1 cup white sugar
- 1½ teaspoons vanilla extract
- 2 eggs
- 1 tablespoon water
- 2 cups flour, sifted
- 2 teaspoons baking powder
- 1 teaspoon salt
- ¾ teaspoon baking soda
- 1½ cups quick oats
- 1½ cups chocolate chips

Preheat oven to 375 degrees. Cream together butter, brown sugar and white sugar. Add vanilla extract, eggs and water. Blend in flour, baking powder, salt and baking soda. Add quick oats and chocolate chips and mix well. Drop by tablespoon on greased baking sheet. Bake for 10 minutes.

Sheridan Sugar Cookies

Yield: 2½ dozen

- 2¼ cups flour
- ½ teaspoon cream of tartar
- ½ teaspoon salt
- ½ teaspoon baking soda
- ½ cup butter
- ½ cup vegetable oil
- ½ cup sugar
- ½ cup powdered sugar
- ½ teaspoon vanilla extract
- 1 egg

Preheat oven to 350 degrees. Sift together flour, cream of tartar, salt and baking soda. Cream together butter, oil and both sugars; add vanilla extract and egg. Add flour mixture. Mix well. To shape cookies, form into round balls and roll in sugar. Place on greased cookie sheet and press with small glass or fork, also dipped in sugar. Bake for 15 minutes, or until light brown.

Florida Orange Gumdrop Cookies

Yield: 3 dozen

- 2 cups flour, sifted
- 2½ cups brown sugar
- 1 teaspoon salt
- 1 tablespoon orange rind, grated
- 1 cup large orange gumdrops, finely chopped
- 1 cup pecans, chopped
- 4 eggs well beaten

Preheat oven to 350 degrees. Mix first 6 ingredients and add well beaten eggs. This makes a solid cookie dough. Spread in well-greased 15x10x1-inch pan. Bake for 15 to 20 minutes. While still warm, cut into squares and roll in powdered sugar. Store at least one day before serving.

Chocolate Chip Pizza Cookie

Serves 14 to 16

1 cup flour, unsifted
½ teaspoon baking powder
½ teaspoon salt
⅛ teaspoon baking soda
½ cup pecans or walnuts, chopped
⅓ cup butter or margarine
1 cup brown sugar, firmly packed
1 egg, slightly beaten
1 teaspoon vanilla extract
1 cup chocolate chips

Glaze:
1 cup powdered sugar, sifted
1 tablespoon hot milk or water

Preheat oven to 350 degrees. Mix flour with baking powder, salt and baking soda; add nuts and set aside. Melt butter in saucepan; remove from heat. Add brown sugar; mix well. Cool slightly; blend in egg and vanilla. Add flour mixture, a small amount at a time, mixing well after each addition. Spread dough in a greased 12-inch pizza pan with ½-inch rim. Sprinkle with chocolate chips and bake for 20 to 25 minutes. Do not over-bake. To prepare glaze, gradually blend 1 tablespoon hot milk or water with powdered sugar. Remove pizza from oven and drizzle with glaze. Cool; then cut into wedges.

Heath Bar Lady Fingers

Serves 8 to 12

2 3-ounce packages lady fingers
2 half-pint cartons whipping cream
10 Heath toffee bars, chopped

Whip cream until stiff. In blender or food processor chop Heath bars and mix into cream. Line 8x8-inch pan with split lady fingers and cover with whipped cream mixture. Add second layer of lady fingers and cover with remaining mixture. Cover and store in refrigerator overnight. Do not freeze.

Louise Gentile's Cream Puffs

Serves 20

1 cup water
½ cup butter
1 cup unbleached, all-purpose flour
¼ teaspoon salt
4 extra-large eggs, beaten

Filling:
1 cup whipping cream
1 to 3 tablespoons confectioner's sugar, sifted
½ teaspoon vanilla extract

20 ripe strawberries

Preheat oven to 400 degrees. Grease and flour 2 baking sheets. Put water and butter into a heavy sauce pan. Bring to a boil. When butter melts and foams, remove from heat and add flour all at once. Stir vigorously to combine. Return pan to very low heat and stir until mixture forms a ball, pulling away from sides of pan, about 1 to 2 minutes. Transfer dough to an electric mixer. Gradually beat in eggs on medium speed until blended. Use buttered teaspoon to shape mounds. Place mounds 2 inches apart on baking sheet; be careful not to squash mounds. Bake 30 minutes or until puffs are golden brown and cooked throughout. Remove from oven; split, removing any soft dough. Cool on wire rack. To make sweetened whipped cream filling, whip 1 cup cream until stiff. Fold in confectioner's sugar and vanilla. Put large spoonful of filling in base of cream puff. Lightly insert a strawberry with pointed end up. Put top on cream puff and serve.

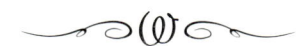

Ann's Green Stuff

Serves 6

1 3-ounce package lady fingers
1 3.4-ounce package pistachio instant pudding
1 8-ounce carton whipped topping
5 Heath toffee bars, crushed

Line a 8x12-inch pan with split lady fingers. Cover with pudding (made according to directions on package). Cover with whipped topping. Sprinkle crushed candy over the top. Refrigerate several hours or overnight.

Aunt Charlotte's Fairy Fluff, 1930

Serves 12

- 2 3¼-ounce packages vanilla pudding (do not use instant)
- 1 20-ounce can crushed pineapple
- ½ pint whipping cream
- 14 regular-size marshmallows
- ½ cup pecans, chopped

Cook pudding according to package directions. Drain pineapple. Whip cream to medium texture; refrigerate. Pour hot pudding over marshmallows in large glass bowl (a trifle bowl is a beautiful serving bowl for this dessert). Stir until melted. While cooling, add drained pineapple and nuts. When completely cooled, add whipped cream. Refrigerate until ready to serve.

Gertrude's Melting Moments

Yield: 18 to 24 cookies

- ¼ pound butter, softened
- 3 tablespoons powdered sugar
- ¾ cup flour
- 1 teaspoon vanilla extract

Preheat oven to 375 degrees. Mix ingredients until light. Form into small balls and place on greased cookie sheet. Press each ball with fork dipped in flour. Bake for 5 to 8 minutes, until lightly browned. When cool, dust lightly with powdered sugar.

Swedish Cream with Strawberries

Serves 8

- 1 envelope Knox plain gelatin
- 2 cups whipping cream
- 1 cup sugar
- 1 pint sour cream
- 1 teaspoon vanilla extract
- 2 cups strawberries or other fruit

Sprinkle gelatin on whipping cream and heat until dissolved. Add sugar. Heat until smooth, about 15 to 20 minutes, but do not boil. Whisk in sour cream and vanilla. Put in custard cups or sherbet glasses; chill for 2 to 3 hours until firm. Serve with fresh strawberries or other fruit.

Frozen Apricot Whip

Serves 8 to 10

Crust:
16 graham crackers
3 tablespoons butter, softened

1 20-ounce can crushed pineapple, drained
2 12-ounce cans Solo apricot filling
1 14-ounce can Eagle Brand Sweetened Condensed Milk
½ cup pecans, chopped
1 8-ounce container Cool Whip

Crush graham crackers and mix with butter. Press into the bottom of a 9-inch springform pan. Blend pineapple, apricot filling, sweetened condensed milk and nuts. Fold in Cool Whip. Spoon over graham cracker crust and freeze. Remove from freezer 15 minutes before serving.

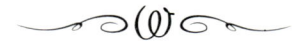

Jeweled Meringues

Serves 25

2 egg whites
⅛ teaspoon salt
½ teaspoon cream of tartar
¾ cup sugar
½ teaspoon vanilla extract
½ cup red hot candies

Preheat oven to 350 degrees. Beat egg whites until foamy. Add salt and cream of tartar. Beat until stiff peaks form, about 7 minutes. Add sugar, 1 tablespoon at a time, beating after each addition. Make sure all sugar is dissolved; if mixture feels grainy when rubbed between fingers, continue beating until smooth. Stir in vanilla extract. Fold in candies. Drop mixture by teaspoon and place 1 to 1½ inches apart on lightly-greased baking sheet. Place in oven and turn off heat. Leave in oven overnight. Do not open oven for at least 2 hours. Meringues do not brown. Remove from baking sheet. Serve.

Frozen Chocolate Frangos

Yield: 18 frangos

- 1 cup butter (not margarine)
- 2 cups powdered sugar
- 4 eggs
- 4 squares chocolate, melted and cooled
- 2 teaspoons vanilla extract
- 1 teaspoon peppermint extract
- 1 16-ounce box vanilla wafers

sliced almonds or small chocolate chips

Cream butter, add sugar and blend well by hand (do not use blender or food processor). Beat in eggs one at a time. Add melted chocolate and flavorings. Put vanilla wafers between 2 sheets of wax paper. Use small rolling pin to roll vanilla wafers into crumbs. Sprinkle ¼-inch layer of crumbs in foil baking (cupcake) cups and place in metal muffin pan. Add chocolate mixture. Sprinkle tops with wafer crumbs and almonds or small chocolate chips. Freeze. Serve frozen.

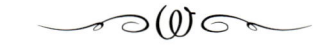

Adeline's Brickle Yummies

Yield: 40 cookies

- ½ pound butter
- 1¼ cups light brown sugar
- 1 egg
- 1 teaspoon vanilla extract
- 2¼ cups all-purpose flour
- ¼ teaspoon salt
- 1 7½-ounce package Heath toffee bar "brickle" chips
- 1 cup pecans, coarsely chopped

Glaze:
- 1 12-ounce package chocolate chips
- 2 tablespoons Crisco

In large mixing bowl, cream butter and sugar. Add egg, then vanilla extract, creaming thoroughly. Combine flour and salt and add to creamed mixture. Stir in "Brickle Chips" and pecans. For easier handling, cover bowl with plastic wrap and refrigerate dough at least 3 hours or overnight. Preheat oven to 375 degrees. Shape rounded spoonfuls of dough into balls, flatten with hand, and place on greased cookie sheets. Bake for 10 to 12 minutes. Cool. Melt chocolate chips and Crisco over low heat. Glaze Yummies.

English Sherry Trifle

Serves 4

1 sponge cake, divided into 4 squares
4 ounces sweet sherry
2 3-ounce packages strawberry Jello
1 16-ounce can peach halves, drained

Custard:
3 eggs, slightly beaten
2 cups milk
¼ cup sugar
1 dash salt
1 teaspoon vanilla

1 cup whipping cream, whipped until stiff
chocolate curls

Put sponge cake squares in bottom of a deep glass serving bowl. Pour sherry over cake and let sit until sherry is absorbed. Cover with half the peaches. Dissolve Jello in boiling water according to package directions. Cool until slightly thickened, then pour over peaches. Add remaining peaches. Chill for 15 minutes or until set. To make custard, combine eggs, milk, sugar and salt in heavy saucepan. Cook and stir over medium heat. Continue cooking until mixture is thick enough to coat a spoon. Let custard mixture cool. Stir in vanilla. Cover top of custard with plastic wax. Cool completely. Cover cake squares with custard; garnish with whipped cream and chocolate curls.

Quick Chocolate~Pecan Fudge

Yield: 60 pieces

½ cup butter or margarine
¾ cup unsweetened cocoa powder
4 cups confectioner's sugar
1 teaspoon vanilla extract
½ cup evaporated milk
1 cup pecan pieces

Microwave butter or margarine in 2-quart microwave-proof bowl on high for 1 to 1½ minutes or until melted. Add cocoa powder slowly, stirring until smooth. Stir in confectioner's sugar and vanilla extract, blending well. Mixture will be dry and crumbly. Stir in evaporated milk. Microwave on high for 30 to 60 seconds until mixture is hot. Stir until smooth, then add pecan pieces. Pour into foil-lined, 8-inch square pan. Cover. Chill until firm. Cut into squares.

Hazelwood Nut Cups

Yield: 24 cookies

An original Hazelwood recipe!

Dough:
- ½ cup butter, softened
- 1 cup cake flour (or unbleached white)
- 1 3-ounce package of cream cheese

Filling:
- ¾ cup walnuts or pecans, ground
- ¾ cup brown sugar, packed
- 1 tablespoon margarine or butter, melted
- 1 egg
- 1 teaspoon vanilla extract

Preheat oven to 325 degrees. Combine softened cream cheese and butter; add flour. For easier handling, chill dough for 30 minutes to 1 hour. Divide dough into 24 balls. Shape into small circles and press into muffin pans. Combine filling ingredients. Put nut mixture into dough cups. Bake for ½-hour until golden brown.

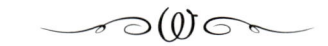

Snow Cap Cheese Cups

Yield: 24 cookies

Shell:
- 2 cups flour
- 1 cup margarine
- ½ cup confectioner's sugar

Filling:
- 1 8-ounce package cream cheese
- ½ cup sugar
- 1 8-ounce container Cool Whip
- 1 21-ounce can cherry or blueberry pie filling

Mix shell ingredients together; dough will be crumbly. Chill for 1 hour. Preheat oven to 350 degrees. Form dough into small, walnut-size balls. Place balls in small muffin pans, pressing them into bottom of cups and along sides. Bake until edges are delicately brown, about 20 to 25 minutes; cool.

To make filling, combine cream cheese and sugar; fold into Cool Whip. Fill baked cups with filling using a pastry bag or cookie press. Top cups with fruit filling, or sprinkle with sugar crystals. Chill, uncovered.

Great Grandmother's Cocoa Drops

Yield: 24 to 30 cookies
- 2 sticks lightly salted butter (*not* margarine)
- 2 cups sugar
- 2 eggs
- 2 teaspoons vanilla extract
- 1 cup evaporated milk (*not* sweetened condensed)
- 3½ cups sifted flour
- 1 cup Hershey's baking cocoa

Frosting:
- 1 stick butter, softened
- 1 1-pound package confectioner's sugar
- 1 teaspoon vanilla extract
- 5 to 6 tablespoons milk (may use leftover evaporated milk)

Preheat oven to 350 degrees. Cream together butter and sugar. Add eggs, vanilla extract and evaporated milk. Beat until smooth. Sift together flour and cocoa. Mix all ingredients together. Drop by teaspoon onto lightly greased cookie sheet. Bake 8 to 9 minutes. Do not over-bake. Cookies should be firm to touch, but not dry. Cool. To make frosting, cream butter. Add confectioner's sugar and beat until smooth; blend in vanilla. Add milk, 1 tablespoon at a time. Frosting should be good spreading consistency. Spread on cooled cookies. Store in single layer.

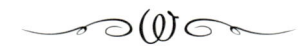

Rum Balls Juanita

Yield: 45 1-inch balls
- 1 16-ounce box vanilla wafers
- 1¼ cups sugar
- 1 cup pecans, finely chopped
- 3 tablespoons cocoa
- ¼ cup rum
- 3 tablespoons corn syrup

Crush wafers, sugar, nuts and cocoa in blender. Remove. Add rum and corn syrup. Roll mixture into 1-inch balls. Roll balls in powdered sugar. Set balls in a tin box for at least 12 hours to ripen.

Lemon Lush

Serves 12 to 16

1st layer:
- 1½ cups flour
- 1½ sticks butter, softened
- 2 ounces walnuts or pecans, chopped

2nd layer:
- 1 12-ounce container Cool Whip
- 1 8-ounce package cream cheese, softened
- 1 cup powdered sugar
- 1 teaspoon vanilla extract

3rd layer:
- 2 3-ounce packages instant lemon pudding
- 3 cups cold milk

Preheat oven to 350 degrees. Mix flour, butter and nuts by hand (save some nuts to sprinkle on top later). Spread mixture with fingers in greased 9x13-inch pan. (If fingers stick to mixture, pat with flour.) Bake for 20 to 30 minutes. Let cool. With an electric mixer, combine two-thirds of a container of Cool Whip with cream cheese, powdered sugar and vanilla extract. Beat well and spread mixture evenly over first layer. Refrigerate for 2 hours. Mix pudding and milk with mixer until completely dissolved. Spread over second layer. Refrigerate for 1 hour. Top with remaining Cool Whip and garnish with chopped walnuts or pecans.

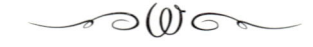

Cherry Delight

Serves 6 to 8

Crust:
- 2 cups vanilla wafers, crushed
- ¼ pound butter, softened
- 1 cup pecans, cut

Filling:
- 1 8-ounce package cream cheese, softened
- 2 tablespoons milk
- 1 cup powdered sugar

Topping:
- 2 boxes Dream Whip, made per package directions
- 1 21-ounce can cherry pie filling

Cherry Delight, *continued on next page.*

Cherry Delight, *continued.*

To make crust, mix together vanilla wafers, butter and pecans; press mixture into greased 8x12-inch glass pan. Refrigerate. Meanwhile, cream together cream cheese, milk and powdered sugar. Spread evenly on top of refrigerated crust. Spread prepared Dream Whip over cream cheese mixture. Top with cherry pie filling. Refrigerate several hours before serving.

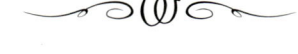

Lemon Delight

Serves 12

Crust:
- ¾ cup margarine or butter, softened
- 1½ cups flour, sifted
- ½ cup nuts

Cream cheese filling:
- 1 cup powdered sugar
- 1 8-ounce package cream cheese, softened
- 1 8-ounce container whipped topping

Lemon filling:
- 3 3-ounce packages instant lemon pudding
- 3 cups cold milk

Topping:
- 1 8-ounce container whipped topping
- ¼ cup nuts, chopped

Preheat oven to 375 degrees. Mix flour, margarine and nuts. (May use 3 sticks melted margarine for a more buttery crust.) Press into greased 9x13-inch baking pan. Bake for 20 minutes or until lightly browned. Cool. Mix together powdered sugar, softened cream cheese and 8 ounces of whipped topping. Spread over cooled crust. Mix 3 packages of instant lemon pudding with 3 cups of milk until thickened. (May use an additional cup of milk in lemon filling.) Spread over cream cheese filling. Cover with whipped topping. Sprinkle with ¼-cup nuts. Chill 4 hours or overnight.

Note: May use other flavors of instant pudding for filling.

Gold Medal Lemon Squares

Serves 10

Crust:
- 1 cup flour
- ½ cup butter, softened
- ¼ cup powdered sugar

- 2 eggs
- 1 cup granulated sugar
- ½ teaspoon baking powder
- ¼ teaspoon salt
- 2 teaspoons grated lemon peel
- 2 tablespoons lemon juice

powdered sugar to sprinkle

Preheat oven to 350 degrees. Combine flour, butter and powdered sugar; mix well. Press evenly into a 8x8x2-inch pan (do not grease), building up half-inch edges. Bake crust for 20 minutes. Beat remaining ingredients, except powdered sugar, until light and fluffy. Pour mixture over hot crust. Bake until no indentation remains when touched in center, about 25 minutes. Sprinkle with powdered sugar. Cool; cut into 1½-inch squares.

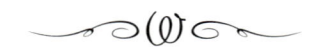

Lemon Squares Lorraine

Yield: 36 bars

Crust:
- 2 cups flour
- ½ cup powdered sugar
- 1 cup butter

- 4 eggs
- 2 cups sugar
- ⅓ cup lemon juice
- ¼ cup flour
- ½ teaspoon baking powder
- ½ cup powdered sugar

Preheat oven to 350 degrees. Mix 2 cups flour with powdered sugar. Cut in butter. Work until crumbly. Place in a buttered 9x13-inch pan and press down with back of a spoon. Bake for 15 to 20 minutes. Beat together eggs, sugar and lemon juice. Set aside. Sift together flour and baking powder. Add to egg mixture. Pour over crust and bake 20 to 25 minutes. While still hot, sprinkle with powdered sugar. Cool before cutting into squares.

Pecan Tiny Tarts

Yield: 24

Crust:
1 3-ounce package cream cheese
½ cup butter
1 cup flour

1 egg
¼ cup brown sugar, packed
1 teaspoon vanilla extract
1 tablespoon butter, softened
1 cup nuts, chopped

Preheat oven to 350 degrees. First, prepare crust. Combine cream cheese, butter and flour; gather mixture into a ball. Cover with wax paper. Chill 4 hours. In a small bowl, combine egg, brown sugar, vanilla extract, butter and nuts. Mix until well blended. Shape pastry into small muffin pans. Fill each with a teaspoon of filling. Bake for 12 to 15 minutes or until brown. Cool. Remove from pan.

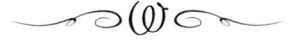

Cherry Tarts

Yield: 24

2 8-ounce packages cream cheese, softened
¼ cup granulated sugar
2 eggs
1 teaspoon vanilla extract
24 vanilla wafers
1 21-ounce can cherry pie filling

Preheat oven to 350 degrees. Beat cheese and sugar until creamy. Add eggs and vanilla extract, and beat until smooth. Line muffin tins with foil and paper cupcake liners. Place a vanilla wafer in each cup, spoon on cheese mixture. Bake 18 to 20 minutes, remove from tins and let cool. Top with cherry pie filling. Chill overnight before serving. Leave in papers to serve.

Fresh Peach or Blueberry Cobbler

Serves 6 to 8

¼ cup plus 2 tablespoons butter or margarine
2 cups peaches, sliced or blueberries
1 cup sugar
¼ teaspoon cinnamon (only if using peaches)
¾ cup all-purpose flour
2 teaspoons baking powder
1 dash salt
¾ cup milk

Preheat oven to 350 degrees. Melt butter in 2-quart baking dish. Layer peaches or blueberries in baking dish. Combine sugar, cinnamon, flour, baking powder, salt and milk. Mix. Drop batter by spoonfuls over melted butter and peaches or blueberries. Do not stir. Bake for 1 hour.

Apple or Peach Streusel Cobbler

Yield: 20 pieces

Dough:
2 cups flour
3 teaspoons baking powder
¼ teaspoon salt
½ cup sugar
3 tablespoons shortening
1 egg, beaten
½ teaspoon vanilla extract
milk

Fruit:
6 to 8 large apples or peaches ~ pitted, cored and thinly sliced
1 cup sugar
2 teaspoons cornstarch
2 tablespoons butter

Streusel:
1½ cups sugar
½ teaspoon cinnamon
1 cup flour
4½ tablespoons butter, melted

whipped cream or ice cream, as topping (optional)

Apple or Peach Cobbler, *continued on next page.*

Apple or Peach Cobbler, *continued.*

Preheat oven to 350 degrees. To make dough, sift dry ingredients and cut in shortening. Put egg in measuring cup. Fill with milk, add to dry ingredients with vanilla extract. Mix well. Put into a 9x12-inch greased pan, after patting sides with butter. Prepare apples or peaches. Combine fruit with sugar and cornstarch. Dot with bits of butter. Arrange apple or peach slices in rows over dough. Mix streusel ingredients, being careful to keep light and crumbly; sprinkle over fruit. Bake for 45 minutes. Top with ice cream or whipped topping.

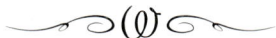

Apple Crunch

Serves 4 to 6

- 2 cups apples, peeled and sliced
- ½ cup granulated sugar
- a few squeezes lemon juice
- ⅓ cup old-fashioned oats
- ¼ teaspoon cinnamon
- ¼ teaspoon nutmeg
- 1 pinch salt
- 4 tablespoons butter or margarine
- whipped cream or ice cream (optional)

Preheat oven to 375 degrees. Place apple slices in an 8x8-inch baking dish or pie plate. Sprinkle with sugar and lemon juice. Mix dry ingredients for topping and cut in butter with two knives until mixture is crumbly. Distribute topping over apples. Bake, uncovered, until bubbly; about 40 minutes. May be served with whipped cream or ice cream.

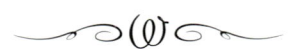

Apple Dump

Serves 10 to 12

- 16 medium-size apples; peeled, cored and quartered
- ¾ cup brown sugar
- 1 dash cinnamon
- ¼ cup pecans, chopped
- 1 18¼-ounce package yellow cake mix
- 1 stick butter
- 1 stick margarine

Preheat oven to 325 degrees. Slice and arrange in rows in greased 9x13-inch baking pan. Sprinkle brown sugar and cinnamon over the apples. Add pecans. Layer dry cake mix over the pecans. Cut up margarine and butter and place on top of cake mix. Bake for 1 hour, or until done.

Glazed Stewed Apple Wedges

Serves 4 to 6

Adapted for your kitchen... from the original Walgreens recipe!

Robin Hood & Briargate Restaurants, 1970's ~ 1980's

- 3 large cooking apples, cored and cut into ½-inch thick wedges
- 3 tablespoons butter or margarine
- 3 tablespoons brown sugar
- 2 teaspoons lemon juice
- ¾ teaspoon cinnamon
- 1 pinch salt

whipped cream, whipped or heavy cream (optional)

In a skillet over medium heat, melt the butter. Add the apples, brown sugar, lemon juice, cinnamon and salt. Cook apples until tender, about 5 to 10 minutes. Divide apples into dessert dishes. Spoon the syrup from the pan over the apples. Garnish with whipped or heavy cream. Serve hot.

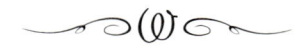

Baked Pears in Cream

Serves 4

- 4 tablespoons butter
- 4 tablespoons sugar
- 2 Bosc pears, cored, but not peeled
- ½ cup heavy cream

Preheat oven to 400 degrees. Butter bottom and sides of a baking dish with 2 tablespoons butter. Sprinkle dish with 1 tablespoon sugar. Cut pears in half. Place pears in dish, cut-side down, and sprinkle with remaining sugar. Dot pears with remaining butter, and bake for 10 minutes. Remove from oven and pour heavy cream over pears. Return to oven and bake another 20 minutes, or until brown.

New England Baked Apples

Serves 6

- 6 large cooking apples, cored, upper half pared (to prevent splitting)
- 6 teaspoons butter or margarine (or more, to taste)
- 6 tablespoons brown sugar, packed or 1-cup maple syrup
- ¾ teaspoon cinnamon (only if using brown sugar)

Preheat oven to 350 degrees. Arrange apples, peeled end up, in a 9x13-inch baking dish. Place 1-teaspoon butter in center of each apple. Then, place 1-teaspoon brown sugar and ⅛-teaspoon cinnamon in center of each apple. Or (instead of brown sugar and cinnamon), pour maple syrup in and around apples. Bake for 1 hour or until tender. Serve hot.

Hot Fruit Compote

Serves 24

- 1 stick margarine
- ½ cup sugar
- 2 tablespoons flour
- 1 cup sherry or a combination of sherry and drained juices from fruits
- 1 20-ounce can sliced or chunk pineapple, drained
- 1 16-ounce can pears, drained
- 1 16-ounce can peaches, drained
- 1 16-ounce can apricots, drained
- 1 16-ounce jar spiced apple rings, drained
- 1 can mandarin oranges, drained

Preheat oven to 350 degrees. Melt margarine; add sugar, flour and sherry. Stir constantly over low heat until thick, about 5 minutes. Arrange drained fruit in 9x13-inch casserole dish. Pour sauce over fruit. Bake 30 minutes.

Taffy Apple Treat

Serves 6 to 8

- 2 8-ounce cans pineapple tidbits
- 4 cups mini marshmallows
- 1 tablespoon flour
- ½ cup brown or white sugar
- 1 egg, well beaten
- 1½ tablespoons white vinegar
- 1 12-ounce container Cool Whip
- 3 large apples, diced (do not peel)
- 1 cup Spanish peanuts, chopped

Drain pineapple; save juice. In a deep glass bowl, mix pineapple with marshmallows. Set aside. In small sauce pan combine juice, flour, brown or white sugar, egg and vinegar. Cook until slightly thickened. Cool. When mixture has cooled, combine with Cool Whip. Fold in marshmallow mixture. Add apples and peanuts (save some peanuts for garnish); mix well. Top with extra peanuts.

Pfeffer's Luchen Kugel ~ Sweet Noodle Pudding

Serves 8 to 10

A sweet and easy traditional Jewish dairy meal ~ perfect for brunches or breakfasts!

- 8 ounces egg noodles, cooked and drained, but not rinsed
- ¼ pound margarine, melted
- 1 small jar pineapple jam
- 1 16-ounce carton cottage cheese
- ½ pint sour cream
- 4 eggs, separated
- ½ to ¾-cup (or to taste) plump white raisins
- 3 teaspoons sugar
- cinnamon, to taste

Preheat oven to 350 degrees. Mix egg noodles, margarine, pineapple jam, cottage cheese and sour cream in large bowl. Stir in 4 egg yolks (set aside egg whites), and add raisins. Whip egg whites until frothy and fold into mixture. Pour mixture into greased (do not use Crisco or any vegetable shortening) 9x13-inch glass pan. Combine sugar and cinnamon for topping, and sprinkle on top. Bake for about an hour, or until toothpick comes out clean.

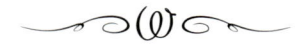

New Orleans Bread Pudding

Serves 16 to 20

- 1 10-ounce loaf stale French bread, crumbled or 6 to 8 cups any bread, crumbled
- 4 cups milk
- 2 cups sugar
- 8 tablespoons butter, melted
- 3 eggs
- 2 tablespoons vanilla extract
- 1 cup raisins
- 1 cup coconut
- 1 cup pecans, chopped
- 1 teaspoon cinnamon
- 1 teaspoon nutmeg

Whiskey sauce:
- ½ cup butter
- 1½ cups powdered sugar
- 2 egg yolks
- ½ cup bourbon, to taste

New Orleans Bread Pudding, *continued on next page.*

New Orleans Bread Pudding, continued.

Combine all pudding ingredients; mixture should be moist, not soupy. Place in buttered 9x13-inch baking dish. Place in a non-preheated oven. Bake at 350 degrees for 1 hour and 15 minutes. To make sauce, cream butter and sugar over medium heat. Remove from heat, blend in egg yolks. Add bourbon gradually to taste, stirring constantly. Sauce will thicken as it cools. Serve sauce warm over warm pudding.

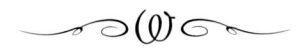

Ris A' Lamande ~ Danish Rice Pudding

Serves 6 to 8

- 2 cups milk
- ⅓ cup long grain rice
- ¼ teaspoon salt
- 2 tablespoons sugar
- 1 teaspoon almond extract
- 1 tablespoon cold water
- 1½ teaspoons unflavored gelatin
- 1 cup whipping cream

Topping:
- 1 cup cherry or raspberry syrup
- 1 teaspoon cornstarch
- 1 tablespoon cold water

In greased medium saucepan, add milk to rice. May preheat milk in microwave for 3 minutes. Simmer for 15 to 20 minutes, stirring occasionally until rice is done. Add salt, sugar and almond extract. Add 1 tablespoon cold water to gelatin in small saucepan. Let stand 1 minute. Stir over low heat until gelatin is completely dissolved, about 1 minute. Cool. Stir constantly while adding to rice mixture. Set aside to cool completely. Whip the cream and slowly add to rice mixture. Refrigerate rice mixture and check after 30 minutes. Stir mixture if rice has settled. Pour syrup into saucepan. If syrup is too concentrated, add an additional ¼-cup of water. Add cornstarch. Stir to dissolve. Heat to boiling, stirring constantly. Refrigerate separately, until ready to serve. Before serving, stir syrup gently into rice mixture, until uniform in consistency.

Strawberry-Banana Gelatin for a Crowd

Serves 28

- 4 3-ounce packages strawberry-banana gelatin
- 3½ cups hot water
- 2 15-ounce container frozen strawberries, thawed
- 4 8-ounce cans unsweetened, crushed pineapple
- 1 8-ounce container sour cream
- 4 ripe bananas, peeled and sliced
- 1 cup whipping cream, whipped

Dissolve strawberry-banana gelatin in hot water. Stir in strawberries and pineapple. Spray an angel food cake pan with non-stick cooking spray. Pour half the gelatin mixture into the pan. Refrigerate until set, about 3 hours. Let remaining gelatin stand at room temperature. Gently spread sour cream in a thin layer over refrigerated gelatin. Add banana slices to room-temperature gelatin; fold in the 1 cup whipped cream to the banana-gelatin mixture. Carefully spoon banana mixture over sour cream. Refrigerate until firm, about 3 hours. Turn gelatin mold upside down on top of platter; banana layer will be on bottom. Chill until serving time. Unmold onto serving plate.

Strawberry Cream Mold

Serves 8 to 10

- 1 3-ounce package strawberry gelatin
- 1 cup hot water
- 1 16-ounce package frozen, sliced strawberries
- 1 3-ounce package lemon gelatin
- 1 cup hot water
- 1 3-ounce package cream cheese, softened
- 1 cup whipping cream, whipped

In a bowl, stir strawberry gelatin into 1 cup of hot water until dissolved. Stir in strawberries, and set aside. In a larger bowl, combine lemon gelatin with 1 cup of hot water. Stir in cream cheese. Refrigerate until partially set, about 45 minutes. Fold whipped cream into lemon gelatin mixture. Refrigerate, again, until partially set, about 1 to 2 hours. Pour strawberry mixture over lemon mixture. Chill several hours until set.

Orange Sherbet Gelatin Mold

Serves 10 to 12

- 3   3-ounce packages orange gelatin
- 3   cups hot orange juice (made from frozen concentrate)
- 1   pint orange sherbet
- 1   cup ginger ale
- 1   16-ounce can mandarin oranges, drained

In a bowl, dissolve gelatin in hot orange juice. Add sherbet and stir until melted. Slowly add ginger ale (it will foam up) and oranges. Pour mixture into a lightly-greased, 8-to-10 cup mold. Chill for several hours, until firm. To unmold, carefully run a knife around the inside edge of the mold; turn mold upside down over serving platter. Put a warm cloth over mold. Shake gently. Mold will fall onto serving platter. Carefully lift mold when all sides are down and mold is fully on serving plate.

Caramel Corn

Serves 10 to 12

- 1   cup popcorn kernels
- 1   cup brown sugar
- 1   stick margarine
- ¼   cup Karo light corn syrup
- ½   teaspoon baking soda

Pop popcorn kernels in microwave or electric popcorn maker. Discard any kernels that do not pop. Combine brown sugar, margarine and Karo syrup in microwave safe bowl. Microwave 2 minutes on high. Mix well. Microwave 1 minute longer Add baking soda. Stir well. Microwave 2 minutes more. In very large covered microwave safe bowl, drizzle mixture over popcorn. Mix well. Microwave covered for 90 seconds. Place on wax paper to cool.

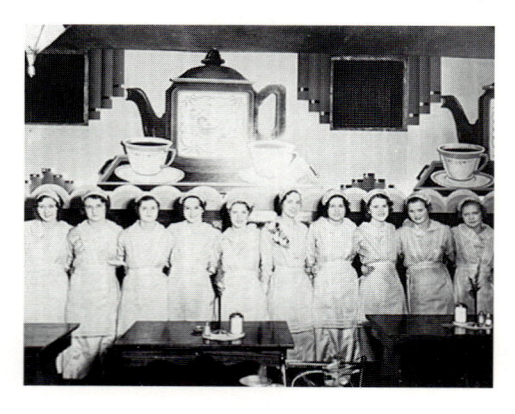

Located in downtown Chicago in the 1940's, Walgreens beautiful in-store "Tea Rooms" rejuvenated the business-weary with first-rate food and service.

Facing Page: (on tray, clockwise from top)
*Refrigerator Pickles, Fancy Beet Relish,
Sweet & Sour Pickles, Nutty Cranberry Relish,
(center) Green Tomato Chow-Chow;
(in jar) Apple, Date & Walnut Chutney*
Photo: Scott Lanza, 1995
Stylist: F. Lynn Nelson

RXCETERA

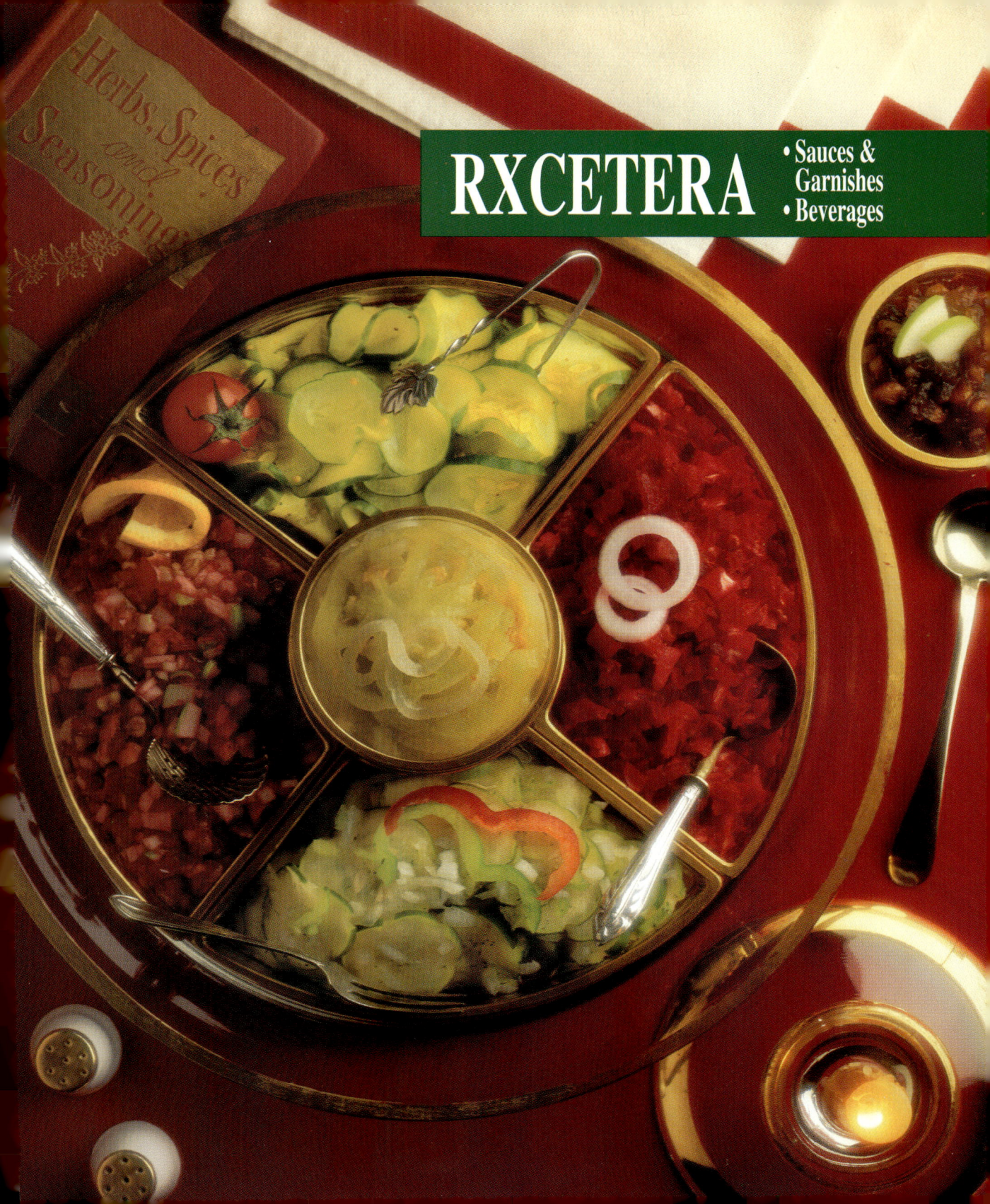

- Sauces & Garnishes
- Beverages

The "Tea Rooms"
Refreshing Respites for the Business-Weary

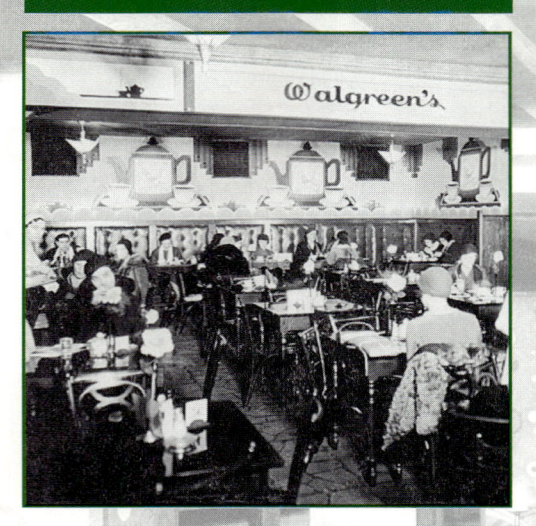

"The modern color and design employed throughout, is a refreshing respite from the noise and bustle of the busy streets above, making it possible to enjoy fine food in relaxing comfort."

From Walgreens employee magazine, Walgreen Pepper Pod, *December 1951.*

Walgreens "tea rooms" (a nickname for the downtown cafeterias) evolved from the soda fountains in the mid 1940's, as a likely response to busy downtown business crowds who wanted a little more than the standard lunch-counter fare. One of the most popular of the tea rooms was located in the basement of Walgreens newly-built State Street Super Store (erected on the site of the old drugstore) at Randolph & State Streets in Chicago, 1940. As part of the famous *Oak Room* restaurant, the tea room featured lavishly-modern decor and the latest technology, which included air conditioning and a remote-controlled phonograph-speaker system that played requests! And...on the main floor above, via escalator, was one of the world's largest soda fountains!

It is interesting to note that, although built as a temporary structure over the site of an old skyscraper, Walgreens present building at Randolph and State is now an historic Chicago landmark thanks to the other famous tenant on the block, the Chicago Theater.

McCulloch's Strawberry~Rhubarb Sauce

Yield: 1½ cups

- 3 cups fresh rhubarb (small, tender stalks), chopped
- ½ cup fresh strawberries, halved or quartered (if large)
- 1 tablespoon water
- ¾ cup sugar (or more, to taste)

Oatmeal crumb topping: (optional)
- ¾ cup oatmeal
- ¾ cup brown sugar
- ½ cup flour
- margarine

To make the sauce, use a double boiler to keep the delicate rhubarb from breaking up. Bring water to a boil in the bottom of the double boiler. In the top of the boiler, carefully blend together the rhubarb, strawberries, water and sugar. Cook until soft, but not mushy, taking care not to break up rhubarb. Taste, adding more sugar if necessary. Serve warm.

McCulloch's Strawberry-Rhubarb Crisp:
To make a dessert crisp, combine the crumb topping ingredients: oatmeal, brown sugar and flour; cutting in margarine (a little at a time) with a knife or pastry blender until mixture is crumbly. Preheat oven to 350 degrees. In 6 individual serving dishes, add enough *Strawberry-Rhubarb* (or *Tangy Rhubarb*) *Sauce* to fill dishes three-quarters full. Top with a generous amount of oatmeal crumb topping to fill dishes. Bake for 15 minutes, or until topping is browned.

McCulloch's Tangy Rhubarb Sauce:
Prepare recipe as directed, substituting the juice and grated rind of 1 orange for the strawberries and water.

Note: May also serve this sauce over fresh, steamed apples (or any firm fruit). It is especially good over vanilla ice cream.

Raspberry or Strawberry Sauce

Yield: 1¼ cups

- 1 pint fresh raspberries or strawberries
- 3 tablespoons sugar
- 1 tablespoon raspberry liqueur
- 1 tablespoon water

Blend all ingredients in food processor until of sauce consistency. Strain sauce to remove seeds.

Pineapple Sauce

Yield: 1 quart

Adapted for your kitchen... from the original Walgreens recipe!

Robin Hood & Briargate Restaurants, 1970's ~ 1980's

2 8-ounce cans crushed pineapple
1 cup sugar
1 quart water
juice of 1 lemon
3 tablespoons cornstarch
¼ cup water, chilled

Drain pineapple and reserve juice. Combine pineapple juice, sugar, water and lemon juice; bring to boil. Dissolve cornstarch in water. Add crushed pineapple to hot syrup. Add liquid cornstarch; bring to boil while stirring.

Raisin Sauce

Yield: 1 quart

Adapted for your kitchen... from the original Walgreens recipe!

Robin Hood & Briargate Restaurants, 1970's ~ 1980's

1 cup light raisins
water to cover and cook raisins
3 tablespoons cornstarch
1½ cups water
¾ cup brown sugar
½ teaspoon salt
⅛ teaspoon nutmeg
3 whole cloves
2 cups pineapple juice
2 tablespoons butter

Wash raisins and cover with water; simmer for 10 minutes until soft. Dissolve cornstarch in 1 cup cold water. Combine all other ingredients except butter and heat to a boil while stirring. Add liquid starch. Cook for 10 minutes, stirring constantly. Add cooked raisins and blend in. Add butter and stir.

Brandy Sauce

Yield: 1 quart

Adapted for your kitchen... from the original Walgreens recipe!

Robin Hood & Briargate Restaurants, 1970's ~ 1980's

- 3 tablespoons cornstarch
- ¼ cup cold water
- 3 cups water
- 1 cup sugar
- 1 cup brown sugar
- ¼ cup lemon juice
- rind, grated, of 1 lemon
- 3 whole cloves
- 1 cinnamon stick
- ½ cup brandy

Dissolve cornstarch in ¼-cup cold water. Combine all other ingredients except brandy, bring to boil and simmer for 15 minutes. Stir and strain. Add liquid cornstarch and bring to boil while stirring. Allow to cool for 20 minutes. Stir in brandy and mix thoroughly.

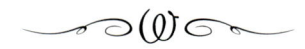

Cinnamon Sauce

Yield: 1 quart

Adapted for your kitchen... from the original Walgreens recipe!

Robin Hood & Briargate Restaurants, 1970's ~ 1980's

- 2 cups water
- 2 cups apple juice
- 1 dash salt
- ¾ cup sugar
- 2 tablespoons cornstarch
- ¼ cup water, chilled
- 1½ teaspoon ground cinnamon

Boil water, apple juice, salt and half the sugar. Dissolve cornstarch in chilled water. Add to boiling syrup while stirring. Mix cinnamon with remaining sugar and add to syrup. Continue to cook and stir until mixture is clear.

"High Dumpsy Dearie" Jam

Yield: 7 pounds

2 pounds cooking apples, peeled, cored and sliced
2 pounds pears; peeled, cored and sliced
2 pounds plums, halved and pitted
juice and rind, grated, of 1 lemon
4½ pounds sugar
1 root of dried ginger, brushed
water

sterilized jars and lids (see *The Sterilizing & Canning Process,* below)

To prepare jam, place all fruit in a large, heavy pan; add just enough water to cover base. Simmer until fruit is tender, 40 to 45 minutes. Remove from heat and add sugar, stirring until dissolved. Add juice, grated rind of lemon and ginger root tied in a muslin bag. Bring mixture to a boil and cook rapidly until setting point of jam is reached, about 15 minutes, or until a candy thermometer reaches 218 to 222 degrees. Skim if necessary. Immediately pour jam into sterilized jars, seal and process in *boiling water bath* (see *The Sterilizing & Canning Process,* below).

The Sterilizing & Canning Process

Sterilizing Jars & Lids

Wash jars and lids in hot, soapy water and rinse well. Stand jars on a rack in a large kettle; add water to cover. Bring water to a full, rolling boil; cover kettle and boil 10 minutes. Jars and closures should stay immersed in hot water until they are needed.

Processing Canned Food in Sterilized Jars

Use a water bath canner, which comes equipped with a wire rack. Fill canner with enough water to cover jars when they are placed on rack. Two processes used to kill microorganisms in canned food are **hot water bath** (180 to 185 degrees), for pickles and preserves; and **boiling water bath** (212 degrees), for fruits and tomatoes. To process, heat or boil water in canner. Lower jars into canner, making sure they do not touch each other or sides of canner. Generally, acid fruits covered by boiling syrup take about 20 to 25 minutes to process. The water in canner must *always* be covering jars; therefore, add water if water level goes down during process.

Vegetables must be canned in a pressure cooker, to prevent botulism.

Home~Canned Pie Filling

Yield: 2½ quarts

- 4 cups sugar
- 1 cup corn starch
- 3 teaspoons cinnamon
- 1 teaspoon nutmeg
- 1 teaspoon salt
- 10 cups water
- 3 tablespoons lemon juice
- 5 to 8 pounds fresh apples or peaches, or 3 to 4 pounds (4 to 5 quarts) cherries or berries

sterilized jars and lids (see **The Sterilizing & Canning Process,** at left)

Cook all ingredients (except lemon juice and fruit) until thickened. Add lemon juice. Fill 7-quart canning jars one-third full with thickened sauce. Prepare fresh fruit (peel, pit, slice, etc.) and smash down into sauce in each jar, until jars are full. (Leave about a ½-inch "head" room, so jars will not explode when fruit boils during sterilizing process.) Put on hot lids and process in *boiling water bath* for 20 minutes (see **The Sterilizing & Canning Process,** at left).

Note: Use for pies or other desserts. Also works well as an ice cream topping.

Strawberry Butter

Yield: 2 cups

- 1 pound unsalted butter, at room temperature
- 1 cup seedless strawberry jam

Using an electric mixer or food processor, mix butter with jam until well-blended. Ready to serve.

Note: Try substituting raspberry jam, or your favorite jam or preserves.

Retz Ranch Chow~Chow

Yield: 7 pints

- 4 cups green tomatoes, coarsely ground
- 4 cups onions, coarsely ground
- 4 cups cabbage leaves, coarsely ground
- 5 cups green peppers, coarsely ground
- 1½ cups sweet red peppers, coarsely ground
- 1 hot pepper, coarsely ground
- ½ cup pickling salt
- 6 cups sugar
- 2 tablespoons mustard seed
- 1 tablespoon celery seed
- 1½ teaspoon turmeric
- 4 cups cider vinegar
- 2 cups water

sterilized jars and lids (see **The Sterilizing & Canning Process,** *this section*)

Mix together green tomatoes, ground onions, cabbage, green peppers, sweet red peppers and hot pepper; sprinkle with pickling salt. Let stand overnight. Rinse, drain and press into saucepan. Add sugar, mustard seed, celery seed, turmeric, cider vinegar and water to mixture. Boil gently for 5 minutes. Pour into sterilized jars, seal and process in boiling water bath for 15 minutes (see **The Sterilizing & Canning Process,** *this section*).

Green Tomato Chow~Chow

Yield: 4 quarts

- 38 medium green tomatoes, sliced
- 3 pounds white onions, peeled and sliced
- ½ cup sea salt
- 3 cups apples, peeled, cored and chopped
- 2 cups white vinegar
- 3½ cups sugar (add more or less, for desired sweetness or tartness)
- ¼ cup pickling spice, tied in cheesecloth bag

sterilized jars and lids (see **The Sterilizing & Canning Process,** *this section*)

Alternate layers of tomatoes and onions in large bowl, sprinkling each layer with salt. Cover and refrigerate overnight. Drain mixture, rinse under cold water and drain again. Combine apples, vinegar, sugar and spices in a double

Green Tomato Chow-Chow, *continued on next page.*

Green Tomato Chow-Chow, continued.

boiler or large saucepan. Add tomato and onion mixture. Bring to a boil, reduce heat and simmer, stirring occasionally, for 30 minutes. Remove spices from mixture. Pour into sterilized jars, seal and process in boiling water bath (see **The Sterilizing & Canning Process,** this section).

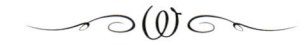

Refrigerator Pickles

Yield: 3 quarts

- 4 cups sugar
- 4 cups vinegar
- ½ cup non-iodized salt
- 1½ teaspoons celery seed
- 1⅓ teaspoons mustard seed
- 1⅓ teaspoons turmeric (or less)
- 3 onions, thinly sliced
- 6 pickling cucumbers, unpeeled

Mix all ingredients together. Do *not* heat! Arrange in layers in sterilized quart-size mason jars, or peanut butter jars. Always keep pickles refrigerated.

Sweet & Sour Pickle Slices

Serves 12

- 7 to 8 cucumbers, thinly sliced
- 10% brine solution (1 quart cold water and 6 tablespoons pickling salt)
- 1 teaspoon salt
- 1 cup white vinegar
- ¼ cup dry sherry
- 2 cups sugar
- 1 cup onion, chopped
- 1 cup green pepper, chopped
- ¼ teaspoon celery salt
- 1 teaspoon dill weed

pepper, to taste

Leave cucumbers in 10% brine solution for 1 hour. Mix remaining pickling ingredients in saucepan. Heat until warm, but *not* hot! Remove cucumbers from brine solution; drain well. Pour heated pickling ingredients over cucumbers. Serve pickles warm or cold.

Spicy Apricot Chutney

Serves 8

- 1 cup dried apricots, chopped
- ⅔ cup raisins
- 2 cups water
- ⅔ cup orange juice
- 1½ tablespoons lime juice
- 1 teaspoon orange zest
- 1 teaspoon lime zest
- 1 small red pepper, chopped
- 1 small green (poblaño) chili pepper, chopped
- ⅓ jalapeño pepper, chopped
- 1⅔ cups sugar

Kathy's "South-of-the-Border" Pork Tenderloin
(see recipe in the *Meats ~ Pork* chapter)

Soak apricots and raisins in water overnight. Pour into pan; add enough water to come half way to top of fruit. Simmer until extremely tender, about 15 minutes, stirring occasionally. Add juices, orange and lime zest, and the 3 different peppers; return to a boil. Add sugar and cook over medium heat, stirring constantly until thick, 20 to 30 minutes, or longer if necessary. Serve with *Kathy's "South-of-the-Border" Pork Tenderloin.*

Apple, Date & Walnut Chutney

Yield: 4 pounds

- 1 pound onions, peeled and chopped
- 2 pounds cooking apples, peeled, cored and chopped
- 1½ pounds dates, pitted and chopped
- ½ cup walnuts, chopped
- 1 teaspoon salt
- 1 teaspoon ground ginger
- 1 teaspoon cayenne pepper
- 1 pint vinegar
- 1 cup dark brown sugar

sterilized jars and lids (see **The Sterilizing & Canning Process,** *this section*)

Put onions in a large, heavy based pan with a little water. Bring to a boil and simmer until soft. Add apples and continue cooking gently for 15 to 20 minutes. Add dates, walnuts, salt, spices and half the vinegar and cook,

Apple, Date & Walnut Chutney, *continued on next page.*

Apple, Date & Walnut Chutney, *continued.*

stirring occasionally, until mixture thickens. Add sugar and remaining vinegar, stirring gently until sugar dissolves. Continue to let chutney simmer, stirring occasionally, until it becomes very thick. Immediately pour chutney into sterilized jars, seal and process in hot water bath (*see* **The Sterilizing & Canning Process,** *this section*).

Fancy Beet Relish

Yield: 6 pints

- 4 cups raw beets, peeled and chopped
- 4 cups raw cabbage, chopped or grated
- 1 cup onion, chopped
- 1½ cups green or red pepper, finely chopped
- 1 4 to 5-ounce jar prepared horseradish (preferably hot)
- 2 cups sugar
- 3 cups white vinegar
- 1 tablespoon salt

Combine all ingredients in 4-quart pan. Simmer for 20 minutes. Cool, and place in sterilized pint jars. Serve cold.

Note: Keeps in refrigerator for 2 weeks.

No~Cook Beet Relish

Yield: 1 quart

**Adapted for your kitchen...
from the original Walgreens recipe!**

Walgreens Cafeterias 1940's ~ 1960's

- 1 15-ounce can beets, finely chopped
- 1½ cups raw cabbage, chopped
- 4 tablespoons green pepper, finely diced
- 3 tablespoons horseradish, grated
- 1 pinch cayenne pepper
- 1 pinch pepper
- ¼ teaspoon salt
- 4 tablespoons sugar
- 3 tablespoons vinegar

Combine beets, cabbage and green pepper in a bowl; mix thoroughly. Add horseradish, cayenne pepper, pepper, salt, sugar and vinegar; mix well. Adjust seasonings to taste, if necessary. Store in refrigerator. Allow to stand at room temperature 30 minutes before serving.

Nutty Cranberry Relish

Serves 12

- 2 cups fresh cranberries
- 1 orange with peel, cut into chunks
- 1 apple with peel, cored and cut into chunks
- ½ cup walnuts, chopped
- 2 cups granulated sugar

sour cream (optional)

Wash fruit. Crush cranberries, orange and apple chunks in food processor until desired consistency. Add walnuts and sugar. Process for a few additional seconds. Refrigerate overnight. May serve with sour cream.

Note: Keeps in refrigerator for 1 week.

Walsh's Welsh Rarebit

Serves 6 to 8

- 4 tablespoons butter or margarine
- 4 tablespoons flour
- 1 pint milk
- 10 ounces sharp cheddar cheese, shredded or finely chopped
- ¼ teaspoon Worcestershire sauce
- 1 tablespoon onion flakes (or, to taste)

salt, to taste

- 1 egg, beaten

6 to 8 English muffins, toasted

Melt butter in top of double boiler. Add flour; while stirring constantly, add milk gradually. Continue stirring; add cheese to milk. When cheese is melted, blend in Worcestershire sauce, onion and salt. To prevent curdling, remove small amount of mixture and blend in beaten egg. Add this to rest of mixture in double boiler. Serve immediately on toasted English muffins.

Cocktail Sauce

Yield: 1 cup

Adapted for your kitchen... from the original Walgreens recipe!

Robin Hood & Briargate Restaurants, 1970's ~ 1980's

1 cup chili sauce
1 to 2 tablespoons horseradish
1 tablespoon lemon juice
2 tablespoons celery, finely chopped
1 to 2 teaspoon(s) vinegar
salt, to taste
1 teaspoon Worcestershire sauce
1 dash hot red pepper sauce (Tabasco)

Combine all ingredients and mix thoroughly. Chill well before serving.

Tartar Sauce

Yield: 1 cup

Adapted for your kitchen... from the original Walgreens recipe!

Robin Hood & Briargate Restaurants, 1970's ~ 1980's

1 tablespoon parsley, finely chopped
1 tablespoon green stuffed olives, finely chopped
1 tablespoon kosher dill pickles, chopped and drained
1 teaspoon onions, finely chopped
1 teaspoon vinegar
1 cup Miracle Whip

Mix parsley, olives, pickles, and onions. Add vinegar. Add Miracle Whip, mix and chill.

Classic Hollandaise Sauce

Yield: 1 cup

- ½ cup butter
- 3 egg yolks
- 1 tablespoon fresh lemon juice, warmed (more if needed)
- 1 tablespoon boiling water
- ¼ teaspoon salt
- 1 pinch white pepper

Melt butter and keep warm. In top of double boiler, whisk egg yolks until they are a light lemon color and thickened. Whisk in lemon juice, boiling water, salt and pepper. Remove from heat and slowly beat in butter in a slow, steady stream. Beat until sauce is thick. If sauce begins to curdle, add additional melted butter and some heated heavy cream. Sauce should be served immediately. It can be held up to 1 hour near a gas pilot light, in a simmering pot or in a pan of tepid (not hot) water.

Note: Hollandaise is usually served over vegetables.

Mock Hollandaise Sauce

Yield: 3 cups

Adapted for your kitchen... from the original Walgreens recipe!

Walgreens Cafeterias 1940's ~ 1960's

- ½ cup butter
- ¼ cup flour
- 1 pinch salt
- 2½ cups milk
- 3 egg yolks, beaten
- 2 tablespoons lemon juice

Using a double boiler, melt half the butter and add flour and salt, making a roux; set aside to cool. Bring milk to a boil and add to cooled roux. Stir constantly until mixture is smooth. Return mixture, in double boiler, to heat; bring to a boil, stirring constantly. Remove from heat. Blend beaten egg yolks with a little of the heated sauce, then add to remaining sauce, stirring constantly. Add remaining butter, a little at a time, stirring each time so butter melts and blends with sauce. Lastly, add lemon juice; mix thoroughly.

Note: When serving sauce with vegetables, do not mix; serve *over* vegetables.

Béarnaise Sauce

Yield: 1½ cups

- ½ cup white wine
- 2 tablespoons tarragon vinegar
- 1 tablespoon shallots or scallions (green onions), finely chopped
- 2 peppercorns, crushed
- 1 to 2 tablespoons fresh tarragon, chopped
- 1 tablespoons fresh parsley, chopped
- 3 to 4 egg yolks
- ½ teaspoon salt
- ½ cup (1 stick) butter, melted

Tenderloin Deluxe (see recipe in the *Meats ~ Beef* chapter)
Mushrooms in Wine Sauce (see recipe in the *Vegetables* chapter)

In saucepan, combine wine, tarragon, vinegar, shallots, crushed peppercorns and parsley; cook until wine is reduced by half and resembles a glaze. Combine glaze with egg yolk and salt in a blender. Heat butter until it is hot and bubbling. Turn blender on and off quickly, and blend ingredients. Turn it on again, and gradually pour in hot, melted butter in a steady stream until sauce thickens. Additional chopped tarragon and parsley may be folded in sauce. Serve with *Tenderloin Deluxe* and *Mushrooms in Wine Sauce*.

Note: Béarnaise is usually served with broiled meat and fish.

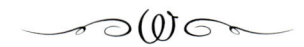

Rémoulade Sauce

Yield: 1¾ to 2 cups

**Adapted for your kitchen...
from the original Walgreens recipe!**

Robin Hood & Briargate Restaurants, 1970's ~ 1980's

- 1 cup mayonnaise
- ¼ cup parsley, chopped
- 1 teaspoon tarragon
- ¼ cup onion, chopped
- 1 garlic clove
- 1 teaspoon Dijon mustard

Combine mayonnaise with the parsley, tarragon, onion, garlic and mustard. Allow to stand 1 hour.

Note: Rémoulade is usually served over cold poultry or fish.

Traditional Creole Sauce

Yield: 1 quart

Adapted for your kitchen…
from the original Walgreens recipe!

Walgreens Cafeterias
1940's ~ 1960's

2	tablespoons vegetable oil
1	cup onions, chopped
2	tablespoons celery, chopped
1½	cups green peppers, chopped
1	14½-ounce can tomatoes, drained and chopped
¾	tablespoon salt
¼	teaspoon pepper
½	tablespoon sugar
¾	tablespoon paprika
1	teaspoon whole, mixed spices, tied in muslin or cheesecloth bag
2½	cups beef stock or bouillon
1½	tablespoon cornstarch, dissolved in 2 tablespoons cold water
¼	tablespoon Lea & Perrins Worcestershire sauce

Heat oil; add onions, celery and green pepper. Sauté slowly, about 1 minute. Add tomatoes, salt, pepper, sugar, paprika, spice bag and stock; simmer over low heat 45 minutes. Remove spice bag. Add dissolved cornstarch to mixture, stirring constantly. Cook 15 minutes. Add Worcestershire sauce. Boil for 3 more minutes.

Spicy Creole Sauce with Mushrooms

Yield: 1½ to 2 cups

2	teaspoons vegetable oil
½	cup celery, chopped
½	cup green pepper, chopped
½	cup onion, chopped
½	cup mushrooms, sliced
1	8-ounce can chopped tomatoes
1	teaspoon salt
½	teaspoon pepper, freshly ground
¼	teaspoon Tabasco sauce

Heat oil in saucepan. Sauté celery, green pepper, onion and mushrooms until lightly browned. Add tomatoes, salt, pepper and Tabasco. Simmer for 15 minutes.

Note: Serve over fish, poultry or meat.

Jardinière Sauce

Yield: 1 quart

Adapted for your kitchen... from the original Walgreens recipe!

Robin Hood & Briargate Restaurants, 1970's ~ 1980's

¼ pound onions, finely chopped
4 tablespoons butter or margarine
2 tablespoons beef base
1½ tablespoons tomato paste
¼ cup flour
1 quart hot stock
½ teaspoon garlic salt
½ teaspoon Worcestershire sauce
1 large carrot, julienne, cooked and drained
1 celery stalk, julienne, cooked and drained
salt and pepper, to taste

Sauté onions and butter or margarine slowly for 30 minutes. Add beef base and cook for 30 minutes. Add tomato paste and cook for 15 minutes. Blend in flour and cook until smooth. Remove from fire and slowly stir in hot stock. Add garlic salt and Worcestershire sauce. Bring to boil, then lower heat. Add cooked vegetables. Salt and pepper to taste.

Note: Like jardinère, the garnish, this vegetable sauce is usually served with meat dishes.

Yogurt~Garlic Sauce or Dip

Yield: 1 quart

1 cucumber, peeled, seeded and diced
6 garlic cloves, minced
½ cup fresh dill, coarsely chopped
½ cup scallions, sliced
4 cups plain yogurt
juice of 2 lemons (about ½-cup)
salt and pepper, to taste

Prepare 1 day before serving, so flavors will blend. To make sauce, combine all ingredients, adding lemon, salt and pepper last. Mix thoroughly. Adjust seasonings to taste.

Note: Serve with grilled chicken or as vegetable dip.

Classic Brown Sauce

Yield: 1½ quarts

Note:
Bordelaise and Brown Mushroom Sauce share Brown Sauce as a common base.

2 pounds shin of beef with bone
1 veal knuckle
1 large onion, stuck with 2 cloves
1 carrot
1 or 2 garlic cloves
1 teaspoon thyme
1 bay leaf
several sprigs parsley
5 cups water
2 tablespoons tomato paste
salt and pepper, freshly ground
6 tablespoons butter
6 tablespoons browned flour

Brown beef and bones in a 450-degree oven for 30 to 45 minutes. Transfer browned meat and bones to a large pot, and add vegetables, garlic, herbs and water. Bring to a boil; reduce heat and simmer covered for 3 hours. Remove cover and simmer for another half hour. Let broth cool. Strain, chill overnight and remove fat. Measure off stock and heat to boiling point. Add tomato paste, taste for salt and correct seasonings. Prepare flour by putting 1 cup in a 250-degree oven and toasting until lightly browned. Prepare roux by melting butter and blending with browned flour. Stir in 2½ cups of stock and continue to simmer very gently until reduced and nicely thickened.

Bordelaise Sauce

Yield: 1½ cups

Adapted for your kitchen... from the original Walgreens recipe!

Robin Hood & Briargate Restaurants, 1970's ~ 1980's

1 cup red wine
¼ cup shallots
1 teaspoon thyme
1 cup *brown sauce* (see **Classic Brown Sauce** recipe, above)
1 tablespoon cognac
1 tablespoon lemon juice
1 cup parsley, chopped

Combine wine with shallots and 1 teaspoon thyme. Reduce over heat to ⅓-cup. Strain into 1 cup brown sauce and add cognac and lemon juice. Simmer for 3 minutes and add chopped parsley.

Note: Bordelaise is brown sauce with wine and seasoning added. Serve over broiled meat.

Yield: 1 quart

**Adapted for your kitchen...
from the original Walgreens recipe!**

Robin Hood & Briargate Restaurants, 1970's ~ 1980's

Brown Mushroom Sauce

1 cup fresh mushrooms, coarsely chopped
5 tablespoons butter or margarine
salt and pepper, freshly ground
1½ cups *brown sauce* (see **Classic Brown Sauce** recipe, at left)
¼ Madeira or sherry

Sauté mushrooms in butter or margarine until soft and dark. Season with salt and pepper. Combine with brown sauce and Madeira or sherry. Simmer for 5 minutes.

Note: Brown mushroom sauce is brown sauce with mushrooms and sherry, thickened with butter and flour.

White Mushroom Sauce

Yield: 1 quart

2 tablespoons butter or margarine
1 cup mushrooms, minced
2 tablespoons flour
1 cup milk
¼ teaspoon salt
1 pinch pepper
2 tablespoons dry sherry

Melt butter or margarine in saucepan; sauté mushrooms for 3 to 5 minutes. Add flour to form a smooth paste. Gradually stir in milk until thickened and smooth. Add seasonings and dry sherry. Let sit 5 minutes, stirring occasionally. If sauce is to be held, transfer to top of double boiler over simmering water. Place piece of wax paper over top of sauce to prevent skin from forming.

Note: White mushroom sauce is béchamel (white sauce) with mushrooms and sherry.

Béchamel ~ Classic White Sauce

Yield: 2½ cups

Adapted for your kitchen...
from the original Walgreens recipe!

Walgreens Cafeterias 1940's ~ 1960's

Note:
Cream Sauce, Mornay, Véloute and White Mushroom Sauce all share Béchamel, or White Sauce, as a common base.

4 tablespoons butter
½ onion, finely chopped
1 celery stalk, finely chopped
4 tablespoons flour
2½ cups hot milk
1 small sprig thyme
½ bay leaf
white peppercorns, to taste
nutmeg, freshly grated, to taste

Melt butter in top of double boiler. Add onion and celery; cook over low heat until onion is soft but not browned. Remove from heat; stir in flour. Cook for 3 to 5 minutes, stirring constantly until flour is absorbed. Add ¼ of the hot milk; return to low heat. As sauce begins to thicken, add remaining milk, stirring constantly until sauce bubbles. Add thyme, bay leaf, peppercorns and nutmeg. Simmer for 15 minutes. Strain through a fine sieve and dot surface with butter.

Note: Serve with meat, fish, eggs, vegetables or noodles.

Cream Sauce

Yield: 2¾ cups

¼ cup heavy cream
2½ cups béchamel (see **Classic White Sauce** recipe, above)
lemon juice

Add cream to béchamel; bring to boil. Stir in a few drops of lemon juice.

Note: Cream sauce is béchamel (white sauce) with heavy cream.

Mornay ~ Cheese Sauce

Yield: 2¾ cups

2 eggs yolks, slightly beaten
heavy cream
2½ cups béchamel (see **Classic White Sauce** recipe, above)
2 to 4 tablespoons butter
2 to 4 tablespoons Parmesan or Swiss cheese, grated

Mornay ~ Cheese Sauce, *continued on next page.*

Mornay ~ Cheese Sauce, continued.

Mix the egg yolks with a little cream; combine with béchamel. Cook, stirring constantly until boiling. Add butter and Parmesan or Swiss cheese.

Note: Mornay is béchamel (white sauce) with Swiss or Parmesan cheese.

American Mornay Sauce

Yield: 2½ cups

Adapted for your kitchen... from the original Walgreens recipe!

Walgreens Cafeterias 1940's ~ 1960's

4 tablespoons vegetable oil
½ cup flour
¾ teaspoon salt
¼ teaspoon white pepper
2½ cups milk, heated to boiling
2 to 4 tablespoons Kraft grated American cheese
1 teaspoon Lea & Perrins Worcestershire sauce
salt and pepper, to taste

Heat oil and blend in flour and seasoning, stirring constantly to make a white roux. Do not allow mixture to brown. Heat until frothy; remove from heat. Pour boiling milk into roux, stirring constantly with a French whip, until smooth. Return mixture to heat. Bring to a boil, stirring constantly. If sauce is too thick, thin by adding hot milk. Blend in cheese, and bring to a boil. Remove from heat. Add Worcestershire sauce. Season to taste.

Velouté Sauce

Yield: 2½ cups

4 tablespoons butter
4 tablespoons flour
2½ cups white broth (chicken or veal), boiling
salt
white peppercorns
4 mushrooms, chopped

Melt butter in saucepan or, preferably, top of double boiler (aluminum pan will discolor sauce). Add flour; cook for a few minutes to form light roux; do not brown. Add boiling broth, salt and pepper. Cook, whisking vigorously. Add mushrooms. Cook slowly, stirring and skimming occasionally, until sauce is reduced to two-thirds and is very thick but light and creamy. Strain through a fine sieve.

Note: Velouté is béchamel (white sauce) with chicken, veal or fish stock thickened with flour and butter. Serve with chicken, fish or veal.

Marinara ~ Classic Red Sauce for Pasta

Yield: 2 quarts

Adapted for your kitchen... from the original Walgreens recipe!

Robin Hood & Briargate Restaurants, 1970's ~ 1980's

- 2 onions, finely chopped
- 1 green pepper, finely chopped
- 4 tablespoons butter or margarine
- 1 6-ounce can tomato paste
- 1 16-ounce can tomato purée
- 1¼ quarts water
- 1½ tablespoons beef base
- 1 tablespoon salt
- 1½ tablespoon sugar
- ¼ teaspoon cayenne pepper
- 1½ teaspoon oregano
- 1 tablespoon paprika
- 2 tablespoons Parmesan cheese, grated
- 1 bay leave
- 1 garlic clove

Sauté onions and pepper in butter or margarine for 10 minutes. Make a spice bag of bay leaves and garlic. Add spice bag and remaining ingredients to pan; simmer for 1½ hours. Stir every 10 minutes. Remove spice bag.

Italian Meat Sauce

Yield: 1½ to 2 quarts

Adapted for your kitchen... from the original Walgreens recipe!

Robin Hood & Briargate Restaurants, 1970's ~ 1980's

- 1 stick butter or margarine
- 2 onions, chopped
- 2 tablespoons beef base
- 1 garlic clove, crushed
- 1 tablespoon salt
- ¼ teaspoon pepper
- ½ teaspoon rosemary
- 1 bay leaf
- 1½ pounds ground beef
- 2 6-ounce cans tomato paste
- ¼ cup flour
- 1 28-ounce can stewed tomatoes
- ½ cup Parmesan cheese, grated
- 1 to 2 cups beef stock or broth (if necessary)
- 4 tablespoons sherry, wine or Chablis wine

Italian Meat Sauce, continued on next page.

Italian Meat Sauce, continued.

In soup or stew pot sauté butter or margarine, onions, beef base, garlic, salt, pepper, rosemary, bay leaves and oregano slowly for 1 hour. Add ground beef and brown lightly. Add tomato paste and cook for 5 minutes. Add flour and blend. Add squeezed stewed tomatoes and stir. Add parmesan cheese. Add stock if needed. Remove from flame and add sherry, wine, or Chablis wine.

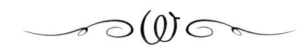

Western Herb Sauce for Steak

Yield: 1½ to 2 cups

- ¼ cup olive oil
- ¼ cup butter
- 2 tablespoons scallions (green onions), chopped
- ½ pound mushrooms, sliced
- 2 tablespoons chives, chopped
- 2 tablespoons tarragon, chopped
- 3 tablespoons parsley, chopped
- ½ cup pickled walnuts, chopped
- 3 tablespoons Diablo sauce
- ½ teaspoon salt

pepper, freshly ground, to taste

Combine olive oil and butter in skillet. Sauté scallions and mushrooms in mixture for 5 minutes. Add remaining ingredients and simmer for 5 minutes. Serve hot.

Note: Serve with broiled steak. This makes a thick sauce; to thin, add ½-cup beef bouillon and simmer an additional 5 minutes.

Garlic~Wine Marinade for Shrimp or Fish

Yield: ½ to ¼ cup

    juice from 3 limes
1   garlic clove, minced
1   splash of wine
1   tablespoon sugar

Blend together all ingredients.

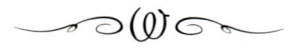

Ginger~Peach Marinade for Chicken

Yield: About 1 cup

1   tablespoon fresh ginger, minced
1   splash of soy sauce
1   shot of Tabasco sauce
1   15-ounce jar spicy peach jam

Stir ginger, soy sauce and Tabasco sauce into jar of spicy peach jam.

Honey~Ginger Marinade for Beef & Chicken

Yield: About 1 cup

½   cup onion, chopped
2   tablespoons sugar
½   cup soy sauce
1½ teaspoons fresh ginger, grated or minced
1   garlic clove, chopped
3   tablespoons honey
¾   cup vegetable oil

Blend ingredients with wire whisk.

Note: Works well with flank steak or chicken.

Wine Marinade for Steaks or Chops

Yield: 3½ to 4 cups

- 1½ cups peanut or cooking oil
- ¾ cup soy sauce
- 2 tablespoons Worcestershire sauce
- 2 tablespoons dry mustard
- 2 teaspoons salt
- 1 teaspoon pepper, freshly ground
- 1 cup dry red wine (Chianti, sherry or Bordeaux)
- 2 teaspoons dried parsley flakes
- ⅓ cup fresh lemon juice

Combine all ingredients in blender. Drain before grilling or baking.

Note: Marinade may be frozen for future use.

Raspberry~Mustard Marinade for Spareribs

Yield: About 1 cup

- 1 8-ounce jar raspberry jam
- 4 tablespoons Dijon mustard
- 2 tablespoons fruit vinegar
- grated peel of half an orange
- sprinkling of dried thyme

Blend together all ingredients.

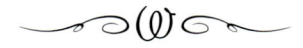

Ham Glaze

Yield: 1¾ cups

- 1 cup grenadine syrup
- ½ cup orange juice
- ¼ cup lemon juice
- ¼ cup sugar
- 1 tablespoon dry mustard
- 2 tablespoons cornstarch

Mix together all ingredients. Heat until thickened. Spread on ham and continue to baste during the last 30 minutes of cooking.

Au Jus ~ Quick or Traditional

Yield: 2 cups

Adapted for your kitchen... from the original Walgreens recipe!

Robin Hood & Briargate Restaurants, 1970's ~ 1980's

Quick:
2   cups boiling water
1   tablespoon beef base

Traditional:
1   cup pan drippings from cooked meat, drained
2   cups water
1   whole onion
1   teaspoon salt
1   tablespoon Kitchen Bouquet
1   teaspoon white pepper
1   tablespoon beef base
2   teaspoon Worcestershire sauce

Quick:
Add beef base to boiling water. Simmer for 15 minutes. Season to taste.

Traditional:
Simmer drippings, water, and onion for 30 minutes. Add all remaining ingredients and cook for an additional 30 minutes. Skim as often as necessary to eliminate grease. Strain and serve.

Chicken Giblet Gravy

Yield: 2 to 3 cups

Adapted for your kitchen... from the original Walgreens recipe!

Robin Hood & Briargate Restaurants, 1970's ~ 1980's

4   tablespoons butter or margarine
1   onion, finely chopped
1   tablespoon chicken base
4   tablespoons flour
cooked roast chicken giblets, coarsely chopped
2 to 3 cups hot stock or broth
salt and pepper

Melt margarine or butter; add onions, chicken base and cook very slowly until onions are soft. Add flour and make roux. Remove from fire and slowly add 2 cups hot stock. Mix using wire whip. Return to fire and bring to boil. Add chopped giblets and bring to boil. If gravy is too thick, add additional cup of stock (or part stock, part cream). Do not allow gravy to separate; constant whipping will prevent that. Salt and pepper to taste.

White Gravy for Chicken

Yield: 2 to 3 cups

Adapted for your kitchen... from the original Walgreens recipe!

Robin Hood & Briargate Restaurants, 1970's ~ 1980's

2	cups hot stock or broth
1	tablespoon chicken base
4	tablespoons butter, margarine or chicken fat, melted
4	tablespoons flour
¼	teaspoon white pepper
¼	teaspoon nutmeg
1	cup scalded milk

salt, to taste

Fortify hot stock as needed with chicken base and bring to boil. Stir and simmer. Combine melted fat with flour and pepper. Cook slowly until roux bubbles. Blend with wire whip; when roux becomes frothy, remove from flame. Slowly add boiling stock to roux, stirring constantly. Add nutmeg and milk. Return to fire and bring to boil, while continually stirring. Season to taste. Strain if needed.

Brown Gravy for Beef

Yield: 1 quart

Adapted for your kitchen... from the original Walgreens recipe!

Robin Hood & Briargate Restaurants, 1970's ~ 1980's

4	tablespoons pan drippings or margarine
4	tablespoons flour
1	14½-ounce can stewed tomatoes, drained and crushed
1	10¾-ounce can tomato purée
1	tablespoon sugar
1	teaspoon salt
½	teaspoon pepper
2	cups beef stock or broth
1	tablespoon Kitchen Bouquet

Slowly cook pan drippings or margarine with flour to make a light brown roux. Combine crushed tomatoes, puree, sugar, salt, pepper and beef stock; bring to a boil. Add to roux. Whip. Simmer for 30 minutes. Continue to whip until velvety smoothness. Strain gravy and serve.

Poultry Stuffing ~ Bread Dressing

Yield: 2 quarts stuffing for 10 to 12-pound turkey

**Adapted for your kitchen...
from the original Walgreens recipe!**

Robin Hood & Briargate Restaurants, 1970's ~ 1980's

1 onion, finely chopped
1 cup celery, finely chopped
½ cup butter or margarine
¼ teaspoon white pepper
½ teaspoon onion salt
¼ teaspoon celery salt
2 teaspoons poultry seasoning
¼ cup parsley, minced
2 quarts dry bread or half bread and half corn bread, chopped
2 cups stock (2 cups water and 2 tablespoons chicken base)
2 to 3 eggs

Sauté vegetables for 15 minutes in butter or margarine. Cool. Combine seasoning and parsley with bread. Toss lightly by hand until mixed. Mix in sautéed vegetable mixture. Add chicken stock gradually until desired consistency. Add eggs one at a time, blending well into mixture. Never pack dressing. Place dressing loosely in a greased pan; cover and bake covered at 325 degrees for 1 hour or until internal temperature reaches 165 to 170 degrees.

Stuffing with Beef ~ Pan Dressing

Serves 8

1 large onion, finely chopped
2 tablespoons butter or margarine
1 cup warm milk
16 ounces white bread, for bread crumbs
1 dozen eggs
½ pound ground beef, more if desired
extra cracker crumbs
turkey gravy, canned or homemade (optional)

Preheat oven to 350 degrees. Sauté chopped onion in butter until bubbly, not brown. Set aside. In large mixing bowl or food processor, mix bread crumbs and 1 cup warm milk. Add cooked onion, 1 dozen eggs, and mix. Add ½-pound raw ground beef and mix. Add cracker crumbs until mixture becomes consistency of hamburger or meat loaf. Put in greased 13x9-inch pan and bake for 45 minutes. (After 30 minutes, cut out one square of dressing to check if it is cooked on the bottom.)

Note: May be made ahead of time and refrigerated. To rewarm, pour gravy over dressing, cover with foil and heat in oven. Gravy is optional, but it keeps dressing moist.

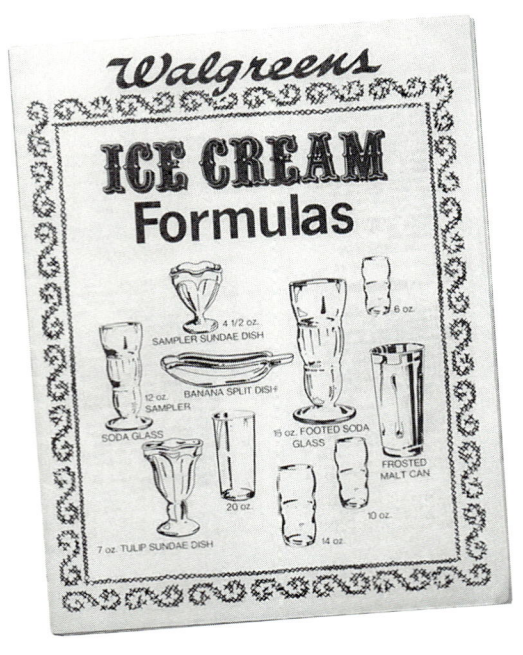

"Property of Walgreen Company ~ Do Not Duplicate" reads the note on this booklet of top-secret formulas for making the famous ice cream treats.

Old~Fashioned Chocolate Malted Milk
(Walgreen Double-Rich Chocolate Malted Milk)

Serves 1

The original recipe...invented at Walgreens!

Walgreens Soda Fountains, 1920's ~ 1960's

Appeared in Wag's "Old-Fashioned Ice Cream Favorites" menu as "Original Thick Malted Milk", 1970's ~ 1980's

2 ounces chocolate syrup
3 rounded scoops vanilla ice cream
4½ ounces milk, cold
1 tablespoon (heaping) malt powder
1 cookie treat
whipped topping

1 malt can, frosted
1 10 to 12-ounce glass

Combine syrup, ice cream, milk and malt powder in a malt can (or in a home blender). Place on malt mixer (or mix in blender) for 90 seconds. Fill glass two-thirds full. Top with whipped topping. Serve on an underliner (small plate) with cookie treat. Serve remainder of malt in malt can. Serve with a straw and a long-handled (ice tea) teaspoon.

Note: Walgreen fountain manager Ivar "Pop" Coulsen invented this recipe, originally known as the legendary Walgreen *Double-Rich Chocolate Malted Milk*, in 1922!

Sampler Thick Shake

Serves 1

The original Walgreens recipe!

Walgreens Soda Fountains, 1920's ~ 1960's

Wag's "Old-Fashioned Ice Cream Favorites", 1970's ~ 1980's

1½ ounces chocolate syrup
2 rounded scoops vanilla ice cream
3 ounces milk, cold
whipped topping
½ teaspoon chocolate shavings
1 cookie treat

1 malt can, frosted
1 12-ounce soda glass

Combine syrup, ice cream and milk in a malt can (or in a home blender). Place on malt mixer (or mix in blender) for 90 seconds. Pour into soda glass. Top with a generous amount of whipped topping and chocolate shavings. Serve on an underliner (small plate) with a straw and long-handled (ice tea) teaspoon. Place cookie treat at an angle in whipped topping.

Brandy Ice

Serves 1

1 cup vanilla ice cream, softened
2 tablespoons brandy
1 cup cognac

Blend softened ice cream with brandy and freeze several hours. (Ice cream will not be firm.) Scoop ice cream into sherbet glasses. Warm cognac, ignite, pour over brandy ice and serve.

Seneca Iced Coffee

Serves 4

1 cup coffee, brewed
2 tablespoons sugar
¼ teaspoon nutmeg
¼ teaspoon cinnamon
¼ teaspoon cloves, ground
4 ounces dark rum (optional)
4 cups ice, crushed
mint sprigs

Pour coffee into blender. Add sugar, nutmeg, cinnamon, cloves and rum (if desired). Blend well. Pour coffee mixture into tall glasses, over crushed ice. Garnish with mint sprigs.

Extraordinary Eggnog

Serves 12

1 quart prepared eggnog
white rum, up to a fifth, to taste
½ pint whipping cream, whipped
1 quart vanilla ice cream

nutmeg, to taste

Mix egg nog and rum. Float spoonfuls of whipped cream and ice cream on top. Add a dash of nutmeg to taste. Prepare about 45 minutes in advance. Stir occasionally.

Note: Equally good without rum.

Spicy, Hot Cider

Yield: 1 gallon

- 1 gallon apple cider
- 1 whole orange, peeled and diced
- 1 whole apple, cored and sectioned
- ¼ cup raisins
- 5 whole allspice
- 5 cinnamon sticks
- 12 whole cloves
- 1 tablespoon candied ginger
- 1 cup brown sugar, packed

Add all ingredients, except brown sugar, to a large saucepan. Bring to a boil. Add sugar. Simmer 20 minutes. Strain. Serve hot, in mugs, with cinnamon stick as garnish.

Airdrie House Hot, Buttered Rum Mix

Yield: 8 cups

- 1 pound butter, softened
- 2 cups light, brown sugar
- 1 tablespoon cinnamon
- ½ teaspoon nutmeg
- ½ teaspoon allspice
- 1 teaspoon vanilla
- dark rum
- boiling water
- cinnamon sticks

Put butter, brown sugar, cinnamon, nutmeg, allspice and vanilla in food processor. Blend until smooth. Put into refrigerator container and keep refrigerated until ready to use. To serve, place 3 tablespoons of mixture into a mug. Add 1-ounce of dark rum per drink, and fill with boiling water. Garnish with cinnamon stick.

Solberg's Glög

Serves 12

1 package Swedish fruit mix
1 quart water
1 quart brandy
1 gallon port wine
1½ pints 90-proof alcohol
1 cup raisins
3 cinnamon sticks
12 whole cloves
4 whole cardamom

Boil fruit mix in water for 30 minutes. Add brandy; let simmer for 15 minutes. Add port, alcohol and spices; let simmer for several hours. Serve hot.

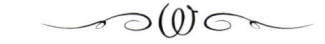

Mint Julip Walgreen

Serves 8 to 10

1 large bunch mint leaves
½ cup sugar
1 bottle 100-proof bourbon

1-gallon jug with screw top

Stuff gallon jug with mint leaves. Add sugar, and fill jug with bourbon. Store in a cool, dark area. Shake once a month for 6 months; then it will be ready to serve. To serve, strain mint leaves from bourbon. Fill a large, tall glass with cracked ice and pour bourbon mixture over it. Garnish with fresh mint sprigs.

Note: This mixture will keep indefinitely.

Raspberry Lime Rickeys

Serves 6

1 cup fresh raspberries
½ cup fresh lime juice
¼ cup sugar
¾ cup light rum
2 cups seltzer water
6 lime wedges

With a spoon, crush raspberries and mix with lime juice and sugar; let stand 10 minutes. Press through sieve into pitcher. Add rum and seltzer. Serve over ice with lime wedges.

Thunderbolt Punch

Serves 60 to 80 drinks

Charles R. Walgreen, Sr. created this special brew, while in a cabin 10,000 feet up in the mountains of Wyoming!
~ August 1934

1	1-fifth bottle (750-ml. or 3 cups) bourbon or scotch
1	1-fifth bottle (750-ml. or 3 cups) sherry
1	1-fifth bottle (750-ml. or 3 cups) cognac
2½	cups orange juice
½	cup lemon juice
½	cup sugar
1	750-ml. bottle (3 cups) champagne, chilled
25	pounds ice

Place ice in punch bowl and add bourbon (or scotch), sherry, cognac, orange juice, lemon juice and sugar. Stir gently and let sit until cool from ice. Add champagne. Serve in punch cups.

Note: Maximum 2 per person recommended!

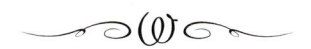

Happy Harry's Bloody Mary

Serves 1

1	lemon wedge
1	tablespoon celery salt
1	jigger (1½ ounces) vodka
½	cup tomato juice
½	teaspoon horseradish sauce
¼	teaspoon garlic salt
½	jigger (¾-ounce) akquavit (a cordial)
1	celery stalk

Rim glass with lemon wedge. Place celery salt in small bowl, and place rimmed glass in bowl, coating edges thoroughly. Add 4 ice cubes to glass; stir in vodka, tomato juice, horseradish and garlic salt. "Float" akquavit on top. Garnish with celery stalk.

Coke or Root Beer Float

Serves 1

The original Walgreens recipe!

Walgreens Soda Fountains, 1920's ~ 1960's

Wag's "Old-Fashioned Ice Cream Favorites", 1970's ~ 1980's

1 rounded scoop vanilla ice cream
8 ounces Coke or root beer
1 beer stein, frosted, or 12-ounce soda glass

Fill stein or glass three-quarters full of Coke. Add a scoop of vanilla ice cream. Serve with a straw and long-handled (ice tea) teaspoon.

Note: May substitute root beer for Coke to make a root beer float. After adding root beer and ice cream, it may be necessary to finish filling glass with a coarse stream of water, to knock down foam.

Julius "Barry"

Serves 1

2 oranges, freshly squeezed
1 banana
½ cup milk
½ cup water
¼ cup sugar
1 teaspoon vanilla
½ cup ice, crushed

Mix all ingredients in blender until well-mixed. Pour into tall glass.

Baby Shower Punch

Serves 15

Ice ring:
1 12-ounce can unsweetened pineapple juice
½ jar maraschino cherries, drained

Punch:
1 1.36 liter (1-quart, 14-ounce) can unsweetened pineapple juice
1 2-liter bottle clear cream soda

To prepare ice ring, put pineapple juice and cherries into a round jello mold ring and freeze.

To prepare punch, combine pineapple juice and cream soda in a punch bowl. Float ice ring on top.

Banana Punch

Yield: 5 quarts

- 7 cups water
- 3½ cups sugar
- 5 bananas, mashed in blender
- 1 6-ounce can frozen orange juice concentrate
- 1 6-ounce can frozen lemonade concentrate
- 1 46-ounce can pineapple juice
- 1 quart ginger ale

Boil water and sugar for 5 minutes. Cool and add all remaining ingredients, except ginger ale. Freeze. Remove from freezer 2 to 3 hours before serving. Mix with ginger ale.

Note: May float assorted fruit in punch bowl. May also add vodka, to taste.

Old~Country Grape Wine

Yield: About 4 gallons per keg or barrel

This original recipe, passed down through the generations, was brought here from Germany and Switzerland in the mid 1880'.

Concord grapes (dark blue), any quantity
sugar (2 pounds per gallon of grape juice)

Take perfectly-ripe grapes from vineyard. Pick off each stem and wash grapes thoroughly. Mash them, breaking skins, and put in a clean vessel (a barrel, with spigot). Let stand for 24 hours. After 24 hours, use a cider press, or other convenient apparatus, to express all the juice.

Put juice in barrel and add 2 pounds of sugar per gallon. Cover top of barrel with a clean piece of muslin to keep dirt and insects out.

Set barrel in a quiet place until cold weather arrives. If allowed to rest perfectly still, it can be drained-off perfectly clear, and ready for use.

Note: One keg or barrel will serve about 4 gallons, lasting through the Christmas holidays. Children would drink grape juice.

Walgreen Food Dictionary

A Manual for Food Preparation in Walgreen Food Service Divisions

Revised and updated ~ from the *Walgreen Cookbook, Your Guide to Good Food*, circa 1945.

á la Broché: Cooked on a skewer (brochette).

á la Carte: Foods prepared to order, each dish priced separately.

á la King: Food prepared in a cream sauce of mushrooms, green peppers and pimentos.

á la Mode: As used in America, ice cream served with pie or cake; also means other dishes served in a special way (á la means "in the manner of"). In French cuisine, braised meat smothered in gravy.

Al Dente: Pasta cooked only long enough to retain a slight bite or crunch.

Amandine: Flavored and garnished with almonds.

Ambrosia: A cold dessert of bananas, oranges and coconut.

Anchovy: A small fish of the herring family.

Antipasto: Assortment of appetizers. (Italian.)

Appetizer: Small, savory foods served before a meal to whet the appetite.

Arrowroot: A nutritious starch obtained from a tropical American plant.

Aspic: A clear gelatin made with meat, poultry or vegetables, and seasoned.

Au Gratin: A dish browned in an oven or broiler, usually topped with buttered bread crumbs or grated cheese, or both.

Au Jus: Meaning "with juices"; a clear, seasoned broth made from meat juices. Usually served with roast beef, as with French-dipped sandwiches.

Bar le Duc: A famous jam made of red or white currants. Gooseberries are also sometimes used.

Béarnaise Sauce: A rich butter and egg sauce, similar to Hollandaise, but also containing wine, vinegar, shallots and herbs. Used on broiled meats and fish.

Béchamel: White ("cream") sauce. Ranging from thin to very thick, this is the most versatile and valuable of all sauces.

Bisque: A creamed soup, usually with a shellfish base.

Blintz: A thin, rolled pancake (crepe) filled with cottage cheese or cream.

Blood Pudding: Also Blood Sausage. A sausage made from cooked swine blood and suet, enclosed in an intestine.

Bordelaise Sauce: A dark brown sauce made from meat stock (marrow bone fat), flour, red or white wine, onions and seasonings. Served with broiled meat.

Bouillon: An unsalted strong beef stock, not as sweet as consommé.

Bouquet Garni: A mix of herbs tied in a cheesecloth; used in soups and stews and then removed.

Bourguignon: A method of culinary preparation for braised meats, eggs, fish and poultry; its main features are a red wine sauce and a garnish composed of mushrooms, small onions and lardoons.

Brisket: Forequarter of beef, below and just behind the foreleg.

419

Broccoli: A cultivated cabbage with an edible flower head; a hardy variety of the cauliflower.

Brown Sauce: Classic French sauce whereby butter and flour are cooked and allowed to brown. This roux is mixed into brown stock or beef broth.

Brown Sugar: The finely crushed molasses of partially-refined cane sugar.

Brussels Sprouts: The edible head of a tiny variety of cabbage.

Buck Rabbit: Welsh rarebit topped with a poached egg.

Burrito: A flour tortilla wrapped around (so as to enclose) a cooked filling of ground meat and cheese and, usually, refried beans and vegetables.

Butterscotch: A mixture of brown sugar and melted butter.

Camembert: A soft, full-flavored cheese made from whole, unskimmed milk. The cheese must be pale yellow, smooth and without holes.

Canapé: Fried or toasted bread, covered with a highly-seasoned spread.

Capon: A rooster that has been castrated and fattened to improve the quality and taste of its meat.

Cappuccino: Espresso with a frothy milk cap. Made by forcing steam through coffee and milk or cream. Invented by the Capuchin monks.

Caramel: Sugar melted over direct heat without moisture and allowed to brown slightly. Water is then added and the mixture is boiled a few minutes. Used for flavoring and coloring.

Carp: A freshwater fish.

Caviar: The eggs (roe) of sturgeon and other large fish, salted and pressed.

Cereal: An edible grain, like corn, wheat or oats. Or a food made from this grain.

Chantilly: Fresh cream beaten to the consistency of a mousse, sweetened and flavored with vanilla or other flavors. Also, a hollandaise sauce to which whipped cream has been added.

Chateaubriand: The center of a beef tenderloin; broiled or grilled and served with a château or Bérnaise sauce.

Cheddar Cheese: A hard, smooth, yellow English cheese; sharp or mild.

Chicken Maryland: Disjointed young chickens, floured, coated with egg and bread crumbs, and baked in an oven or deep-fried. Served with a cream gravy.

Chicory: A green of the endive family. The leaves are used for salad; the roots, as a cooked vegetable.

Chiffonade: A French salad dressing made with chopped eggs, onions, parsley and red bell peppers. Also, a mixture of sorrel and lettuce cut into julienne strips and cooked in butter.

Chow-Chow: A relish made of mustard and chopped, pickled vegetables, such as green tomatoes.

Chowder: A thick soup or stew made with shellfish (clam) meat, fish or vegetables to which salt pork, milk, diced vegetables, and even bread and crackers may be added. Often contains chopped potatoes.

Chutney: A pungent, chunky relish of fruits, spices and herbs. (Indian.)

Cocktail: A mixed, alcoholic drink, stirred or shaken with ice and served cold in cocktail glasses; or a special appetizer, usually made with seafood (shrimp).

Coffee Latté: Coffee with steamed milk added.

Compote: A dessert stew of fresh or dried fruit. Usually served cold and sprinkled with Kirsch or other liqueur.

Condiment: A relish, sauce or seasoning used to flavor food at the table (like catsup or mustard).

Conserve: Mixed fruit jam with nuts and raisins.

Consommé: A meat stock which has been enriched, concentrated or clarified.

Cream Cheese: A soft, mild-flavored white cheese made from cream and milk.

Creole Sauce: A spicy sauce prepared with sautéed tomatoes, green peppers and onions. (Louisiana origin)

Crepe: A very thin pancake.

Croissant: A rich, flaky, tender crescent roll made with puff pastry or leavened dough.

Croquette: A small cake or ball of minced food combined with a white or brown sauce, coated with egg and bread crumbs, and deep-fried. There are also sweet croquettes made with milk, rice, semolina or with a salpicon of fruit combined with French pastry cream.

Deviled: Method of preparation usually for poultry. The bird is grilled first, breaded and browned. Or other pieces of meat or poultry coated with mustard, dipped in beaten egg and rolled in bread crumbs.

Dijon Mustard: Prepared mustard made with white wine. (Dijon, France.)

Drawn Butter Sauce: A roux of butter and flour moistened with water or consommé and simmered with seasonings.

Duchess Potatoes: Potatoes mashed with butter, eggs, spices and squeezed through a pastry tube; brushed with beaten egg and browned in an oven. They also serve as borders for dishes.

Dumpling: A small ball of dough or potato, cooked in a soup or stew.

Éclair: A tubular or finger-shaped pastry filled with French pastry cream or custard, often iced with fondant icing. (French.)

Edam: A hard, yellow-red, Dutch cheese.

Eggnog: A beverage made from beaten eggs, sugar, brandy or rum, and milk.

En Casserole: Food served in the same dish in which it is baked, as with casseroles or pot pies.

Enchiladas: Thinly rolled, open-ended tortillas stuffed with meat or cheese and served with a chili pepper sauce.

Endive: A curly salad green.

Entrée: Generally refers to the main dish or course.

Escargot: An edible snail served in its shell.

Espresso: A strong, full-flavored coffee brewed by forcing pressurized steam over the beans.

Fillet: Boneless strips cut from meat or fish.

Filet Mignon: Tenderloin of beef; usually broiled with a strip of bacon fastened around each steak.

Finnan Haddie: Haddock which has been cured with smoke and soaked in tepid water to remove saltiness. (Scottish.)

Flambé: To serve food covered with a flammable liquor, usually brandy, and ignited.

Flank: The hindquarter of beef below the sirloin.

Fondue: Chafing dish of melted cheese used for dipping bread chunks. Chocolate is also used for dipping cake cubes and fruits.

Forcemeat: Chopped meats combined with ground vegetables, bread crumbs and seasonings; used for stuffing and dressings.

French Dressing: A salad dressing containing oil, vinegar or lemon juice and seasonings.

French Drip: Coffee brewed by filtering boiling water through finely ground beans.

French-Fried Potatoes: Raw, julienne potatoes fried in deep fat.

French or German Toast: Bread dipped in egg and milk batter and fried.

Fricassee: A stew of chopped chicken or veal served with a thick gravy, often in the company of vegetables.

Fritter: A ball of food dipped in a batter and deep-fried.

Gazpacho: A chilled soup of tomatoes, green peppers, other vegetables and herbs. (Spanish.)

German-Fried Potatoes: Boiled potatoes thinly sliced and fried in a heavy frying pan until brown.

Gherkin: A small, green cucumber gathered for pickling and used as a condiment.

Glacé: Glazed, iced or candied. Glacé fruit is fruit which has been dipped in syrup and cooked to the hard-crack stage.

Goulash: A stew of meat (beef) and vegetables, seasoned with paprika. (Hungarian.)

Grenadine: A syrup made from pomegranates or red currants; used for flavoring.

Grits: Coarsely ground grain; usually hulled, dried corn (hominy). Often made into porridge.

Gruyère: A Swiss type of cheese made in France and Switzerland.

Gumbo: A stew made with okra, chicken, onions, green peppers and tomatoes. (Louisiana.)

Haggis: Minced sheep or calf heart, lungs and liver, mixed with suet, oatmeal and seasonings, and baked in the stomach. (Scottish.)

Hollandaise Sauce: A creamy, yellow sauce made with egg yolks, butter, water and lemon juice; usually served over vegetables.

Hard Sauce: A sauce of creamed butter and powdered sugar with brandy or rum and vanilla.

Head Cheese: Jellied, spiced, pressed meat from the head of a hog.

Hors D'Oeuvres: Appetizers.

Italienne: Served Italian style.

Jam: A thick spread or preserve made by boiling whole or chopped fruit with sugar.

Jardinière: A dish prepared with a variety of vegetables, glazed and sauced; used as a garnish.

Jelly: A clear, gelatinous spread made by boiling sugar, fruit pectin, fruit acid and fruit juice.

Kebab: Also Kabob. See Shish Kebab.

Kielbasa: Polish sausage. Made from beef and pork, and seasoned with garlic.

Kohl Rabi: A type of turnip cabbage.

Küchen: German cake, not necessarily sweet.

Kugel: A sweet, baked pudding made with noodles, preserves, cottage cheese, sour cream and raisins. A traditional Jewish dairy meal.

Lard: Pork fat; preferred as a shortening because of its soft texture and rich, almost nutty, flavor. Also, a preparation in which strips of pork fat are threaded into large cuts of meat by means of a larding needle.

Lemon-Parsley Butter Sauce: A sauce of creamed or melted butter, lemon juice and finely chopped parsley. Also called maître d'hôtel sauce.

Liederkranz Cheese: A soft, rich, strong cheese.

Limburger Cheese: A semi-hard, fermented, rich and odorous cheese. (Belgium.)

Lyonnaise: Famous cooking region in France, well known for a potato dish cooked with onions.

Maître d'Hôtel: Head of a restaurant or food service. Also a lemon-parsley butter sauce.

Manhattan Clam Chowder: Clam chowder made with tomatoes.

Marinade: A solution of vinegar or wine, oil and seasonings, in which meat or fish is allowed to stand before cooking.

Marinara: A seasoned, Italian tomato sauce, often with cheeses, chopped peppers, onions or mushrooms; usually served over pasta.

Marmalade: A jelly, usually citrus, made with bits of fruit and fruit peel.

Marzipan: A sweet almond paste used in making desserts and candy.

Marmite or Petit Marmite: An iron or earthenware pot or casserole; or the French preparation combining chicken, beef and vegetables in a clear broth.

Matzo: Unleavened bread; thin and cracker-like.

Mayonnaise: A dressing made from raw egg yolks, oil, vinegar or lemon juice and seasonings. Used on salads or as a spread; also used for binding ingredients together.

Melba Toast: Very thinly sliced, crisp toast.

Menu: Bill of fare.

Meringue: Egg whites, with sugar added, stiffly-beaten to a froth or standing peaks; usually baked or dried.

Meunière: With a lemon-parsley butter sauce.

Mincemeat: A mixture of finely chopped apples, currants, raisins, spices, and occasionally, meat.

Minute Steak: A thin sirloin butt steak without the bone.

Mixed Grill: Usually broiled lamb chop, bacon and pineapple; or any three grilled items.

Mocha or Moka: A coffee flavoring; used in cakes, fillings, frosting and ice cream.

Morel: A wild mushroom with a spongy, conical cap; valued for its flavor and is usually sold dried.

Mornay Sauce: White sauce (béchamel) enriched with Swiss or Parmesan cheese and seasonings.

Mousse: Cold dessert of whipped cream, beaten egg whites and gelatin, sweetened and flavored; there is also savory mousse made with meat or fish purée.

Mush: Boiled cornmeal, sliced and pan fried.

Mushroom Sauce: A brown sauce base with seasonings and sliced mushrooms, sautéed in butter. For roast meat, chicken and casseroles.

Mutton: The meat of a full-grown sheep.

Nectarine: A smooth skinned halfbreed of plum and peach.

Nesselrode: A sauce or pudding mixture of candied fruit and nuts flavored with rum; used in making desserts.

Newburg: A sauce made with cream, egg yolks, butter, wine and nutmeg; used on seafood. Also, a dish cooked with Newburg sauce, such as lobster or seafood Newburg.

New England Clam Chowder: Clam chowder made with milk.

Noodles: A pasta made from flour, eggs and water into dried, flat, narrow strips of dough.

Omelette or Omelet: A mixture of eggs, milk and seasonings fried in butter and folded over.

Parfait: A dessert of fruit layered with ice cream, whipped cream, syrup and sometimes, cake.

Parmesan Cheese: A hard, sharp Italian cheese; served grated on soups, pasta and vegetables.

Pasta: Dried or fresh paste or dough made from Durham wheat or semolina flour, sometimes with egg. Available in long strips or other shapes. Examples: spaghetti, linguini, fettuccini, macaroni, lasagna, manicotti and rotini. (Italian.)

Pastrami: Highly-seasoned, smoked beef. Usually shoulder or breast cuts.

Pastry: A food, usually a dessert, made from a baked paste (crust) of flour, water and shortening. The dough, itself, is used to make a dessert or savory pie.

Pâté: A paste or thick spread made from meat, fish, cheese or vegetables. Bound with eggs, whipping cream, cognac or wine, and spices.

Patty: A small pie or pastry shell in which foods are served.

Petit Fours: Small, fancy cakes and biscuits.

Phyllo Dough: Dough rolled into paper-thin sheets; often layered to make flaky pastry crusts.

Picante Sauce: Spicy-hot sauce used in Mexican and Latin American dishes. Sometimes prepared chunky like salsa.

Piccalilli: A relish of sweet red and green peppers, green tomatoes, onions and spices.

Pigeon Peas: The edible, brown seeds of a tropical shrub.

Pilaf: Steamed, seasoned rice with chopped meat, seafood or vegetables.

Planked Steak: Small or quick cooking cuts of meat or fish on a plank and broiled under a flame.

Plantains: Starchy banana-shaped fruit. Used as a staple for cooking in the tropics. Served as a starch.

Polenta: A porridge-like cornmeal mush, served with sauce or as a side dish to meat. (Italian.)

Porridge: A boiled cereal (edible grain), often oatmeal cooked in water, and usually served with milk.

Porterhouse Steak: The choice steak; taken from the loin, with the largest portion of tenderloin.

Postum: The trade name of a coffee substitute made from grain.

Pot Pourri: A Spanish stew of meats and spices.

Prawn: A large shrimp or shrimp-like crustacean.

Prosciutto: Cured Italian ham. Deep-red and very spicy. Served in very thin slices.

Quiche: A pie made from eggs, cream, seasonings and often cheese, onions and spinach, in a crust.

Ragout: A seasoned stew of meat and vegetables.

Rasher of Bacon: One to three slices of bacon.

Rémoulade: A creamy, cold sauce made with mayonnaise, chopped pickles, capers, anchovies and herbs. Served over cold poultry or fish.

Risotto: Seasoned rice cooked in a broth. (Italian.)

Rissolé: Pastry with filling of different sorts of forcemeat, made in the shape of a turnover and deep fried.

Roquefort Cheese: Semi-hard, white, crumbly cheese streaked with green mold.

Roquefort Dressing: A French salad dressing made with Roquefort cheese.

Roulade: A thin slice of meat wrapped around a filling rolled into a sausage and cooked.

Round Steak: The top of the beef hindquarter.

Roux: A cooked mixture of fat and flour used for thickening sauces and stews.

Saccharin: A white, crystalline powder used as a sweetener. A coal-tar product.

Salami: A highly-spiced sausage of beef or pork. Hard or soft in consistency.

Salsa: A mild-to-hot, chunky Mexican garnish; usually made with chopped jalapeño or chili peppers, tomatoes, cilantro and spices. Salsa verde ("green salsa") is made with green chili peppers.

Saltine: Also called soda cracker. A thin, crisp cracker topped with salt.

Sauerkraut: Pickled cabbage.

Scallion: A small green onion with long, slender green leaves intact.

Scotch Broth: Lamb or mutton broth with barley, carrots and onions.

Scrapple: Meat from the hogshead cooked slowly with corn meal, buckwheat flour and herbs.

Scrod: A young cod or haddock.

Shallots: Vegetable of the onion family; similar to an onion in flavor and shape.

Shepherd's Pie: Casserole of cooked, cubed lamb or beef, topped with mashed potatoes and gravy.

Sherbet: Sweetened and flavored ice mixed with milk and beaten egg whites or gelatin.

Shish Kebab: Cubed meat or vegetables, cooked (usually grilled) on a skewer. (Turkish.)

Sirloin: Hindquarters of beef, first rib of quarter to hip or rump.

Sizzling Steak: Steak served on a heated platter which has been dotted with pieces of chopped suet so that steak and juices sizzle.

Smorgasbord: A large, varied spread of buffet-style dishes. (Swedish.)

Sorbet: An ice served between courses of a meal.

Soy Sauce: A dark, thin oriental sauce made from fermented soybeans and seasonings. Used to heighten the flavor of various dishes.

Spare Ribs: Pork trimmed from bacon sides.

Spoon Bread: Corn meal, butter, eggs and milk; this custard-like corn meal pudding makes a good potato substitute.

Squab: A very young pigeon.

Strata: A layered casserole; usually made with bread slices, cheese, milk and eggs.

Strudel: A flaky pastry usually filled with apple, butter, currants and chopped almond, flavored with cinnamon and a little brandy.

Succotash: A mixture of corn and lima or green beans with butter and seasonings.

Suet: Hard fat from beef.

Sweetbreads: The thymus gland of a calf.

Swiss Steak: A round or shoulder steak pounded with flour and seasonings, and braised.

Taco: A folded, crispy-fried corn tortilla stuffed with ground meat, shredded cheese and often fresh, chopped vegetables; served with chili sauce.

Table d'Hôtel: A full-course, fixed-price meal.

Tamale: A cornhusk spread with cornmeal paste, stuffed with a highly-seasoned meat and chili pepper mixture; then rolled, tied and steamed.

Tapas: An assortment of appetizers served with wine, often sherry, and other drinks. (Greek.)

Tapioca: A clear, beady starch product from cassava roots; used in pudding and for thickening.

Tartar Sauce: A sauce made with mayonnaise, vinegar, chopped pickles, onions, olives and capers; served over fish.

T-Bone Steak: Similar to a porterhouse, but with a "T"-shaped bone and less tenderloin.

Tenderloin: The most tender part of the loin of beef or pork. Resembles a fillet.

Terrapin: A saltwater turtle.

Thousand Island Dressing: A salad dressing made with mayonnaise, chili sauce, sweet pickles, onions, hard-boiled eggs and seasonings.

Tabasco: The trade name for a red pepper sauce.

Tofu: Soybean curd cakes, soft or hard; often used as a substitute for eggs or meat in dishes.

Tortilla: A thin, unleavened bread or pancake, made from flour or cornmeal. (Mexican.)

Tostada: A corn tortilla fried crisp and flat. Served with a refried bean or meat topping.

Tournedos: Slices of steak fillet, cut from the center of a beef tenderloin.

Truffle: An edible, underground fungus, considered a delicacy. Also, a fancy chocolate candy.

Tutti Frutti: A mixture of fruit flavors.

Velouté Sauce: A white sauce (béchamel), made with chicken, veal or fish stock.

Venison: Deer meat.

Vinaigrette: A sauce or dressing with a base of vinegar and oil mixed with herbs and seasonings.

Welsh Rarebit or Rabbit: Melted cheese scraps, highly seasoned, and served on toast or crackers.

White Sauce: Also called béchamel or "cream" sauce. A simple sauce made with milk, butter, flour and white pepper, the preparation varying the degree of thickness.

Wiener Schnitzel: Veal cutlet breaded and browned in hot fat and served with anchovy fillets and a slice of lemon. (German.)

Worcestershire Sauce: A pungent, spicy sauce made from soy, vinegar, spices and often, anchovy paste. (Worcester, England.)

Yams: A red, starchy root (tuber) similar to a sweet potato. (South and West Indies.)

Yeast: Microorganisms (one-celled fungi) which ferment carbohydrates (like breads), releasing carbon dioxide (gas bubbles) and alcohol, causing dough to rise.

Yogurt: A custard-like product made from milk fermented with special bacteria cultures. Plain or flavored; slightly acidic or tart in taste.

Yorkshire Rarebit: Welsh rarebit with bacon.

Yorkshire Pudding: A baked pudding made from batter, eggs, flour, milk and roast beef drippings.

Zest: The outermost, colored part of the citrus rind, which is grated and used for flavoring.

Zwieback: A highly-sweetened, crispy bread; twice-baked and sliced. (German.)

Zucchini: A variety of squash with a smooth, green skin and elongated shape.

Spices, Herbs & Seasonings

A Manual for Food Preparation in Walgreen Food Service Divisions
Originally titled: "Spices ~ A Modern Definition"
Revised and updated ~ from the *Walgreen Cookbook, Your Guide to Good Food*, circa 1945.

True Spices: Those products of aromatic, tropical plants; like peppers and cloves.

Herbs: The leaves of temperate-zone plants; like sage and oregano.

Aromatic Seed: Seeds used for seasoning or flavoring; like anise and caraway.

Miscellaneous Dry Seasonings: Seasonings which can be dried; like garlic, onion or celery. Also liquid or semi-liquid seasonings.

Buying Spices: Strength and quality of flavor are the most important considerations in buying spices. It is well worth the money to purchase higher quality spices.

Keeping Spices: Buy spices in moderation, and do not keep any spice more than six months. (It should not be necessary to keep most spices much more than a month.) Avoid prolonged exposure to air, excessive heat or moisture by keeping jar tightly closed when the spices are not being used. If the spices are left open, or placed in a warm location, they will lose their strength as the volatile flavor oils escape into the air. Excessive moisture also causes some spices to cake. Spices should be kept on a rack or shelf, away from stove or oven heat, or dishwashers.

Using Spices: Spices should be used to *enhance* flavor of food, not disguise it. If no formula is available, start with one-quarter teaspoon of spice ~ except red pepper ~ per pint of sauce, gravy, soup or vegetables; or per each pound of meat, fowl or fish. And increase the amount "to taste." In food preparation, ground spices should be added at the same time as salt. For *cooked* dishes that take longer to prepare, such as stews and soups, add the ground spices at the time of serving. Conversely, in foods that are *not cooked*, spices should be added well before serving. Spiced preparations that are refrigerated, such as salad dressings, should be allowed to stand at room temperature at least one hour before serving so that the flavors can properly blend.

Origins and Descriptions:

Allspice: Spice. West Indies, particularly Jamaica and Mexico. A pea-sized, green fruit that grows in small clusters on a tree; it is cured brown. As its name implies, Allspice is reminiscent of several spices, like cinnamon, nutmeg, and cloves.

Annatto Seeds: (Achiote.) Aromatic Seeds. From a tropical, American tree. Used for cooking, making oil and making a yellowish-red dye.

Anise: (Aniseed.) Aromatic Seeds. Small, oval, gray-brown seeds. Pungent, licorice flavor. Used in baking, and in making candy.

Basil: (Sweet Basil.) Herb. India and United States. From the mint family. Clean, dried leaves and tender stems; with an aromatic flavor. Used in tomato dishes, vegetables and meats.

Bay Leaves: Herb. Mediterranean. Smooth, oblong, dried leaves of an evergreen tree. Sweet, spicy flavor. Used for pickling, stews and soups.

427

Black Pepper: Spice. India and Indonesia. The small, dried berry of the pepper vine. A *peppercorn* is the whole pepper. Warm, pungent, aromatic flavor. Used frequently, in most dishes.

Capers: Herb. Mediterranean. Flower buds of the caper shrub; pickled or dried. Tart, acidic flavor. Used in salads, sauces, seafoods, and as a garnish.

Caraway Seeds: Aromatic Seed. Northern Europe and Asia. Curved, spiky seeds with a warm, sweet, sharp taste. Delicately licorice and nutty. Used in rye bread and vegetable dishes.

Cayenne Pepper: Spice. Africa. A mixture of powdered pods and seeds from hot red peppers. Very hot, savory flavor. Used with meats, sauces.

Celery Seed: Aromatic Seed. India and Southern Europe. A tiny, olive-brown seed. Flavor resembles celery, but is stronger. Used in pickling, salads and dressing. Celery salt is the ground seed mixed with fine salt.

Chervil: Herb. Dried or fresh. Fresh leaves resemble parsley. Delicate, tarragon-like flavor. Used as a fine, subtle seasoning with fish, eggs, cream sauces.

Chili Powder: Spice. Made from dried Mexican chili peppers, cumin seed and other spices. Used in chili con carne, seafood cocktails, omelettes.

Cilantro: (Chinese Parsley.) Aromatic Seed. The leaves of fresh coriander. Resembles parsley. Tangy, minty flavor. Used in salsa, pasta dishes.

Cinnamon: Spice. Southeast Asia. The dried, aromatic bark of a bushy evergreen (cassia) that grows 30 to 50-feet high. Sweet, spicy flavor. Sold in sticks or ground. Used in desserts and drinks.

Cloves: Spice. East Indies. The dark-brown or reddish-brown, unopened flower buds of an evergreen tree. Flavor is sweet and mildly spicy. Used in ham, roasts and pickling.

Coriander: Aromatic Seed. Mediterranean. An herb, the seeds of which are used for seasoning. See *Cilantro*.

Cumin: Aromatic Seed. Mediterranean Islands and Morocco. Small and oblong with a strong, caraway-like flavor. Chief ingredient of chili and curry powders. Used in soups and meats.

Curry Powder: Spice. India. A bright yellow, blended condiment containing cumin, coriander, turmeric, other spices. Used with fish and meat.

Dill: Herb. Fresh dill or dill weed has feathery, fern-like leaves. The tan seeds are tiny and oval. Used in pickling and with fish and cucumbers.

Garlic: A pungent, edible bulb of the lily family. The cloves are minced and used to flavor meats, salads and sauces. Garlic salt is ground, dried garlic mixed with fine salt.

Fennel: Herb. Tiny, yellow-brown seeds with a licorice-like flavor. Used in vegetable dishes.

Ginger: Spice. Jamaica, West Africa, India, and the Orient. The pungent, aromatic root of a tropical Asian plant. Yellow-orange on the outside, and yellow-brown on the inside. Flavor is warm and pungently spicy. Used in cakes, pumpkin pie, pot roast, canned fruit and India pudding.

Mace: Spice. East and West Indies. The orange-red, fleshy growth between the nutmeg shell and outer husk. Flavor resembles nutmeg. Used whole (called Blade) in fish sauce, pickling and gingerbread batter, or ground in cakes and chocolate.

Marjoram: Herb. Europe and South America. Small, gray-green leaves. Related to oregano, with an aromatic, spicy-bitter taste. Used in stews, soups, sauces, fish and lamb roast.

Mint: Herb. United States. A perennial herb with soft, fuzzy, green leaves. Pungent and aromatic. Used as a garnish and with meat, vegetables, salads. The oil extract flavors gum, candy, jelly.

Mustard: Spice. United States. A brown, black, yellow or white seed. Very pungent flavor. Powdered or prepared as a condiment. Used with salads, meats, fish and vegetables.

Nutmeg: Spice. East and West Indies. The seed of the nutmeg fruit that resembles an apricot; it grows on a 40-foot high, bushy tree. Sweet, spicy, nutty flavor. Used in eggnog, sauces, puddings and meat pies.

Onions: A pungent, fleshy, edible bulb of the lily family. Used to flavor soups, chowders, meat and relishes. Scallions are small green onions, diced and used as a garnish or seasoning. Onion salt is ground, dried onion mixed with fine salt.

Oregano: (Mexican Sage.) Herb. Italy and Mexico. Similar to marjoram in flavor, but stronger. Used for pork dishes, beef stews, meat sauces, gravies and salads.

Paprika: Spice. Spain, Hungary and United States. Sweet red pepper, diced and ground after the seeds and stems have been removed. Spanish variety is mild; Hungarian variety is slightly spicy, aromatic and sweet. Used as a colorful, red garnish for any pale food such as fish, salad dressings, vegetables, meats, gravies and goulash.

Parsley: Herb. United States. A green biennial herb with a stalk and tiny, tree-like leaves. Used as a garnish, and with meat, vegetables and salads.

Pepper: See *black, red, white, or Cayenne.*

Pickling Spice: United States. An assortment of a dozen or more whole spices such as bay leaves, dill seed, allspice, cinnamon, ginger and mustard seed. Used for pickling and in sauces.

Pimento: The fleshy fruit of the Spanish paprika. Sold canned or bottled, usually chopped or diced. Used in meats, vegetables and salads; and stuffed into green olives.

Poppy Seeds: Aromatic Seeds. Netherlands. The tiny, crunchy, black seeds of the poppy plant. Nut-like flavor. Used as a topping for breads, cakes, cookies, buttered noodles, and as a pastry filling.

Poultry Seasoning: A mixture of herbs and spices such as sage, thyme, and marjoram. Used for poultry, veal, pork, fish, stuffings and meat loaf.

Pumpkin Pie Spice: A mixture of spices, such as cinnamon, cloves and ginger. Used for pumpkin pie, spiced cookies and gingerbread.

Red Pepper: Spice. United States. Pungent and very hot. Used as flakes or whole, chopped. Used in relishes, hot sauces, highly-spiced meat dishes.

Rosemary: Herb. Southern Europe. The leaves and flowers of the Rosemary evergreen plant. Flavor is sweet, fresh and lemony. Used with fish, stews, lamb, pork, stuffings and boiled potatoes.

Saffron: Spice. Mediterranean. The world's most expensive spice, Saffron is the orange stigma of a flower similar to a crocus. Used for its rich, orange-gold color and its agreeable, slightly bitter, vanilla-like flavor. Used in baking and to color rice.

Sage: Herb. The best comes from Yugoslavia, but it is also grown in Greece. Long, slender, velvety leaves. Sage is a perennial shrub about 2-feet high. Flavor is minty and spicy. Used with pork, fish, poultry, stuffings and Manhattan clam chowder.

Savory: Herb. France and Spain. *Summer* (more common, used in early American cooking) or *winter* varieties. An herb, the leaves of which have a mild, mint flavor, resembling thyme. Used in dressings and stuffing, poultry, meat, fish, sauces.

Sesame Seeds: Aromatic Seeds. Asia. Small honey-colored seeds. The best grade is a fancy orange variety from Turkey. A rich, toasted-nut flavor. Baked on rolls, breads and buns.

Shallot: An edible, bulbous plant, related to the onion, but with a milder flavor.

Tarragon: Herb. Spain and France. A small perennial plant which forms tall stalks about 1½-yards high. Flavor is minty and anise-like. Used in salads, sauces and vinegar.

Thyme: Herb. Southern Europe. Thyme is the leaves and stems of a 1-inch high shrub. Flavor is strong, distinct and tea-like. Used in stews, soups, poultry stuffing, clam chowder, stewed tomatoes and fricassee.

Turmeric: Spice. India. The aromatic, powdered root of the turmeric plant. Used as a condiment and as a yellow dye.

White Pepper: Spice. India and Indonesia. The black peppercorn with the outer pulp fiber removed. Milder in taste and finer in texture than black pepper. Used in soups and white sauces.

Abbreviations & Equivalents

Revised and updated ~ from the *Walgreen Cookbook, Your Guide to Good Food*, circa 1945.

F.G.	=	Few Grains	°C	=	Degrees Centigrade
t or tsp.	=	Teaspoon	°F	=	Degrees Fahrenheit
T or Tbsp.	=	Tablespoon	1 Tablespoon	=	3 Teaspoons
C.	=	Cup	1 Cup	=	16 Tablespoons
Pt.	=	Pint	1 Pint	=	2 Cups
Qt.	=	Quart	1 Quart	=	4 Cups or 2 Pints
Gal.	=	Gallon	1 Gallon	=	4 Quarts
Pk.	=	Peck	1 Peck	=	8 Quarts
Bu.	=	Bushel	1 Bushel	=	4 Pecks or 32 Quarts
Gm.	=	Gram	1 Ounce	=	28.35 Grams
Oz.	=	Ounce	1 Pound	=	16 Ounces
Lb. or #	=	Pound	1 Fluid Quart	=	32 Ounces
No.	=	Number	1 Fluid Pint	=	16 Ounces
A.P.	=	As Purchased	1 Fluid Cup	=	8 Ounces
E.P.	=	Edible Portion	½ Fluid Ounce	=	1 Tablespoon

The formulas above are based
on the following:

Standard level measures:
- Set of Measuring Spoons
- 8 Ounce Measuring Cup
- Quart Measure

Plus:
- An Accurate Scale

Cooking Terms Defined

A Manual for Food Preparation in Walgreen Food Service Divisions

Revised and updated ~ from the *Walgreen Cookbook, Your Guide to Good Food,* circa 1945.

FOOD PREPARATION

Bard: To cover (lean) meat with a thin layer of fat before roasting, thus retaining its moisture.

Baste: To brush, spoon or squeeze melted fat, drippings or seasoned sauce over food while cooking, moistening it and adding flavor.

Beat: To mix rapidly, incorporating air into mixture, thus making it smooth and light.

Blend: To thoroughly mix, either by hand or in a blender, two or more ingredients to make a uniform mixture.

Bone: To remove the bones from meats, fish or poultry.

Bread: To coat food with bread crumbs, cracker crumbs or cornmeal. An egg and milk coating are usually used first to help crumbs adhere.

Bruise: To partially crush food, such as garlic cloves, thus releasing their flavor.

Chop: To coarsely cut food into small pieces with a knife or other sharp tool; chopped foods are coarsely cut.

Clarify: To separate solids from a liquid, making it clear. Clarified butter is the clear, yellow liquid that separates from the butter when it is melted; it is used for cooking (because it does not burn or spoil easily) and seasoning.

Cream: To beat ingredients, usually butter or other fat alone or with sugar, until smooth and creamy.

Crimp: To make a fluted, sealed edge by pinching together edges of a pie or pastry.

Cube: To cut food into equally-sized, square chunks, at least ½-inch thick. Also, to tenderize meat by cutting the top in a checkerboard pattern, as with cube steak.

Cure: To preserve meat, fish or cheese by salting, smoking or drying (aging).

Cutting or Cut In: To mix shortening (or any solid fat) into dry ingredients, using a pastry blender or knives, until texture is coarse and mealy.

Devein: To remove the spine from shrimp.

Deglaze: To mix pan drippings (leftover glaze and meat bits) with a liquid, then heat or reduce the mixture to form a natural sauce.

Degrease: To remove grease from food, particularly soups and gravies, by skimming it off the top with a spoon or skimmer; or by chilling food until fat solidifies and then lifting it off.

Dice: To cut into small cubes, usually ⅛ to ¼-inch thick.

Dot: To sprinkle butter bits over food, which adds flavor and keeps food moist while baking.

Draw: To remove the entrails of poultry, fish or meat.

Dredge: To cover food with a dry ingredient, such as flour or sugar, by dredging, shaking or sifting.

Dress: To mix food with a dressing or sauce. Also, to clean poultry, fish or meat.

Drizzle: To sprinkle food lightly with liquid.

Dust: To sprinkle food lightly with a dry or powdery mixture.

Eviscerate: See "Draw."

Flute: To make small, decorative indentations or scallops on a piecrust or vegetables.

Fold: To mix an ingredient into another by gently turning it with a spatula. Usually refers to mixing a light substance, such as whipping cream or beaten egg whites, with a heavier substance to help it retain volume.

Garnish: To decorate food with colorful herbs and seasonings, sliced fruit, or vegetables before serving.

Glaze: To cover food with a shiny coating.

Grate: To shred food by rubbing it using a metal utensil (grater) with sharp-edged holes.

Grind: To process or crush food into fine particles.

Julienne: To cut into long, thin strips. Also, often refers to vegetables and meats prepared in this manner.

Knead: To manipulate dough with a pressing motion accompanied by a rhythmic pressing-folding-turning pattern until smooth and shiny.

Larding: To insert strips (lardons or lardoons) of pork fat into lean meat to give it a richer flavor and keep it moist and succulent throughout cooking.

Macerate: To soak fruits and vegetables in a liquid, usually a liqueur, to add flavor and soften.

Marinate: To soak meats, poultry or fish in a spicy liquid (marinade), to add flavor and tenderize.

Mask: To enhance or improve the appearance or flavor of a food with a spice or sauce.

Mince: To cut food into pieces, finer than chopping, but not as fine as grinding.

Mix: To stir together using a circular motion.

Mold: To pour food into a decorative pan (mold) and steaming, baking or chilling it to make food retain shape.

Pare: To shave off the outer skin of a fruit or vegetable.

Pasteurize: To destroy bacteria in dairy foods and fruit juices by heating. This allows the product to be kept fresh for longer periods of time.

Peel: To remove the skin (peel) of fruits or vegetables.

Pickle: To preserve or flavor food in a seasoned brine or vinegar mixture.

Pipe: To push soft, smooth food (such as icing) through a pastry tube to make decorative shapes or a border (piping) on cakes or other foods.

Plump: To soak dried fruits in a liquid, causing them to swell.

Proof: To test the potency of yeast in a warm, dry spot.

Purée: To make a smooth, thick pulp or paste by putting food through a food processor, blender or food mill. Usually refers to vegetables or fruit, but can also be meat.

Reconstitute: To restore concentrated food to its natural liquid state, usually by adding water.

Refresh: To revive or cool boiled food by plunging it into cold water to set color and flavor.

Scallop or Escallop: 1. To bake in cream or a cream sauce underneath a bread crumb topping. 2. To make a fluted edge (usually on a piecrust). 3. A small, thin slice of meat. 4. A species of bivalve shellfish (scallop).

Score: To cut shallow slits in the surface of a food to tenderize it and help it keep its shape during cooking. Also, to decorate food.

Shred: To cut or grate food into thin slivers (shreds) using a knife or grater.

Shuck: To remove oyster, clam or other bivalve shellfish meat from its shell. Also, to remove husks from corn.

Sift: To remove lumps from dry ingredients, such as flour and baking powder, by putting them through a sifter. Also, to add volume.

Skim: To remove melted fat or accumulated particles (scum) from the surface of a liquid.

Slice: To cut a food into thin pieces.

Stir: To mix ingredients in a circular motion with a spoon or whisk.

Truss: To tie-up or bind the legs and wings of poultry with string or skewers before cooking, to retain shape during cooking.

Unmold: To turn a food out of its mold while retaining its molded (decorative) shape.

Whip: To beat liquid food rapidly with a whisk or rotary or electric beater. This lightens mixture with air (aerate) and increases its volume.

Whisk: To beat or mix liquid food using a utensil made of looped wires (a whisk or whip).

METHODS OF COOKING

Bake: To cook with continuous dry heat, usually in a gas or electric oven. Before baking, the oven is usually preheated.

Barbecue: To cook food on a grill over a live fire of charcoal or wood. Also refers to the preparation by which grilled food is covered with a seasoned "barbecue" sauce.

Blanch: To boil (usually vegetables) in water for a very short time; this loosens skin, seals in juices, sets color and destroys bacteria when canning or freezing.

Boil: To cook by boiling in liquid or water; or to heat liquid until it bubbles rapidly (212 degrees at sea level). Slowly-boiling water is as effective as rapidly-boiling water, with less steam (heat loss).

Braise: To brown in fat, then cook slowly (at a low temperature) in a covered pan, using a small amount of liquid. Braising is done in an oven or over direct heat.

Broil: To cook in a broiling (at its hottest setting) oven, under strong, direct heat. Food is placed on a special pan or grill which allows fat or liquid to drip through.

Brown: To sear meat at the highest heat level in a broiler, skillet or oven, locking in juices and giving it color before adding it to a stew or other dish.

Caramelize: To heat sugar over low heat until it melts and turns a golden-brown color. Also, to glaze food with caramelized sugar.

Coddle: To carefully poach food in water that is below the boiling point (barely simmering).

Deep-Fry or French-Fry: To cook (usually breaded) food covered in a deep layer of hot fat (animal or vegetable oil), usually about 360 degrees, until food is light-brown and crispy textured. Also called "deep-fat frying."

433

Fricassee: To gently stew food, usually poultry or small game. The pieces are first dredged and browned; then cooked and covered in liquid or sauce, often in the company of vegetables.

Frizzle: To fry thinly sliced food in a small amount of fat, turning it crispy and brown.

Fry: To cook food in a skillet with fat, without pouring off drippings. Deep-fat frying or panfrying are variations of frying.

Grill: To cook food on a grill, commonly over charcoal, over intense heat.

Hard-Cooked or Hard-Boiled: A food cooked to a solid consistency (usually an egg in its shell).

Panbroil: To fry food in its own fat in an uncovered skillet, over high heat. Accumulated fat is poured off.

Panfry: To fry food in a small amount (for sautéing) or layer (for browning) of hot fat, or in its own fat (for panbroiling).

Parboil: To partially cook (precook) food, by boiling it in water or in its own juices.

Parch: To dry corn or other starchy vegetables by roasting.

Poach: To cook submerged in simmering liquid.

Pressure Cook: To cook by steam at a pressure from 5 to 30 pounds and at a temperature of 228 to 274 degrees.

Reduce: To decrease the volume of a liquid by boiling it rapidly, uncovered, so that the excess water evaporates and flavor is concentrated.

Render: To liquefy fat by heating it, such as with cooking fatty meat to produce liquid fat. Rendered lard is smooth and creamy, almost pure fat.

Roast: To cook uncovered with dry heat. See "Bake."

Sauté: To cook food quickly in a pan, over direct heat, using a small amount of fat.

Scald: To heat liquid (usually milk) just to the boiling point until bubbles begin to gather around the edge of the pan. Also, to dunk solid food into boiling water very briefly to loosen its skin.

Sear: To heat or brown meat quickly at a very intense heat, to seal in juices and intensify flavor.

Simmer: To heat liquid to about 185 degrees, just until bubbles begin to form. Also, to cook food in simmering liquid.

Steam: To cook food over boiling water without touching the water, allowing the steam formed in the pan to do the cooking.

Steep: To pour boiling water over a food (such as tea) and letting it soak, extracting flavor and color.

Stew: To cook food submerged in liquid for long period of time, at a low temperature. Also refers to food cooked in this manner.

Stir-fry: To quickly cook thinly sliced food in a small amount of vegetable oil in a skillet or wok while stirring constantly. This Chinese style of cooking preserves food color, texture and flavor.

Toast: To brown bread by heating.

Fat Substitutes

Fat Substitute	Fat	Use in	Saves up to
Prune or apple butter, or apple sauce	Butter, margarine or oil ~ *all but 1 tablespoon* with prune or apple butter, or *up to ½-cup* with apple sauce	Baked goods ~ like cakes, breads, muffins or brownies	40 calories and 5 grams fat per serving (1 brownie, for example)
Liquid egg substitutes	Whole eggs	Most recipes ~ *except* where beaten egg whites are needed (meringues)	50 calories, 5 grams fat and 200 milligrams cholesterol per egg
Low-fat or fat-free cottage cheese ~ sweetened and puréed	Heavy cream ~ sweetened and whipped	Dessert topping	40 calories and 5 grams fat per tablespoon (using low-fat cottage cheese)
Fat-free or low-fat cream cheese	Regular cream cheese	Cheesecake ~ to prevent cracking, beat cream cheese well before adding egg; don't over-beat	160 calories and 22 grams fat per serving (1 slice, using fat-free cream cheese)
Non-stick cooking spray	Butter, margarine, or oil	Dish or pan bottoms ~ when sautéing or baking (instead of greasing)	30 calories and 4 grams fat
Low-fat or fat-free plain yogurt	Sour cream ~ replace half or entire amount with yogurt	Most recipes ~ on stovetop, use low heat to prevent curdling; for more stability, add 1 tablespoon cornstarch to 1 cup yogurt	40 calories and 5 grams fat per serving (1 slice coffee cake, for example, using low-fat plain yogurt)
Balsamic vinegar and vegetable oil ~ mix 1 part to 1 part	Vinegar and oil ~ the standard combination: 1 part vinegar to 2 parts oil	Salad dressings	20 calories and 2 grams fat per tablespoon
Skim or low-fat (1%) milk	Whole milk	Most recipes ~*except* puddings, sauces and custards	50 calories and 6 grams fat per cup of milk
Low-sodium chicken broth ~ 2 tablespoons	Cooking oil ~ 1 tablespoon	Vegetable dishes ~ stir-fried or sautéed	115 calories and 13 grams fat

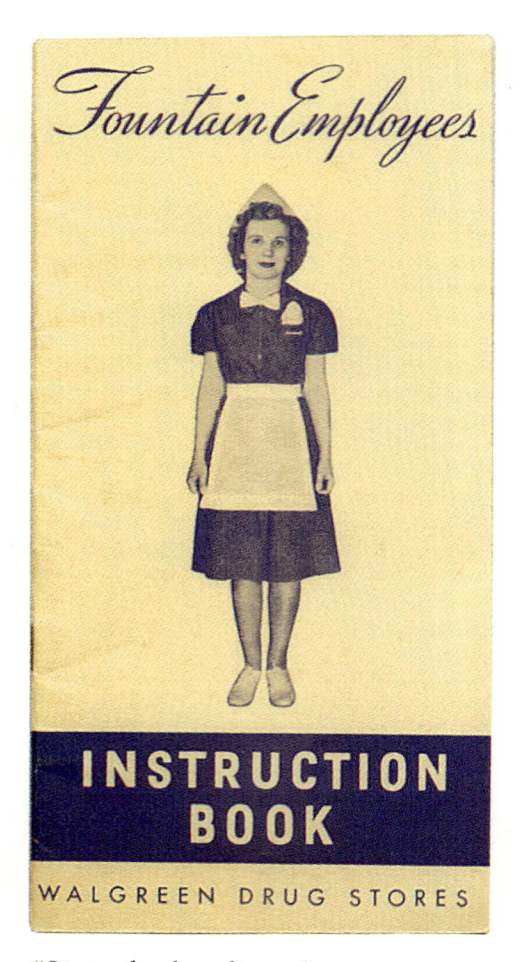

"Since the founding of our company, millions of folks have come to know our slogan, 'You're Always Welcome at Walgreens.' It is part of your task to give life to this slogan to every customer, whether the request be great or small."

Charles R. Walgreen, Jr. addressed his new fountain employees in this 1942 instruction book.

Personal Appearance & Conduct
A Behavior Guide for Walgreen Food Service Divisions
Unedited ~ from the *Walgreen Cookbook, Your Guide to Good Food*, circa 1945.

A Word to the Wise...

We are dealers in commodities of luxury, catering to those desiring refreshing deliciousness. **Taste, Eye Appeal** and a uniformally high standard of **Quality** and **Service** are necessary. A concentrated effort must be made to satisfy these before you can hope to bring your customers back and back again.

COURTEOUS SERVICE

Service creates good will, and good will defined, is the disposition of a person to return to the place where they have been well served. Courteous attention without the prevailing accommodation attitude, is vital. There is no excuse for an indifferent attitude.

Service to *every* customer at a Walgreen Fountain *must* include:

A. Greeting the customer by name, if possible, with a cheery greeting such as: "Good morning, Mr. —" or "How do you do? What may I serve you?" Never say, "What's yours?" or "Yours?"

B. In approaching a customer, always be sure counters or tables are clean and dry.

C. A glass of water with cracked ice, and a fresh napkin.

D. Present open menu to customer and when there seems to be doubt or hesitation in deciding an order, an intelligent suggestion should be offered in a courteous and helping manner. For example, at lunch time, suggest the feature luncheon or sandwich luncheon; in the afternoon, a sandwich, malted milk, cake á la mode or a sundae; in the evening, a sandwich luncheon, a hot dish or a special sundae, etc.

E. Refill glass of water. The fact that other people do not refill water glasses will make the customer appreciate it when we do it at our Fountains. Keep water decanter on table.

F. Give the customer his check promptly and immediately after serving the last item of his order. A sincere and clearly spoken "thank you" must accompany the giving of each check.

G. Before customer leaves, ask very pleasantly if the food was satisfactory, and if there is any other service you can give him.

With a sincere effort on the part of every fountain employee to make each customer feel that his patronage is appreciated, and that there is a sincere desire to give him the best possible service, there is no limit to the success of this fountain.

PERSONAL APPEARANCE

Table Girls ~ Before Going on Duty

1. Clean hands and neatly manicured finger nails. BRIGHT POLISH ON NAILS PROHIBITED.
2. Have hair net carefully adjusted over neatly combed hair.
3. Have clean head band on so it holds ends of hair snugly.
4. Use powder, rouge, lipstick sparingly.
5. SMILE.
6. Do not chew gum on duty at any time.
7. Avoid bad breath; use mouth wash regularly.
8. Be ready to speak pleasantly to customer.
9. Have clean towel, neatly folded.
10. Remove all jewelry except bar pin to hold neck of dress properly closed. Never use safety pins; conceal pins used in adjusting uniform. The pins must never show.
11. Use some deodorant to prevent body odors. Bathe daily.
12. Be sure handkerchief is clean before putting it in pocket.
13. Wear a clean apron and be careful not to have it too short.
14. Clean stockings neatly adjusted.
15. Well polished shoes.
16. Wear rubber heels.
17. Memorize menus and prices.

Soda Men ~ Before Going on Duty

1. Clean hands and fingernails.
2. Clean face and clean shave.
3. Comb hair neatly; have hair cut regularly.
4. Have clean soda cap on straight and properly.
5. Brush teeth twice daily.
6. Avoid bad breath; use mouth wash regularly.
7. Do not chew gum on duty.
8. SMILE.
9. Be ready to speak pleasantly to customer.
10. Wear clean shirt. White shirt only.
11. Wear Walgreen standard bow tie properly.
12. No body odors. Use deodorant. Bathe daily.
13. Wear badge on left side properly.
14. Clean soda jacket properly buttoned.
15. Wear rubber heels.
16. Have shoes polished.
17. Have clean bar towel folded on creamer.
18. Memorize menus and prices.

PERSONAL CONDUCT

➤ Always have a place for everything and everything in its place. Take as much personal pride in yourself and surroundings as if it were your own business.

➤ On duty as well as off duty, soda men should be gentlemen. There is nothing to be gained by using slang or profanity or by being abusive and noisy.

➤ Never put your hands into a glass or cup except to wash it. All glassware and dishes must be clean and spotless. Never give water glass or coffee cup to customer with fingers touching the rims. Hold tumbler near the bottom and cup by the handle.

➤ Don't lean on the counter.

➤ Don't refuse anyone a glass of water.

➤ Don't let a customer leave dissatisfied; make the drink again, or make something else if desired.

➤ Don't deviate from formulas definitely decided upon.

➤ Don't sneeze over or around food; use a clean folded handkerchief.

➤ Don't reach in front of the customer, but if unavoidable, say, "Pardon, please."

➤ Don't wear caps and head bands at an angle; put them on straight.

➤ Don't argue with a customer.

➤ Don't eat or drink behind the counter.

➤ Don't vary portions; all portions should be the same to all customers.

➤ Don't visit over the counter or back of the counter with your co-workers.

➤ Don't use code in giving orders; call a sundae, soda, etc. by their proper name.

➤ Don't have B.O. (Body Odor.)

➤ Don't smell or sniff a customer's food.

➤ Don't wear old sloppy shoes, frayed or dirty pants.

Walgreen Alumni Acknowledgements

We thank the following Walgreen Alumni, family and friends
for their gracious support and recipe contributions.

Allen, Carl A.	Campbell, Helen	Gaspard, Patti
Allen, Gigi	Campbell, Kathleen	Gentile, Annette
Allen, Katie	Campbell, Linda	Gentile, Louise
Amirouche, Ginger	Caplan, Roberta	Gentile, Marsha Bartholomei
Anderson, Florence	Carlson, Helen	Gerdes, Gladis
Anglade, Hank	Celozzi, Carol	Gilroy, Ethel J.
Aspinall, Scott	Celozzi, Roseanne	Gladys, Green
Atlas, Judy	Cohen, Shelley	Good, Marlene
Baer, Rosemary	Commo, Kathryn	Graham, William
Balkany, Ella	Conway, Genevieve	Graham, Kyong
Ball, Evelyn R.	Corey, Marie M.	Grassie, Colin S.
Banks, Maxine	Correia, Robert W.	Grassie, Jorie
Barry, Christina Hudson	Coryell, Louise	Grassie, Lilias
Barry, Nell	Coryell, Robert E.	Green, Barb
Beckman, Penny Edger	Cramer, Mrs. Alvin	Grejczyk, Gary
Berg, Irene	de Frank, John	Hackworth, Lula Mae
Bernauer, Mary	de Frank, Mrs. P.	Hagen, Clare A.
Bernier, Therese	de Frank, Sandi	Haines, Margaret Pennebaker
Biek, Ann	DeRosa, Eric	Hamilton, Deborah A.
Biek, Tara L.	Dilts, Anne McCulloch	Heller, Janet Haines
Boerner, Laura	Dimitriou, Chris	Hickman, Carolyn L.
Boldt, Lucille M.	Duncan, Lillie M.	Holm, Betty
Bonk, Marie D.	Dwyer, Jerene M.	Holvay Family
Bonsignore, Albert J.	Dwyer, Patra N.	Horak, Millie
Bonsignore, Eve	Earnest, Gayle	Hudson, Phyllis
Bonsignore, Louis J.	Eckstaedt, Martha Bonk	Hunter, Joy
Bonsignore, Vicki	Engelmann, Erin	Hyatt, Betty
Bonsignore, Vincent	Erbacci, Yolanda	Jacobs, Julie
Borek, Pauline	Erickson, Donna	Jacobsen, Lorraine
Boucher, Jerry	Faragia, Mary	Johnson, Frances
Boyles, Fay	Fedor, Gertrude	Jorndt, Pat
Brandenburg, Esther	Fink, Gertrude	Karl, Jane Boyd
Brown, Mary	Flori, Mildred Bartholomei	Karlin, Carol
Brunner, Sharon	Fordonski, Lillian	Kerstner, Jane
Bucaro, Kaitlin Rose	Freeman, Merelyn M.	Kramer, Kathy
Bucaro, Michelle Gentile	Frey, Audrey	Kraska, Jamie
Bucaro, Rosemary	Fritsch, Judy	Kraska, Judee
Buerger, Karen	Galioto, August C.	Lichtman, Gloria H.
Campbell, Dorothy	Gammon, Bev	Liphardt, Florence

Continued...

Locy, Grace
Lucas, Dolly
Lyskawa, Jo
Malcoun, Penny
Meinke, Richard
Merrifield, Carolyn
Meyer, Laurie
Meyers, Maureen Walsh
Miller, Kay
Mitchell, Allyson
Mitchell, Bob
Molnar, Lydia
Moore, Judy
Nachman, Cathy
Nachman, Ros
Navis, Lorraine
Neumiller-Heller, Cathie
Neumiller, Joan Dilts
Newman, Mrs. Barney
Nickels, Jim
Norman, Angela
Novak, Louise
Oettinger, Sheila
Pankey, Ella
Pankros, Matilda
Patitz, Doris
Pawlak, Josephine
Peralta, Edwardo
Perlstein, Evelyn
Pfeffer, Lisa B.
Pippert, Loraine Doelger
Polark, Bobbi

Powelson, Katie L.
Powers, Jean L.
Press, Rhoda
Przybylski, Frank R.
Raaber, Violet
Repke, Anna Mae
Retz, Marcy
Reuther, Betty
Roby, Ann H.
Romps, Betty
Rubino, Ronnie
Sachrison, Marie S.
Sandberg, Adeline
Sanner, Fern
Sanner, Lou
Schluckwerder, Ralph L.
Schwemm, Nan
Sensyk, Emily
Shank, Bill
Sheridan, Eileen
Shiel, Laurie
Sikorski, Halina
Simon, Bernece
Sinclair, Craig M.
Sinclair, Gloria
Sipple, Joyce
Small, Nancy
Smith, Connie
Smith, Gloria
Smith, Martin D.
Spata, Rose A.
Starmann, Madge
Steele, Roberta
Stoddard, Audrey

Stolzman, Agnes
Sutherland, Dan
Teeters, Marion
Theisen, Betty
Thomas, Judy
Ulinski, Katie
Umbach, Irene
Umbach, Richard
Urban, Peggy
Waits, W. Dawson
Walder, Mrs. Robert
Walgreen Family
Walgreen, Alexis
Walgreen, Brooke
Walgreen, Buffy
Walgreen, Charles R., Jr.
Walgreen, Mrs. Charles R., Jr.
Walgreen, Charles R., III
Walgreen, Charles Richard
Walgreen, Chris P.
Walgreens, Estelle G.
Walgreen, Kathleen B.
Walgreen, Kevin P.
Walgreen, Les
Walgreen, Nadia
Walker, Steve
Waters, Ward
Williams, Betty
Wilson, Bodil
Wirsing, Mary L.
Wisler, Ethel
Wolff, Rachel
Zelazny, Sandy
Zygmun, Patricia

Recipe Index

A

Angel Hair Pasta (Capellini), *See "Pasta"*
APPETIZERS
    Artichoke Balls…31
    Artichoke Dip Bucaro…31
    Artichoke Dip, Jean's…31
    Basil Pâté, Marlene's…21
    Breadsticks, Becky's Bacon…36
    Broccoli, Spicy Spread…35
    Bruschetta…28
    Caviar Cream Cheese Spread…28
    Ceviche…98
    Cheese Dip, Italian…21
    Cheese on Rye…20
    Cheese Spread, Hungarian…20
    Cheese Spread, Liptoi…20
    Cheese Things, Emergency…21
    Chili Dip, Hot…27
    Clam Dip, Chris'…25
    Crab Meat Dip…24
    Crab Meat Spread…25
    Crab, Hot, Fondue…24
    Curry Spread or Dip…29
    Fruit Spread, Healthy…19
    Garlic Cloves, Roasted…19
    Girls' Day Out Dip…27
    Guacamole…26
    Ham, Deviled, Cornucopias…35
    Meatballs Bourguignon…37
    Meatballs, Beefy…36
    Meatballs, Crazy…37
    Meatballs, Swedish…38
    Mexican Dip…27
    Mushroom Turnovers…32
    Mushrooms, Crisp, Golden…32
    Mushrooms, Stuffed…33
    Nacho Dip…26
    Party Mix, TV…33
    Quesadillas…38
    Salmon Spread…25
    Sandwiches, Cucumber…19
    Sandwiches, Kentucky Hot Brown…30
    Sausage & Sauerkraut Bites…29
    Shrimp in Cocktail Sauce…23
    Shrimp Mold…22
    Shrimp, Bacon-Wrapped…23
    Shrimp, Cheese & Bacon Delight…22
    Shrimp, Louisiana Mustard Sauce…23
    Spinach Strudel…34
    Spinach, Balls…34
    Steak Tartare…39
    Sweet Brie…39
    Water Chestnuts in Bacon…30
    Welsh Rarebit, Walsh's…392
Apple(s), *See "Fruit(s)"*
Apricot(s), *See "Fruit(s)"*
Artichoke(s), *See "Vegetables"*
Asparagus, *See "Vegetables"*
Au Jus, *See "Sauce(s)"*
Avocado(s), *See "Vegetables"*

B

Bacon, *See "Meat(s)"*
Baked Beans, *See "Vegetables, Bean(s)"*
Banana(s), *See "Fruit(s)"*
Barbecue Recipes
    Beef, Emily's Barbecued…136
    Chicken, Oven-Barbecued…193
    Sauce…136, 159
    Shrimp, Barbecued…112
    Spareribs, Barbecued…159
Barley, *See "Grain(s)"*
Bars, *See "Desserts"*
Batter
    Beer, for Fish…97
    Tempura…109
Bean(s), *See "Vegetables"*
Beef, *See "Meat(s)"*
Beer, Batter, for Fish…97
Beet(s), *See "Vegetables"*
BEVERAGES
    Bloody Mary, Happy Harry's…415
    Brandy Ice…412
    Cider, Spicy, Hot…413
    Coffee, Iced, Seneca…412
    Eggnog, Extraordinary…412
    Float, Coke or Root Beer…416
    Glög, Solberg's…414
    Julius "Barry"…416
    Lime Rickeys, Raspberry…414
    Malted Milk, Old-Fashioned Chocolate…411
    Mint Julip Walgreen…414
    Punch, Baby Shower…416
    Punch, Banana…417
    Punch, Thunderbolt…415
    Rum, Hot, Buttered Mix, Airdrie House…413
    Shake, Sampler Thick…411
    Wine, Grape, Old-Country…417
Black-Eyed Pea(s), *See "Vegetables"*
Blueberry(ies), *See "Fruit(s)"*
Bran, *See "Grain(s)"*
BREAD(S)
    Applesauce Nut, One-Bowl…302
    Armenian, Amarillo…303
    Banana, Saint John…300
    Bonanza…301
    Cheese Caraway Batter…307
    Cheese Loaf, Pull-Apart…300
    Cranberry…11
    Irish Soda…307
    Mandel…306
    Oatmeal, Molasses…306
    Pineapple Date-Nut…302
    Poppy Seed, Almond, Conway's…305
    Poppy Seed, Lydia's, Circa 1950…305
    Pumpkin…11
    Zucchini, Deluxe…304
    Zucchini, Eve's…304
Breadsticks
    Bacon, Becky's…36
Coffee Cake(s)
    Apricot, Refrigerator…308
    Cowboy…308
    Sour Cream, Lola's…309
Croissant(s)
    Wag's Breakfast…178
French Toast
    Day-Before…310
Hushpuppies
    Baton Rouge…312
Muffin(s)
    Blueberry Buttermilk…297
    Bran, Pear…298
    Bran, Refrigerator…299
    Corn, Pecan…296
    Cranberry-Nut…297
    Lemon…298

Pancake(s)
    Crepe Cups, Florentine...230
    "Russian," Zina's...311
    Apple, Zygmun Inn...310
    Peach Popover...311
    Potato, New-Style...287

Popover(s)
    Nana's...312
    Pancake, Peach...311

Pretzel(s)
    Salad, Pie...85
    Soft...299

Pudding(s)
    New Orleans...376
    Yorkshire, London...313
    Yorkshire, Peggy's...313

Roll(s)
    Butterscotch, Bev's Easy...294
    Butterscotch, Nutty Scotsburn...294
    Cinnamon, Swedish...293
    Danish, Cheese...293
    Pumpkin...295
    Twists, Cinnamon...292
    Twists, Pecan, Sweet Roll Dough for...291
    Twists, Sour Cream...292

Scone(s)
    Blueberry Oat, Sandra's...296
    English Tea...295

BREAKFAST & BRUNCH
    Breakfast Strata, Christmas...176
    Casserole, Egg-Sausage...177
    Casserole, Sunday Brunch...175
    Croissant, Wag's Breakfast...178
    Eggs, Texas...179
    Kugel, Luchen, Pfeffer's ~ Sweet Noodle Pudding...376
    Omelette, Ham & Cheese...180
    Omelette, Spinacheese...180
    Omelette, Western...181
    Quiche, Kathy's...179
    Quiche, Sweet Onion...178
    Sausage with Biscuits & Gravy, Country...175
    Soufflé, Egg-Sausage...176
    Soufflé, Pennebaker's "Little Pig"...177
    Welsh Rarebit, Walsh's...392

Broccoli, *See "Vegetables"*
Brownie(s), *See "Desserts"*
Brunch, *See "Breakfast & Brunch"*
Bulgar, *See "Grain(s)"*

Burger(s)
    Barbecue Beef, Emily's...136
    Patty Melt, The Famous...123
    Salsa, Hot-Mouth...135
    Sloppy Joes, Crock Pot...137

Butter, *See "Spread(s)"*

Butterscotch
    Pie, Cream Cheese...325
    Rolls, Bev's Easy...294
    Rolls, Nutty Scotsburn...294

C

Cabbage, *See "Vegetables"*
Cake(s), *See "Desserts"*
Cake(s), Coffee, *See "Bread(s)"*
Canning & Sterilization Process...386
Capellini, *See "Pasta, Angel Hair"*
Caramel Corn, *See "Desserts"*
Carrot(s), *See "Vegetables"*

Casserole(s)
    Barley, Nutty Bake...269
    Bean, "21-Bean"...247
    Beef & Cabbage...143
    Beef & Cheese, Gladys'...144
    Broccoli...9
    Carrot, Knox County...243
    Chicken & Rice...207
    Chicken, Crescent Roll...208
    Chicken, Miracle...208
    Chicken-Green Bean...207
    Corn, Fort Myers...235
    Crab Custard...114
    Egg-Sausage...177
    Enchiladas, Marie's...134
    Lentil with Sausage...249
    Mexican, Penny's...144
    Noodle, Green...260
    Onion, Heavenly...228
    Pork Chop...154
    Pork Tenderloin...154
    Potato Bake, Adeline's Cheesy...284
    Potato Bake, Cheese & Bacon...285
    Potato Bake, Cream Cheese...283
    Potato, Boldt...281
    Potato, Mashed, Creamy...280
    Potato, Peggy's...281
    Rice-Noodle...272
    Roman...240
    Rutabaga Bake, Galesburg...225
    Salmon, Creamed, with Peas...101
    Shrimp, Gulf Coast...113
    Spinach & Egg...231
    Squash, Yummy Yellow...226
    Sunday Brunch...175
    Sweet Potato...9
    Turkey, Margaret's Terrific...209
    Vegetable...239
    Veggie Brown Rice Bake, Wild...270
    Wild Rice, Pecan...270
    Wild Rice, Wisconsin...271

Caviar, *See "Fish"*
Celery, *See "Vegetables"*

Cheese
    Beef, Chipped, and Noodles au Gratin...135
    Bread, Caraway Batter...307
    Cake, Ricotta...346
    Cheddar, Baked Chicken Soufflé...205
    Danish...293
    Dressing, Blue Cheese...69
    Dressing, Blue Cheese, KBW's World-Famous...88
    Dressing, Blue Cheese-Yogurt...88
    Jarlsberg, Chicken Breasts, with Dressing...204
    Macaroni &, President Reagan's Favorite...253
    Meat Loaf Stuffed with...149
    Omelette, Ham &...180
    Omelette, Spinacheese...180
    Pie, Spinach-Cheddar...230
    Potato Bake, Adeline's Cheesy...284
    Potato Bake, Bacon &...285
    Potato Skins, with Bacon...279
    Ricotta Filling...263
    Ricotta-Spinach Filling...262, 264
    Cheese(s)
    Brie, Sweet...39
    Dip, Girl's Day Out...27
    Dip, Hot Chili...27
    Dip, Italian...21
    Dip, Mexican...27
    Dip, Nacho...26
    Emergency Things...21
    on Rye...20
    Pâté, Marlene's Basil...21
    Sauce, Mornay...400
    Sauce, Mornay, American...401
    Spread, Hungarian...20

Cheese, continued
    Spread, Liptoi…20
    Welsh Rarebit, Walsh's…392
Cheesecake, See "Desserts"
Cherry(ies), See "Fruit(s)"
Chicken, See "Poultry"
Chickpeas (Garbanzo Beans),
    See "Vegetables, Bean(s), Garbanzo"
Chili
    Albuquerque…139
    con Carne and Beans…139
    Dip, Hot…27
    Firehouse…138
    Mac…137
    Marie's Red No-Beans…138
    Turkey…210
    Vegetarian, in a Tortilla
        Bowl…224
Chocolate
    Cake, Orange-Chocolate Chip,
        1945…335
    Bars, Cherry…353
    Bars, Mississippi Mud…355
    Brownie, Drops…356
    Brownies, Nutty Chocolate
        Chip…356
    Brownies, One-Bowl…355
    Cake, Auntie Netta's Every-
        Party…327
    Cake, Chocolate Chip Fudge,
        "Killer"…328
    Cake, Chocolate, Fudge-
        Drenched…329
    Cake, Chocolate~Covered
        Cherry…327
    Cake, Deluxe Zucchini…330
    Cake, Earthquake…338
    Cake, Eclair, No~Bake…326
    Cheesecake, Cocoa…349
    Cookies, Chocolate Chip
        Pizza…360
    Cookies, Oatmeal-Chocolate
        Chip…358
    Drops, Cocoa, Great
        Grandmother's…367
    Fudge, Chocolate-Pecan,
        Quick…365
    Pie, Cream…323
    Pie, Mousse…322
Chow Mein
    Beef…133
    Chicken ~ Shanghai Style…192
    Pork ~ Shanghai Style…192

Chow-Chow, See "Relish(es)"
Chowder, See "Soup(s)"
Chutney, See "Relish(es)"
Cider, See "Beverages"
Cinnamon
    Rolls, Swedish…293
    Twists…292
Clams, See "Seafood"
Cobbler, See "Desserts"
Coconut
    Bars, Cherry…353
    Bars, Dream…352
    Cake, "Rave About It"…340
    Cake, Earthquake…338
    Cake, Oatmeal-Raisin,
        "Coco-Nutty"…343
Coffee Cake(s), See "Bread(s)"
Coffee, See "Beverages"
Coleslaw, See "Salad(s)"
Compote, See "Desserts"
Conch, See "Seafood"
Consommé, See "Soup(s)"
Cookies, See "Desserts"
Corn, See "Vegetables",
    also see "Grain(s), Cornmeal"
Cornish Hens, See "Poultry"
Cornmeal, See "Grain(s)"
Cottage Cheese
    German…83
Couscous, See "Pasta"
Cowpea(s), See "Vegetables,
    Black-Eyed Pea(s)"
Crab, See "Seafood"
Cranberry(ies), See "Fruit(s)"
Crawfish (Crayfish), See "Seafood"
Cream Puffs, See "Desserts"
Crepe(s), See "Bread(s), Pancake(s)"
Croissant(s), See "Bread(s)"
Cucumber(s), See "Vegetables"
Curry, Spread or Dip…29

D

Danish(es), See "Bread(s), Roll(s)"
Date(s)
    Bread, Pineapple, Nut…302
    Chutney, Apple, & Walnut…390
Dessert(s), See also "Bread(s)"
DESSERTS
    Ann's Green Stuff…361
    Apple, Taffy, Treat…375
    Apple Crunch…373
    Apple Dump…373

Apples, Baked, New
    England…374
Apples, Glazed Stewed,
    Wedges…374
Balls, Rum, Juanita…367
Banana Split,
    Old~Fashioned…317
Bars
    Butter Pecan Turtle…354
    Cheesecake, Lemon…351
    Cherry-Coconut, 1950…353
    Chocolate-Cherry…353
    Coconut Dream…352
    Cookie, Magic…352
    Toffee, Easy…354
    Mississippi Mud…355
Brandy Ice…412
Brickle Yummies, Adeline's…364
Brownie(s)
    Drops…356
    Mississippi Mud Bars…355
    Nutty Chocolate Chip…356
    One-Bowl…355
Cake(s)
    Apple, Danish,
        Gudrun's…343
    Apple, Kathy's…344
    Apple, One-Bowl…345
    Apple, Roberta's Fresh…345
    Best-Ever…341
    Carrot, Helen's
        Hazelwood…333
    Carrot, Pecan-Filled…332
    Cheese, Ricotta…346
    Cherry Streusel…341
    Chocolate Chip Fudge,
        "Killer"…328
    Chocolate Eclair,
        No~Bake…326
    Chocolate Fudge-
        Drenched…329
    Chocolate, Auntie Netta's
        Every~Party…327
    Chocolate-Covered
        Cherry…327
    Chocolate-Deluxe
        Zucchini…330
    Earthquake…338
    Fruit, Old~Fashioned…342
    Grandmother's…338
    Imperial, Esther's…340
    Oat, Cape Breton…358
    Oatmeal-Raisin, "Coco-
        Nutty"…343

Cake(s), continued
    Orange Candy...334
    Orange, Fresh, Mother's
        Favorite...334
    Orange-Chocolate Chip,
        1945...335
    Pistachio, Chicago,
        1970...336
    Pound, Cherry...347
    Pound, Cream Cheese...347
    Pound, Sophie's, 1929...348
    Pound, Sour Cream...346
    Raspberry, Heavenly...339
    "Rave About It"...340
    Rum, Dark...337
    Rum, Pecan,
        Conjurer's...336
    Spice, Iced...331
    Streusel, Cherry...341
    Sunshine...339
    Trifle, English Sherry...365
    Wacky, Rhoda's...337
Caramel Corn...379
Cheesecake
    Bars, Lemon...351
    Cocoa...349
    Des Plaines...349
    Gloria's Excellent...348
    Rubly...350
    Squares...351
    Tarts...350
Cobbler, Apple or Peach
    Streusel...372
Cobbler, Peach or Blueberry,
    Fresh...372
Compote, Hot Fruit...375
Cookie(s)
    Chocolate Chip Pizza...360
    Oat, Cape Breton...358
    Oatmeal-Chocolate
        Chip...358
    Orange Gumdrop,
        Florida...359
    Seven~Layer,
        Grandma's...357
    Sugar, Sheridan...359
    Zucchini...357
Cream Puffs, Louise
    Gentile's...361
Cream, Swedish, with
    Strawberries...362
Crisp, Strawberry-Rhubarb
    McCulloch's...383

Cups, Cheese, Snow Cap...366
Cups, Nut, Hazelwood...366
Delight, Cherry...368
Delight, Lemon...369
Drops, Cocoa, Great
    Grandmother's...367
Fairy Fluff, Aunt Charlotte's,
    1930...362
Frangos, Frozen Chocolate...364
Fudge, Quick Chocolate-
    Pecan...365
Gelatin
    Orange Sherbet, Mold...379
    Strawberry-Banana for a
        Crowd...378
    Strawberry Cream Mold,
        Fresh...378
Ice Cream
    Banana Split, Old-
        Fashioned...317
    Brandy Ice...412
    Egg Nog...412
    Float, Coke or Root
        Beer...416
    Malted Milk, Old-Fashioned
        Chocolate...411
    Milk Shake, Sampler
        Thick...411
    Sundae, Hot Fudge...317
    Vanilla, French,
        Homemade...13
Kugel, Luchen, Pfeffer's...376
Lady Fingers, Heath Bar...360
Lush, Lemon...368
Malted Milk, Old-Fashioned
    Chocolate...411
Melting Moments,
    Gertrude's...362
Meringues, Jeweled...363
Milk Shake, Sampler Thick...411
Pears, Baked, in Cream...374
Pie(s)
    Apple Slices...320
    Apple, Sugar~Free...320
    Banana Split...322
    Blueberry Torte...318
    Butterscotch Cream
        Cheese...325
    Cherry, Raaber...318
    Chocolate Cream...323
    Chocolate Mousse, Oreo-
        Lovers'...322
    Cream Cheese...324

    Crust, Never-Fail...326
    Filling, Home-Canned...387
    Mother's Ice Box...321
    Peach, Ethel's Supreme...319
    Peanut Butter, New Orleans
        Café...325
    Pecan, Georgia...12
    Pretzel Salad...85
    Pumpkin, Old-Fashioned,
        with Brandy...13
    Rhubarb-Strawberry...319
    Ritz Cracker...324
Pound Cake
    Cherry-Nut...347
    Cream Cheese...347
    Sophie's, 1929...348
    Sour Cream...346
Pudding
    Bing-Banana Salad...84
    Bread, New Orleans...376
    Pistachio Salad with
        Sherbet...84
    Rice, Danish ~ Ris A'
        Lamande...377
    Sweet Noodle...376
Salad(s)
    Bing-Banana...84
    Layered Jello...84
    Pineapple-Mandarin
        Fruit...83
    Pistachio with Sherbet...84
    Pretzel Pie...85
    Taffy Apple...85
Sauce(s)
    Brandy...385
    Cinnamon...385
    Pineapple...384
    Raisin...384
    Raspberry...383
    Rhubarb, Tangy,
        McCulloch's...383
    Strawberry...383
    Strawberry-Rhubarb,
        McCulloch's...383
Squares
    Cheesecake...351
    Lemon, Gold Medal...370
    Lemon Lorraine...370
Sundae, Hot Fudge...317
Tarts
    Cheesecake...350
    Cherry...371
    Pecan Tiny...371

Desserts, *continued*
    Trifle, English Sherry…365
    Whip, Frozen Apricot…363
Dip(s)
    Artichoke, Bucaro…31
    Artichoke, Jean's…31
    Cheese, Italian…21
    Clam, Chris'…25
    Cocktail Sauce, Shrimp in…23
    Crab Meat…24
    Curry…29
    Fondue, Hot Crab…24
    Guacamole…26
    Nacho…26
    Shrimp, Louisiana Mustard Sauce…23
    Yogurt-Garlic…397
Dough
    Manicotti, Aunt Netta's…261
    Piecrust, Never-Fail…326
    Sweet Roll, for Pecan Twists…291
Dressing(s), *See "Salad Dressings"* or *"Stuffing"*
Duck, *See "Poultry"*
Dumplings
    Potato, Mama Kozol's Polish…287

E

EGG(S)
    Casserole, Sausage &…177
    Casserole, Spinach &…231
    Casserole, Sunday Brunch…175
    Croissant, Wag's Breakfast…178
    Omelette, Ham & Cheese…180
    Omelette, Spinacheese, Fresh…180
    Omelette, Western…181
    Quiche, Kathy's…179
    Quiche, Sweet Onion…178
    Soufflé, Broccoli de Norman…236
    Soufflé, Broccoli, Sandy's…236
    Soufflé, Chicken, Cheddar-Baked…205
    Soufflé, Cornmeal Spoon Bread…277
    Soufflé, Pennebaker's "Little Pig"…177
    Soufflé, Sausage &…176
    Strata, Christmas Breakfast…176
    Texas…179
Eggnog, *See "Beverages"*
Eggplant(s), *See "Vegetables"*

Enchiladas
    Chicken, Suiza…190
    Chicken, Swiss…191
    Marie's Casserole…134

F

Fajitas
    Chicken, Potatoes…188
    Southwestern…134
Fettuccine, *See "Pasta"*
FISH
    Beer Batter…97
    Caviar, Spread, Cream Cheese…28
    Ceviche…98
    Chowder, Northumberland White…46
    Chowder, Nova Scotia Seafood…46
    Marinade, Garlic-Wine…404
    Mustard-Baked Fillets…98
    Sauce, Tartar…393
    Singapore Steamed…96
Flounder
    Fillet with Onions…95
Haddock
    Finnan Haddie, Granny Gunn's…97
Halibut
    Baked, Greek Style ~ Plaki…94
    Creole…95
    with Crumb-Nut Topping…94
Salmon
    Broiled, with Grapes…99
    Broiled, with Tarragon Butter…102
    Chowder…47
    Creamed, with Peas…101
    Honey Fillet…99
    Loaf, Alaskan, with Creole Sauce…102
    Loaf, Michigan Farmhouse…103
    Scotch-Mustard…103
    Spread…25
    Terrine, with Shrimp…100
    with Cilantro Oil & Mango Salsa…100
    Vermouth White Sauce…93
Sole
    with Lemon and Capers…96

Swordfish
    in Citrus-Ginger Marinade…93
Trout
    Baked, with Dill Sour Cream…105
    Brook, Broiled Amandine…104
Tuna
    Salad Niçoise…69
    Spaghetti with, & Lemon…259
Turbot
    Chowder, Northumberland White Fish…46
Walleye
    Baked, in Wine Sauce…104
Flounder, *See "Fish"*
Fondue(s)
    Hot Crab…24
French Toast, *See "Bread(s)"*
Fritters
    Conch…118
FRUIT(S)
    Cake, Old~Fashioned Fruit…342
    Citrus-Marinated Pork Chops…151
    Compote…375
    Fruited Pot Roast…128
    Jam, "High Dumpsy Dearie"…386
    Pie Filling, Home-Canned…387
    Salad, Fruit & Nut…82
    Salad, Myrtle's…12
    Salad, Pineapple-Mandarin…83
    Salad, Waldorf Raisin…83
    Salsa, Citrus…200
    Spread, Healthy…19
Apple(s)
    Bake, Rutabaga, Galesburg…225
    Baked, New England…374
    Bread, One-Bowl Applesauce…302
    Cake, Danish, Gudrun's…343
    Cake, Kathy's…344
    Cake, One~Bowl…345
    Cake, Roberta's Fresh…345
    Chutney, Date & Walnut…390

Apple(s), continued
    Cobbler, Streusel...372
    Cran-Apple Salad Mold...67
    Crunch...373
    Dump...373
    Glazed Stewed, Wedges...374
    Pancake, Zygmun Inn...310
    Pie, Slices...320
    Pie, Sugar~Free...320
    Pork Chops with, Rings...153
    Salad, Taffy...85
    Taffy, Treat...375

Apricot(s)
    Chutney, Spicy...390
    Coffee Cake, Refrigerator...308
    Glazed Cornish Hens...211
    Whip, Frozen...363

Banana(s)
    Bread, Bonanza...301
    Bread, Saint John...300
    Julius "Barry"...416
    Pie, Split...322
    Punch...417
    Split, Old-Fashioned...317
    Strawberry, Gelatin for a Crowd...378

Blueberry(ies)
    Cheese Cups, Snow Cap...366
    Cheesecake, Gloria's Excellent...348
    Cobbler, Fresh...372
    Muffins, Buttermilk...297
    Pie, Torte...318
    Scones, Oat, Sandra's...296

Cherry(ies)
    Bars, Chocolate...353
    Bars, Coconut...353
    Cake, Chocolate-Covered...327
    Cake, Pound, Nut...347
    Cake, Streusel...341
    Cheese Cups, Snow Cap...366
    Cheesecake, Gloria's Excellent...348
    Cheesecake, Squares...351
    Delight...368
    Pie Raaber...318
    Pork Chops...153
    Tarts...371

Cranberry(ies)
    Salad, Red Raspberry Relish, Grace's...75
    Bread...11
    Cran-Apple Salad Mold...67
    Muffins, Nut...297
    Relish...10
    Relish, Nutty...392
    Salad, Spinach, with Orange...74
    Salad, Waldorf...82

Grape(s)
    Salmon, Broiled with...99
    Wine...417

Lemon(s)
    Cheesecake Bars...351
    Chicken Breasts, Sautéed...202
    Delight...369
    Lush...368
    Muffins...298
    Squares, Gold Medal...370
    Squares, Lorraine...370

Mango(s)
    Salsa...100

Orange(s)
    Cake, Candy...334
    Cake, Chocolate Chip, 1945...335
    Cake, Fresh, Mother's Favorite...334
    Cookies, Gumdrop...359
    Julius "Barry"...416
    Salad, Spinach, with Cranberry...74
    Sauce, Roast Duckling with...210
    Sherbet Gelatin Mold...379

Papaya(s)
    Salsa...100

Peach(es)
    Cobbler, Fresh...372
    Cobbler, Streusel...372
    Pancake, Popover...311
    Pie, Ethel's Supreme...319

Pear(s)
    Baked, in Cream...374
    Muffins, Bran...298

Pineapple(s)
    Date-Nut Bread...302
    Fairy Fluff, Aunt Charlotte's...362
    Ham, Baked...161

    Punch, Baby Shower...416
    Sauce...384

Raisin(s)
    Sauce...384

Raspberry(ies)
    Cake, Heavenly...339
    Dressing, Poppy Seed...87
    Salad, Red, Cranberry Relish, Grace's...75
    Sauce...383
    Vinaigrette...73

Rhubarb
    Pie, Strawberry...319
    Sauce, Strawberry, McCulloch's...383
    Sauce, Tangy, McCulloch's...383

Strawberry(ies)
    Banana Gelatin for a Crowd...378
    Butter...387
    Cheesecake, Squares...351
    Cream Mold...378
    Cream Puff's, Louise Gentile's...361
    Pie, Rhubarb...319
    Sauce...383
    Sauce, Rhubarb, McCulloch's...383
    Swedish Cream with...362

Fudge, See "Desserts"
Fusilli, See "Pasta"

G

Garbanzo Beans (Chickpeas), See "Vegetables, Bean(s)"

Garlic
    Cloves, Roasted...19
    Dressing, Creamy House...86
    Roasted Pork Loin...156
    Yogurt Sauce or Dip...397

Gazpacho, See "Soup(s)"

Gelatin
    Cran-Apple Salad Mold...67
    Jello, Layered Salad...84
    Orange Sherbet, Mold...379
    Red Raspberry-Cranberry Relish Salad, Grace's...75
    Strawberry Cream Mold, Fresh...378
    Strawberry-Banana, for a Crowd...378

Glaze, *See "Sauce(s)"*
GRAIN(S)
- **Barley**
  - Bake, Nutty...269
  - Soup, Scotch...54
- **Bran**
  - Muffins, Pear...298
  - Muffins, Refrigerator...299
- **Bulgar**
  - Spanish, Zesty...269
- **Corn, Cornmeal**
  - Caramel Corn...379
  - Muffins, Pecan Corn...296
  - Polenta, Chicken with...188
  - Polenta, Parmesan...276
  - Spoon Bread...277
- **Oat(s), Oatmeal**
  - Bread...306
  - Cake, Raisin, "Coco-Nutty"...343
  - Cookies or Cakes, Cape Breton...358
  - Cookies, Chocolate Chip...358
  - Scones, Blueberry, Sandra's...296
- **Rice**
  - Bake, Wild Veggie Brown Rice...270
  - Basmati, Ratatouille...271
  - Beef Stew Deluxe...147
  - Casserole, Chicken &...207
  - Noodle Casserole...272
  - Pilaf ~ Three Ways...274
  - Pudding, Danish ~ Ris A' Lamande...377
  - Puerto Rican Chicken with...196
  - Risotto Erbacci...276
  - Risotto Milanese...275
  - Sausage, Spanish with...174
  - Soup, Hearty Tomato...51
  - Southern Paint Yellow...273
  - Spanish, Kay's...273
  - Spanish, Rochester, with Beef...272
  - Steamed, Szechwan Chicken Over...191
  - Veal, Creamed, with...167
- **Wheat (Whole)**
  - Bread, Bonanza...301

Wild Rice
- Casserole, Pecan...270
- Casserole, Wisconsin...271
- Chicken with Artichokes &...196
- Lamb, Crown Roast of, with...169
- Wild Veggie Brown Rice Bake...270

Grapes, *See "Fruit(s)"*
Gravy, *See "Sauce(s)"*
Guacamole...26

H

Haddock, *See "Fish"*
Halibut, *See "Fish"*
Ham, *See "Meat(s)"*
Hamburger(s), *See "Burger(s)"*
Hash
- Corned Beef...131

Hens, Cornish, *See "Poultry"*
Hors d'oeuvres, *See "Appetizers"*
Hushpuppies, *See "Bread(s)"*

I

Ice Cream
- Banana Split, Old-Fashioned...317
- Brandy Ice...412
- Egg Nog...412
- Float, Coke or Root Beer...416
- Malted Milk, Old-Fashioned Chocolate...411
- Milk Shake, Sampler Thick...411
- Sundae, Hot Fudge...317
- Vanilla, French, Homemade...13

J

Jam, *See "Spread(s)"*

K

Kebabs (Kebobs), *See "Shish Kebabs"*
Kosher/Jewish
- Cabbage, Stuffed...143
- Kugel, Luchen, Pfeffer's...376

L

Lamb, *See "Meat(s)"*
Lasagne, *See "Pasta"*

Lentil Beans, *See "Vegetables, Bean(s)"*
Lima Bean(s), *See "Vegetables"*
Linguine, *See "Pasta"*
Liver, *See "Meat(s), Beef"*
Loaf, *See "Meat Loaf"*
Lobster, *See "Seafood"*

M

Macaroni, *See "Pasta"*
Mango, *See "Fruit(s)"*
Manicotti, *See "Pasta"*
Marinade(s), *See "Dressing(s)" or "Sauce(s)"*
Meatballs
- Beefy...36
- Bonsignore's Italian Chicken Soup with...62
- Bourguignon...37
- Crazy...37
- Sauce, Grandma Katie Romano's...266
- Spaghetti &...258
- Swedish...38

Meat Loaf
- Cheese-Stuffed...149
- Ham...160
- Meat & Vegetable...148
- Monday...149
- Salmon, Alaskan, with Creole Sauce...102
- Salmon, Michigan Farmhouse...102

MEAT(S)
- Sauce, Grandma Katie Romano's...266
- Sugo, Nona's Tuscana...256
- **Bacon**
  - Beef Roulades...124
  - Breadsticks, Becky's...36
  - Chicken Breasts Wrapped in...198
  - Dip, Girl's Day Out...27
  - Lamb Patties with...171
  - Liver & Onions with...145
  - Potato Bake, Adeline's Cheesy...284
  - Potato Bake, Cheese &...285
  - Potato Skins, with Cheese...279
  - Potatoes, Baked, with, & Scallions...282
  - Quiche, Kathy's...179

Bacon, continued
    Sandwiches, Kentucky Hot
        Brown…30
    Shrimp, Cheese, Delight…22
    Soup, Bean, Spanish…60
    Soup, Lima Bean…55
    Spaghetti Carbonara…258
    Veal Cutlets, Paprika…165
    Water Chestnuts in…30
    Wrapped Shrimp…23

Beef
    Barbecue, Emily's…136
    Bourguignon…124
    Braised, with Noodles…131
    Brisket of…130
    Burgers, Hot-Mouth
        Salsa…135
    Cabbage Casserole…143
    Cabbage, Stuffed Rolls…142
    Cabbage, Stuffed,
        Kosher…143
    Casserole, Cabbage…143
    Casserole, Mexican,
        Penny's…144
    Casserole, with Cheese,
        Gladys'…144
    Chili con Carne and
        Beans…139
    Chili Mac…137
    Chili, Albuquerque…139
    Chili, Firehouse…138
    Chili, Marie's Red
        No-Beans…138
    Chipped, with Noodles
        au Gratin…135
    Chow Mein…133
    Corned…130
    Corned, Hash…131
    Enchiladas, Marie's
        Casserole…134
    Fajitas, Southwestern…134
    French Dip au Jus…126
    Goulash, Gigi's…140
    Gravy, Brown…407
    Hash, Corned Beef…131
    Liver Stew, Uncle
        Louie's…145
    Liver, Bacon & Onions…145
    Loaf, Ham…160
    Marinade, Honey-
        Ginger…404
    Marinade, Wine, for
        Steaks…405

    Meat & Vegetable Loaf…148
    Meat Loaf, Cheese-
        Stuffed…149
    Meat Loaf, Monday…149
    Meatballs, Spaghetti &…258
    Meatballs, Swedish…38
    Mexican Casserole,
        Penny's…144
    Mexican Roast, a la
        Sanborns…125
    Patty Melt, The
        Famous…123
    Pepper Steak…133
    Plantains, Stuffed, Ripe ~
        Canoas…141
    Pot Roast, American, with
        Noodles…129
    Pot Roast, Fruited…128
    Ribs, Short, Roasted with
        Vegetables…123
    Rice, Spanish,
        Rochester…272
    Risotto Erbacci…276
    Roast, au Jus…126
    Roast, Louise…125
    Roast, Mexican, a la
        Sanborns…125
    Roulades…124
    Salad, Mexican Corn
        Chip…78
    Salad, Red-Bean Taco…78
    Sauce, Au Jus ~ Quick or
        Traditional…406
    Sauce, Herb, Western for
        Steak…403
    Sauce, Meat, Italian…402
    Sloppy Joes, Crock Pot…137
    Soup, Bean, Spanish…60
    Soup, French Market…59
    Soup, Petite Marmite…58
    Soup, Pigeon Peas with,
        Puerto Rican…57
    Spiced, Texas…136
    Steak Tartare…39
    Stew, Deluxe…147
    Stew, Easy, Oven-
        Baked…146
    Stew, Hunter's…148
    Stew, Over Noodles…146
    Stew, with Fresh
        Vegetables…147
    Stroganoff…128
    Stuffing, with ~ Pan

        Dressing…408
    Swiss Steak, Mrs. B's…132
    Swiss Steaks in Pan
        Gravy…132
    Tenderloin Deluxe…127
    Zucchini, Stuffed…140

Ham
    Croissant, Wag's
        Breakfast…178
    Croquettes…161
    Deviled, Cornucopias…35
    Glaze…405
    Loaf…160
    Meat Loaf, Cheese-
        Stuffed…149
    Omelette, Cheese &…180
    Omelette, Western…181
    Pineapple-Baked…161
    Prosciutto, Chicken
        Saltimbocca…186
    Sandwiches, Kentucky Hot
        Brown…30
    Scalloped, & Potatoes…160
    Soup, Bean, Spanish…60
    Soup, Bean, U.S. Senate…58
    Soup, Black Bean,
        Cuban…61
    Soup, Scotch Barley…54
    Soup, Split Pea…56

Lamb
    Croquettes…171
    Patties with Bacon…171
    Roast Leg of…170
    Roast of, Crown, with Wild
        Rice…169
    Stew, Spring, with Fresh
        Vegetables…168

Pork
    Casserole, Egg-Sausage…177
    Casserole, Sunday
        Brunch…175
    Chop, Casserole…154
    Chops in Spicy Mustard
        Sauce…152
    Chops with Apple
        Rings…153
    Chops, Cherry…153
    Chops, Citrus-
        Marinated…151
    Chops, Supreme…152
    Chops, with Sage &
        Onion…151

Pork, *continued*
- Chow Mein ~ Shanghai Style…192
- Loaf, Ham…160
- Loin, Garlic-Roasted…156
- Loin, Roasted, with Gravy…156
- Loin, with Rice & Pigeon Peas…155
- Marinade, Raspberry-Mustard for Spareribs…405
- Marinade, Wine, for Chops…405
- Meatballs, Swedish…38
- Sausage, Country, with Biscuits & Gravy…175
- Soufflé, Egg-Sausage…176
- Soufflé, Pennebaker's "Little Pig"…177
- Soup, Mofongo Dumpling…63
- Spareribs & Sauerkraut…159
- Spareribs, Barbecued…159
- Spareribs, Breaded, in Mustard Gravy…158
- Spareribs, Honey, Zygmun…158
- Steaks a la Criolla…157
- Strata, Christmas Breakfast…176
- Tenderloin, Casserole…154
- Tenderloin, Kathy's South-of-the-Border…155

Sausage
- & Sauerkraut Bites…29
- Calzone ~ Italian Easter Pie…173
- Casserole, Egg &…177
- Casserole, Lentil…249
- Casserole, Sunday Brunch…175
- Country, with Biscuits & Gravy…175
- Meal-in-One…173
- Smoked, & Sauerkraut…174
- Soufflé, Egg &…176
- Soufflé, Pennebaker's "Little Pig"…177
- Soup, Italian…43
- Soup, Lentil, Bavarian…60
- Soup, Portuguese Potato…48
- Spanish, with Rice…174

Strata, Christmas Breakfast…176

Veal
- Chops, with Mushrooms in Cream Sauce…166
- Creamed, with Rice…167
- Cutlets in Marsala Wine…165
- Cutlets, Paprika…165
- Fricassee of, with Morels…164
- Osso Buco ~ Vincent…168
- Piccata de Hudson…163
- Piccata, Santina's…163
- Scallopini…166

Meringue(s)
- Jeweled…363
- Topping…323

Microwave Recipes
- Potato Bake, Adeline's Cheesy…284
- Chicken Fajita Potatoes…188

Molasses, Bread, Oatmeal…306

Mold(s)
- Cran-Apple Salad…67
- Jello, Layered Salad…84
- Orange Sherbet Gelatin…379
- Red Raspberry-Cranberry Relish Salad, Grace's…75
- Salmon & Shrimp Terrine…100
- Shrimp…22
- Spinach, Sea Breezer…231
- Strawberry Cream…378
- Strawberry-Banana Gelatin for a Crowd…378

Mousse, Pie, Chocolate, Oreo Lovers…322
Muffin(s), *See* "Bread(s)"
Mushroom(s), *See* "Vegetables"
Mussels, *See* "Seafood"

N

Navy Bean(s), *See* "Vegetables, Bean(s)"

O

Oat(s), Oatmeal, *See* "Grain(s)"
Oil, Cilantro…100
Onion(s), *See* "Vegetables"
Orange(s), *See* "Fruit(s)"
Oysters, *See* "Seafood"

P

Pancake(s), *See* "Bread(s)"
Papaya, *See* "Fruit(s)"
Party Mix, TV…33

PASTA
- Salad, Artichoke & Shrimp…77
- Salad, Spicy Szechwan Noodle…73
- Salad, Summer…76
- Sauce, Marinara, Classic Red…402
- Sauce, Meat, Grandma Katie Romano's Luria…266
- Sauce, Meat, Italian…402
- Soup, Strega Nana's Pasta & Fagioli…64
- Soup, Tortellini…64

Angel Hair (Capellini)
- Arrabiata Sauce with…259

Couscous
- Chicken with…185

Fettuccine
- Alfredo Tomaselli…257
- Nona's Tuscana Sugo with…256
- Pesto Francesca…257

Fusilli
- with Cottage Cheese Pesto & Broccoli…254

Lasagne
- Rolls, Spinach…265
- Two-Sauce ~ Red & White…264

Linguine
- Artichoke Sauce, with…255
- Pesto, with, Jorie's…254
- White Clam Sauce, with…255

Macaroni
- Casserole, Turkey, Margaret's Terrific…209
- & Cheese, President Reagan's Favorite…253
- Chili Mac…137

Manicotti
- Aunt Netta's…261
- Spinach-Stuffed…260

Noodle(s)
- Beef Bourguignon…124
- Beef Stew…146
- Beef Stew Deluxe…147
- Beef Stroganoff…128
- Beef, Braised…131

Beef, Chipped, au
   Gratin...135
Casserole, Green...260
Chicken, Chopped
   with...206
Chow Mein, Beef...133
Pot Roast, American...129
Pudding, Sweet...376
Rice Casserole...272
Rotini
   Vegetable & Olive in
      Mustard Sauce...253
Shells (Conchiglie/Conchiglioni)
   Jumbo, Spinach- Stuffed
      ...262
   Ricotta-Stuffed...263
   Stuffed, Fast Version...262
Spaghetti
   Carbonara...258
   Chicken Cacciatore...186
   & Meatballs Spectacular
      ...258
   with Tuna & Lemon...259
Tortellini
   Alfredo Primavera...267
Pâté, Basil, Marlene's...21
Patty Melt, The Famous...123
Pea(s), See "Vegetables"
Peach(es), See "Fruit(s)"
Peanut(s)
   Pie, Peanut Butter, New Orleans
      Café...325
   Soup, Schwemm House...43
Pear(s), See "Fruit(s)"
Pecan(s)
   Butter, Turtle Bars...354
   Cake, Carrot, Filled...332
   Cake, Rum, Conjurer's...336
   Muffins, Corn...296
   Muffins, Cranberry-Nut...297
   Pie, Georgia...12
   Twists, Sweet Roll Dough
      for...291
Pheasant, See "Poultry"
Pickle(s)
   Refrigerator...389
   Slices, Sweet & Sour...389
Pie(s), See also "Pie(s), Desserts"
   Crust, Never-Fail...326
   Filling, Home Canned...387
   Italian Easter ~ Calzone...173
   Onion, Auntie's...229
   See also "Desserts, Pie(s)"...318

Spinach-Cheddar...230
Turkey-Broccoli...209
Pigeon Peas, See "Vegetables"
Pineapple(s), See "Fruit(s)"
Pizza
   Chocolate Chip Cookie...360
   Mexican Black Bean...223
Plantain(s), See "Vegetables"
Polenta, See "Grain(s), Cornmeal"
Popover(s), See "Bread(s)"
Pork, See "Meat(s)"
Pot Roast, See "Meats, Beef"
Potato Salad, See "Salad(s)"
Potato(es), See "Vegetables"
POULTRY
   Chicken
      a la King...197
      Artichokes & Wild Rice
         with...196
      Breast Cutlets, Texas...199
      Breasts in Sour Cream &
         Sherry...202
      Breasts in White Wine...201
      Breasts, Alpine-Dressed...203
      Breasts, Bacon-Wrapped...198
      Breasts, California
         Crunch...203
      Breasts, Crisp, Baked...205
      Breasts, Divan, Julie's...200
      Breasts, Jarlsberg, with
         Dressing...204
      Breasts, Lil's No-Peek...199
      Breasts, Marinated, Grilled,
         with Citrus Salsa...200
      Breasts, Sautéed
         Lemon...202
      Cacciatore ~ A Garlic
         Lover's Recipe...186
      Casserole, Crescent
         Roll...208
      Casserole, Green-Bean
         &...207
      Casserole, Miracle...208
      Casserole, Rice &...207
      Chive Crescent
         Squares...204
      Chopped, with
         Noodles...206
      Chow Mein ~ Shanghai
         Style...192
      Cinnamon, with
         Couscous...185
      Crab-Stuffed, Smith's...198

      Creamed, on a Biscuit...206
      Deep-Fried...194
      Dixie Fried...194
      Enchiladas Suiza...190
      Enchiladas, Swiss...191
      Fajita Potatoes...188
      Gravy, Giblet...406
      Gravy, White...407
      Hot Dish...192
      Italian, with Polenta...188
      Marinade, Ginger-
         Peach...404
      Marinade, Honey-
         Ginger...404
      Meal, Papa's Only...187
      Milanese...187
      Oven-Barbecued...193
      Puerto Rican, with
         Rice...196
      Robin Hood...195
      Salad Niçoise...69
      Salad, Chinese...72
      Salad, Hot...71
      Salad, Spicy Szechwan
         Noodle...73
      Salad, Summer...71
      Saltimbocca...186
      Soufflé, Cheddar-
         Baked...205
      Soul, Stir-Fry with Black-
         Eyed Peas...193
      Soup, Bonsignore's Italian
         with Meatballs...62
      Soup, Dad's Homemade...63
      Soup, Petite Marmite...58
      Stuffing ~ Bread
         Dressing...408
      Szechwan, Over Steamed
         Rice...191
      Tacos...189
      Tortilla, Crisp...190
      Totopo Jalisciense...190
   Duck
      Roast Duckling with Orange
         Sauce...210
   Pheasant
      Donna Erickson's...211
   Rock Cornish Game Hens
      Apricot~Glazed...211
   Turkey
      Casserole, Margaret's
         Terrific...209
      Chili...210

Turkey, continued
    Pie, Broccoli…209
    Roast, with Giblet Gravy…7
    Sandwiches, Kentucky Hot Brown…30
Pound Cake, *See "Desserts"*
Pretzel(s), *See "Bread(s)"*
Pudding, *See "Desserts"*
Pumpkin, *See "Vegetables"*
Punch, *See "Beverages"*

Q

Quesadillas…38
Quiche(s), *See "Egg(s)"*

R

Raisin(s), *See Fruit(s)*
Raspberry(ies), *See "Fruit(s)"*
Relish(es)
    Beet, Fancy…391
    Beet, No-Cook…391
    Chow-Chow, Green Tomato…388
    Chow-Chow, Retz Ranch…388
    Chutney, Apple, Date & Walnut…390
    Chutney, Spicy Apricot…390
    Cranberry…10
    Cranberry, Nutty…392
Rhubarb, *See "Fruit(s)"*
Ribs, *See "Meat(s), Beef or Pork"*
Rice, *See "Grain(s)"*
Rock Cornish Game Hens, *See "Poultry"*
Roll(s), *See "Bread(s)"*
Rotini, *See "Pasta"*
Rutabaga(s), *See "Vegetables"*

S

Salad Dressing(s)
    Blue Cheese…69
    Blue Cheese, KBW's World-Famous…88
    Blue Cheese-Yogurt…88
    Caesar…68
    Dill, Spicy…89
    French, A-1…89
    Garlic, Creamy House…86
    Honey, for Fruit Salad…87
    Marinade, Cider…70
    Pepper, Creamy…86

Raspberry-Poppy Seed…87
Vinaigrette…74, 82
Vinaigrette, Apple Cider…69
Vinaigrette, Honey-Mustard…70
Vinaigrette, Mustard…79
Vinaigrette, Mustard-Wine, with Pecans…87
Vinaigrette, Raspberry…73
Vinaigrette, Red Wine…67-68
Vinaigrette, Red Wine-Mustard…77
Vinaigrette, Sesame…72-73
Vinaigrette, Sweet-Sour…81
Vinaigrette, White Wine…79
Vinaigrette, White Wine-Honey…74
Western, Tara's…89
SALAD(S)
    Bing-Banana…84
    Caesar, Blackstone…68
    Chicken, Chinese…72
    Chicken, Hot…71
    Chicken, Summer…71
    Chinese Chicken…72
    Chinese Vegetable, Hawthorn Club…72
    Coleslaw, "Dressed-Up"…80
    Coleslaw, "Sis W"…81
    Coleslaw, Yacht Club…80
    Cottage Cheese, German…83
    Cran-Apple Mold…67
    Cucumbers, Sweet & Sour…81
    Endive & Escarole with Raspberry Vinaigrette…73
    Fruit & Nut Tossed…82
    Fruit, Myrtle's…12
    Fruit, Pineapple-Mandarin…83
    Honey-Pear Tossed…70
    Insalata La Famillia…67
    Jello, Layered…84
    Kidney Bean, Madge's…80
    Korean Spinach…74
    Niçoise…69
    Noodle, Spicy Szechwan…73
    Pasta, Artichoke & Shrimp…77
    Pasta, Summer…76
    Pistachio, with Sherbet…84
    Potato, Mom's…76
    Potato, Sour Cream…77
    Pretzel Pie…85
    Red Raspberry-Cranberry Relish, Grace's…75

Spinach, Crunch…75
Spinach, Korean…74
Spinach, with Cranberry and Orange…74
Szechwan Noodle, Spicy…73
Taco, Mexican Corn Chip…78
Taco, Red-Bean…78
Taffy Apple…85
Three-Bean with White Wine Vinaigrette…79
Three-Bean, Jean's Mustard…79
Tomato, Greek…68
Tomatoes, Sliced, with Blue Cheese Dressing…69
Vegetable, Calico…70
Vegetable, Chinese, Hawthorn Club…72
Waldorf Raisin…83
Waldorf, Cranberry…82
Salmon, *See "Fish"*
Salsa
    Citrus…200
    Mango or Papaya…100
    Sofrito…196
Salt, Chef's…201
Sandwich(es)
    Cucumber…19
    Emergency Cheese Things…21
    Kentucky Hot Brown…30
    The Famous Patty Melt…123
    Wag's Breakfast Croissant…178
SAUCE(S)
    Alfredo…257, 267
    Amandine…104
    Arrabiata…259
    Artichoke…255
    Au Jus ~ Quick or Traditional…406
    Au Jus, French Dip Beef…126
    Au Jus, Roast Beef…126
    Barbecue…136, 159
    Béarnaise…395
    Béchamel ~ White, Classic…400
    Bordelaise…398
    Brandy…385
    Brown…398
    Cheese…135
    Cheese, Mornay…400
    Cheese, Mornay, American…401
    Cherry…153
    Cinnamon…385
    Clam, White…255

Cocktail…393
Cocktail, Shrimp in…23
Cream…400
Creole…95
Creole, Spicy, with
    Mushrooms…396
Creole, Traditional…396
Criolla…157
Curry…110
Dill Sour Cream…105
Fudge, Hot…329
Ginger-Apple…153
Glaze, Ham…405
Gravy, Brown, for Beef…407
Gravy, Chicken Giblet…406
Gravy, Giblet…7
Gravy, Mustard…158
Gravy, White, for Chicken…407
Herb, for Bay Scallops…118
Herb, Western, for Steak…403
Hollandaise, Classic…394
Hollandaise, Mock…394
Honey…99
Honey-Soy…158
Jardinière…397
Marinade, Brown Sugar,
    Spicy…155
Marinade, Citrus…151
Marinade, Citrus-Ginger…93
Marinade, Garlic-Wine for Shrimp
    or Fish…404
Marinade, Ginger-Peach for
    Chicken…404
Marinade, Honey-Ginger, for Beef
    & Chicken…404
Marinade, Indian…108
Marinade, Raspberry-Mustard for
    Spareribs…405
Marinade, Red Wine…170
Marinade, Scotch-Mustard…103
Marinade, Sherry…112
Marinade, Wine, for Steaks or
    Chops…405
Marinara…258, 266
Marinara, Classic Red, for
    Pasta…402
Meat, Italian…402
Mornay ~ Cheese Sauce…400
Mornay, American…401
Mushroom, Brown…399
Mushroom, White…399
Mustard…114, 152, 253
Mustard, Shrimp, Louisiana…23

Mustard-Ginger Basting…170
Orange…210
Pesto…254, 257
Pesto, Cottage Cheese…254
Pineapple…384
Raisin…384
Raspberry…383
Red, Marinara…264, 402
Rémoulade…395
Rhubarb, Tangy,
    McCulloch's…383
Sofrito…196
Strawberry…383
Strawberry-Rhubarb,
    McCulloch's…383
Sugo, Nona's Tuscana (with
    meat)…256
Syrup, Brown Sugar…225
Tartar…393
Tempura…109
Tomato…142
Tomato, Greek…94
Tomato, Kosher…143
Tomato-Wine, Spicy…168
Velouté…197, 206, 401
Vinaigrette, Red Wine…232
Welsh Rarebit, Walsh's…392
Whiskey…376
White…97, 101, 161, 167, 171,
    231, 239, 243, 264
White, Classic, Béchamel…400
White, Vermouth…93
Yogurt-Garlic…397
Sauerkraut, See "Vegetables, Cabbage"
Sausage, See "Meat(s)"
Scallops, See "Seafood"
Scone(s), See "Bread(s)"
SEAFOOD
    Chowder, Nova Scotia…46
    Marinade, Garlic-Wine…404
    Sauce, Cocktail…393
    Sauce, Tartar…393
    Clams
        Chowder, Creamy…45
        Chowder, Mike's…45
        Dip, Chris'…25
        Gazpacho, Clamato…44
        Sauce, White, Linguine
            with…255
    Conch
        Fritters…118
    Crab
        Cakes, in Tangy Mustard

            Sauce…114
        Cakes, Kerstner's Fresh…115
        Casserole, Custard…114
        Chicken, Stuffed,
            Smith's…198
        Dip, Meat…24
        Fondue, Hot…24
        Spread, Meat…25
        Stuffed, Deviled…116
    Crawfish (Crayfish)
        Éttouffée, Cajun…108
    Lobster
        Fresh, North Atlantic…107
        Nova Scotia-Style…107
    Mussels
        Marinere…119
    Oysters
        Scalloped…119
    Scallops
        Bay, Herb Basted…118
        in Parchment…117
        Oven-Fried…116
    Shrimp
        Bacon-Wrapped…23
        Barbecued…112
        Casserole, Gulf Coast…113
        Cheese & Bacon
            Delight…22
        Creole Allen…112
        Curry…110
        de Jonghe…111
        Indian-Broiled…108
        Kebabs with Curry
            Butter…113
        Mold…22
        Salad, Artichoke &
            Pasta…77
        Sauce, Cocktail…23
        Sauce, Mustard,
            Louisiana…23
        Tempura…109
        Terrine, with Salmon…100
Shellfish, See "Seafood"
Shells, Pasta (Conchiglie/
    Conchiglioni), See "Pasta"
Shish Kebabs, Shrimp, with Curry
    Butter…113
Short Ribs, See "Meat(s), Beef"
Shrimp, See "Seafood"
Sloppy Joes, See "Meat(s), Beef"
Sole, See "Fish"
Soufflé(s), See "Egg(s)"

453

Soul Food
    Soul Chicken Stir-Fry with Black-Eyed Peas...193

SOUP(S)
    Asparagus, Cream of...53
    Barley, Scotch...54
    Bavarian Lentil...61
    Bean, U.S. Senate...58
    Beef with Pigeon Peas, Puerto Rican...57
    Broccoli, Swiss...50
    Cabbage, Polish...52
    Cabbage, Sweet & Sour...52
    Celery, Cream of...53
    Chicken, Bonsignore's Italian with Meatballs...62
    Chicken, Dad's Homemade...63
    Chowder, Clam, Creamy...45
    Chowder, Clam, Mike's...45
    Chowder, Salmon...47
    Chowder, Seafood, Nova Scotia...46
    Chowder, Vegetable, Halifax...47
    Chowder, White Fish, Northumberland...46
    Consommé, Swiss Mushroom...57
    Corn, Cheesy...50
    Cuban Black Bean...60
    Cucumber, Low-Fat...54
    French Market...59
    Gazpacho, Clamato...44
    Gazpacho, Good's...44
    Lima Bean & Bacon...55
    Mofongo Dumpling...63
    Onion, French...56
    Pasta & Fagioli, Strega Nana's...64
    Pea, Split...56
    Peanut, Schwemm House...43
    Petite Marmite...58
    Potato, German...49
    Potato, Gourmet...48
    Potato, Janet Ann's Best...49
    Potato, Portuguese...48
    Pumpkin...10
    Sausage, Italian...43
    Spanish Bean...60
    Tomato, Ten-Minute...51
    Tomato-Rice, Hearty...51
    Tortellini...64
    Vegetable, Diet...55

Spaghetti, *See "Pasta"*

Spareribs, *See "Meat(s), Pork"*
Spinach Salad, *See "Salad(s)"*
Spinach, *See "Vegetables"*

Spread(s)
    Broccoli, Spicy...35
    Butter, Strawberry...387
    Caviar Cream Cheese...28
    Cheese, Hungarian...20
    Cheese, Liptoi...20
    Clam, Chris' Dip...25
    Crab Meat...25
    Curry...29
    Fruit, Healthy...19
    Jam, "High Dumpsy Dearie"...386
    Pâté, Basil, Marlene's...21
    Salmon...25
    Welsh Rarebit, Walsh's...392

Squash, *See "Vegetables"*
Steak, *See "Meat(s), Beef"*

Stew(s)
    Beef, Deluxe...147
    Beef, Easy, Oven-Baked...146
    Beef, Over Noodles...146
    Beef, with Fresh Vegetables...147
    Hunter's...148
    Lamb, Spring, with Fresh Vegetables...168
    Liver, Uncle Louie's...145

Strawberry(ies), *See "Fruit(s)"*

Stuffing
    Apple Corn Bread...8
    Beef, with ~ Pan Dressing...408
    Poultry ~ Bread Dressing...408

Sweet Potato(es), *See "Vegetables"*
Swordfish, *See "Fish"*
Syrup, *See "Sauce(s)"*

Szechwan
    Chicken Over Steamed Rice...191
    Salad, Noodle, Spicy...73

T

Taco(s)
    Chicken...189
    Salad, Mexican Corn Chip...78
    Salad, Red-Bean...78

Tarts, *See "Desserts"*

Toffee
    Ann's Green Stuff...361
    Bars, Easy...354
    Brickle Yummies, Adeline's...364
    Lady Fingers, Heath Bar...360

Tomato(es), *See "Vegetables"*

Topping, Crumb-nut...94
Tortellini, *See "Pasta"*

Tortillas
    Chicken, Crisp ~ Totopo Jalisciense...190

Trifle, *See "Desserts"*
Trout, *See "Fish"*
Tuna, *See "Fish"*
Turbot, *See "Fish"*
Turkey, *See "Poultry"*
Twists, *See "Bread(s), Roll(s)"*

V

Veal, *See "Meat(s)"*

VEGETABLES
    Beef Stew...147
    Beef Stew Over Noodles...146
    Beef, Easy, Oven-Baked Stew...146
    Casserole...239
    Casserole, Roman...240
    Chicken, Szechaun, Over Steamed Rice...191
    Chili, Vegetarian, in a Tortilla Bowl...224
    Chow-Chow, Retz Ranch...388
    Chowder, Vegetable, Halifax...47
    Chow Mein, Chicken or Pork...192
    Lamb Stew, Spring...168
    Meat & Vegetable Loaf...148
    Pizza, Mexican Black Bean...223
    Pot Roast, American...129
    Ratatouille, Basmati Rice...271
    Risotto Milanese...275
    Rotini, in Mustard Sauce...253
    Salad Niçoise...69
    Salad, Calico...70
    Salad, Chinese, Hawthorn Club...72
    Salad, Spicy Szechwan Noodle...73
    Salad, Summer Pasta...76
    Short Ribs, Roasted...123
    Soup, Diet...55
    Soup, French Market...59
    Soup, Gazpacho, Clamato...44
    Soup, Gazpacho, Good's...44
    Soup, Petite Marmite...58
    Tortellini Alfredo Primavera...267

Artichoke(s)
    Balls…31
    Chicken with, & Wild
        Rice…196
    Dip Bucaro…31
    Dip, Jean's…31
    Salad, Pasta & Shrimp…77
    Sauce, Linguine with…255
    Spinach with, Dish…234
    Stuffed…234

Asparagus
    a la Hazelwood…238
    Cold, with Walnuts…238
    Sesame…239
    Soup, Cream of…53

Avocado(s)
    Guacamole…26

Bean(s)
    Baked, Boston…246
    Baked, Calico…247
    Black, Soup, Cuban…61
    Casserole, "21-Bean"…247
    Casserole, Chicken,
        Green…207
    Casserole, Lentil with
        Sausage…249
    China, Bake…246
    Garbanzo, Soup,
        Spanish…60
    Garbanzos, Baked…248
    Lentil Casserole with
        Sausage…249
    Lentil, Soup, Bavarian…60
    Navy, Soup, French
        Market…59
    Navy, Soup, U.S.
        Senate…58
    Pizza, Mexican Black
        Bean…223
    Salad, Jean's Mustard Three-
        Bean…79
    Salad, Madge's Kidney
        Bean…80
    Salad, Three-Bean with
        White Wine
        Vinaigrette…79
    Soup, Strega Nana's Pasta &
        Fagioli…64
    Texas, Chicago Style…248

Beet(s)
    Hot, Spiced…235
    Relish, Fancy…391

    Relish, No-Cook…391

Black-Eyed Pea(s)
    Chicken, Soul, Stir-Fry
        with…193

Broccoli
    Casserole…9
    Chicken Breasts Divan,
        Julie's…200
    Fusilli with Cottage Cheese
        Pesto &…254
    Party…237
    Pie, Turkey…209
    Ring with Carrots…237
    Soufflé de Norman…236
    Soufflé, Sandy's…236
    Soup, Swiss…50
    Spread, Spicy…35

Cabbage
    Casserole, with Beef…143
    Colcannon…285
    Creamed, The Best…241
    Meal-in-One…173
    Red, Dutch…241
    Sauerkraut, Crazy
        Meatballs…37
    Sauerkraut & Sausage
        Bites…29
    Sauerkraut, Sherwood
        Forest…242
    Sauerkraut, Smoked Sausage
        &…174
    Sauerkraut, Spareribs
        &…159
    Soup, Diet Vegetable…55
    Soup, Polish…52
    Soup, Sweet & Sour…52
    Stuffed, Kosher…143
    Stuffed, Rolls…142

Carrot(s)
    Bourbonade…242
    Broccoli Ring with…237
    Cake, Helen's
        Hazelwood…333
    Cake, Pecan-Filled…332
    Casserole, Knox
        County…243
    Casserole, Vegetable…239
    Marmalade-Glazed,
        Mary's…242
    Mint-Glazed…243

Celery
    Soup, Cream of…53

Corn
    Casserole, Fort Myers…235
    Creole…235
    Parmesan Polenta…276
    Soup, Cheesy…50

Cucumber(s)
    Salad, Sweet & Sour…81
    Sandwiches…19
    Soup, Low-Fat…54

Eggplant(s)
    Casserole, Roman…240

Lima Bean(s)
    Soup, with Bacon…55

Mushroom(s)
    Crisp, Golden…32
    Crumb-Topped…245
    in Wine Sauce…244
    Morels, Fricassee of Veal
        with…164
    Soup, Swiss Consommé…57
    Stuffed…33
    Supreme…245
    Swiss Baked…244
    Turnovers…32
    Veal Chops with, in Cream
        Sauce…166

Onion(s)
    Balsamic, Roasted…228
    Casserole, Heavenly…228
    Fish Fillet with…95
    Liver & Bacon with…145
    Pie, Auntie's…229
    Pork Chops & Sage
        with…151
    Quiche, Sweet…178
    Scallions, Baked Potatoes
        with, & Bacon…282
    Soup, French…56
    Sweet, & Potatoes Au
        Gratin…279
    Sweet, Roasted…229

Pea(s)
    Creamed Salmon with…101
    Rice Pilaf with, and
        Mint…274
    Soup, Split Pea…56

Pigeon Peas
    Pork Loin with Rice &…155
    Soup, Beef with Pigeon Peas,
        Puerto Rican…57

Plantain(s)
    Mofongo ~ Plantain
        Pudding…249

Plantain(s), *continued*
  Soup, Mofongo
    Dumpling...63
  Stuffed, Ripe ~ Canoas...141

Potato(es)
  Au Gratin, Sweet Onions
    &...279
  Baked, Paprika, Fans...282
  Baked, with Bacon &
    Scallions...282
  Boiled New...280
  Casserole, Boldt...281
  Casserole, Mashed,
    Creamy...280
  Casserole, Roman...240
  Casserole, Vegetable...239
  Cheese & Bacon Bake...285
  Cheesy Bake, Adeline's...284
  Chicken Fajita...188
  Colcannon...285
  Cream Cheese, Bake...283
  Dumplings, Mama Kozol's
    Polish...287
  French-Style,
    Grandmother's...286
  Ham, Scalloped with...160
  Hashed, in Cream...286
  Mashed, Creamy...8
  Meal-in-One...173
  Pancakes, New-Style...287
  Party...284
  Peggy's Casserole...281
  Penn Dutch...280
  Salad, Mom's...76
  Salad, Sour Cream...77
  Skins, Cheese & Bacon...279
  Slices, Grandma's
    Crunchy...285
  Soup, German...49
  Soup, Gourmet...48
  Soup, Janet Ann's Best...49
  Soup, Portuguese...48
  Twice-Baked...283

Pumpkin
  Bread...11
  Roll...295
  Soup, Beef with Pigeon Peas,
    Puerto Rican...57
  Pie, Old-Fashioned, with
    Brandy...13
  Soup...10

Rutabaga(s)
  Bake, Galesburg...225

Spinach
  Appetizer Balls...34
  Artichoke with, Dish...234
  Casserole, Egg &...231
  Crepe Cups, Florentine...230
  Lasagne Rolls...265
  Lasagne, Two-Sauce ~ Red &
    White...264
  Manicotti, Stuffed...260
  Mold, Sea Breeze...231
  Omelette, Spinacheese...180
  Pie, Cheddar &...230
  Salad, Crunch...75
  Salad, Korean...74
  Salad, with Cranberry and
    Orange...74
  Shells, Stuffed...262
  Strudel...34
  Tomatoes, Stuffed...232

Squash
  Casserole, Yummy
    Yellow...226
  Patty Pan, Supreme...226
  Rings, Glazed...227
  Zucchini Bread, Deluxe...304
  Zucchini Bread, Eve's...304
  Zucchini Cake,
    Chocolate~Deluxe...330
  Zucchini Cookies...357
  Zucchini with Green Pepper
    & Dill...227
  Zucchini, Fried...227
  Zucchini, Stuffed...140

Sweet Potato(es)
  Candied...225
  Casserole...9

Tomato(es)
  Chow-Chow, Green...388
  Chow-Chow, Retz
    Ranch...388
  Fire & Ice...232
  Green, Fried...233
  Salad, Greek...68
  Scalloped...233
  Sliced, with Blue Cheese
    Dressing...69
  Soup, Hearty, Rice...51
  Soup, Ten-Minute...51
  Spinach-Stuffed...232

Water Chestnuts
  in Bacon...30

Yam(s)
  with Grand Marnier...224

W

WALGREEN RECIPES
Cafeterias
Alaskan Salmon Loaf with
  Creole Sauce...102
American Mornay
  Sauce...401
American Pot Roast with
  Noodles...129
Barbecued Spareribs...159
Béchamel ~ Classic White
  Sauce...400
Beef Stew with Fresh
  Vegetables...147
Braised Beef with
  Noodles...131
Chicken a la King...197
Chili Con Carne and
  Beans...139
Chipped Beef and Noodles au
  Gratin...135
Creamed Salmon with
  Peas...101
Creamed Veal with
  Rice...167
Creole Corn...235
Deep-Fried Chicken...194
Ham Croquettes...161
Hot, Spiced Beets...235
Lamb Croquettes...171
Lamb Patties with
  Bacon...171
Meat & Vegetable Loaf...148
Mock Hollandaise
  Sauce...394
No-Cook Beet Relish...391
Paprika Veal Cutlets...165
Scalloped Ham &
  Potatoes...160
Spareribs with
  Sauerkraut...159
Spinach & Egg
  Casserole...231
Spring Lamb Stew with Fresh
  Vegetables...168
Stuffed, Deviled Crab...116
Swiss Steaks in Pan
  Gravy...132
The Famous Patty Melt...123
Traditional Creole
  Sauce...396

Vegetable Casserole…239
Corky's
   Dixie Fried Chicken…194
Corporate Cafeteria
   Bavarian Lentil Soup…60
   Chicken or Pork Chow Mein
      ~ Shanghai Style…192
   Cuban Black Bean Soup…61
   French Market Soup…59
   Lima Bean & Bacon
      Soup…55
   Petite Marmite Soup…58
   Sautéed Lemon Chicken
      Breasts…202
   Spinach Lasagne Rolls…265
   Sweet & Sour Cabbage
      Soup…52
   Szechaun Chicken Over
      Steamed Rice…191
   Vegetarian Chili in a Tortilla
      Bowl…224
Puerto Rican Grills
   Mofongo Dumpling
      Soup…63
   Mofongo ~ Plantain
      Pudding…249
   Pork Loin with Rice &
      Pigeon Peas…155
   Pork Steaks a la Criolla…157
   Puerto Rican Beef Soup with
      Pigeon Peas…57
   Puerto Rican Chicken with
      Rice…196
   Spanish Sausage with
      Rice…174
   Stuffed, Ripe Plantains ~
      Canoas…141
Robin Hood & Briargate
   Au Jus ~ Quick or
      Traditional…406
   Bordelaise Sauce…398
   Boston Baked Beans…246
   Brandy Sauce…385
   Brisket of Beef…130
   Broiled Brook Trout
      Amandine…104
   Brown Gravy for Beef…407
   Candied Sweet
      Potatoes…225
   Chicken Giblet Gravy…406
   Chicken Robin Hood…195

Cinnamon Sauce…385
Cocktail Sauce…393
Corned Beef…130
Corned Beef Hash…131
Cream of Celery Soup…53
Creamy Garlic House
   Dressing…86
Dixie Fried Chicken…194
Dutch Red Cabbage…241
French Onion Soup…56
Glazed Stewed Apple
   Wedges…374
Italian Meat Sauce…402
Jardinière Sauce…397
Marinara ~ Classic Red
   Sauce for Pasta…402
Mint-Glazed Carrots…243
Mushroom Sauce…399
Pineapple Sauce…384
Pineapple-Baked Ham…161
Raisin Sauce…384
Rémoulade Sauce…395
Roasted Pork Loin with
   Gravy…156
Scalloped Tomatoes…233
Scotch Barley Soup…54
Sherwood Forest
   Sauerkraut…242
Split Pea Soup…56
Tartar Sauce…393
Veal Scallopini…166
White Gravy for
   Chicken…407
Sanborns
   Ceviche…98
   Chicken Salsa Suiza…191
   Chicken Tacos…189
   Mexican Roast Beef a la
      Sanborns…125
   Totopo Jalisciense ~ Crisp
      Chicken Tortilla…190
Soda Fountains
   Coke or Root Beer
      Float…416
   Hot Fudge Sundae…317
   Old-Fashioned Banana
      Split…317
   Old-Fashioned Chocolate
   Malted Milk (Double-Rich
      Chocolate Malted
      Milk)…411

Sampler Thick Shake…411
Wag's & Humpty Dumpty
   Cheese & Bacon Potato
      Skins…279
   Coke or Root Beer
      Float…416
   Ham & Cheese
      Omelette…180
   Hot Fudge Sundae…317
   Liver, Bacon & Onions…145
   The Famous Patty Melt…123
   Old-Fashioned Banana
      Split…317
   Original Thick Malted
      Milk…411
   Sampler Thick Shake…411
   Spinacheese Omelette…180
   Wag's Breakfast
      Croissant…178
   Western Omelette…181
Walleye, *See "Fish"*
Water Chestnuts, *See "Vegetables"*
Welsh Rarebit (or Rabbit),
   See "Spread(s) or Sauce(s)"
Wheat (Whole), *See "Grain(s)"*
Wild Rice, *See "Grain(s)"*
Wine, *See "Beverages"*

Y

Yam(s), *See "Vegetables"*
Yorkshire Pudding(s), *See "Bread(s)"*

Z

Zucchini, *See "Vegetables, Squash"*